A Cancer

Source Book

for Nurses

Julie Moran
6363 Sherman R,
Lockport, NY
14094

434-7620

A Cancer Source Book for Nurses

SIXTH EDITION

Edited By
Susan B. Baird, RN, MPH, MA
Director of Nursing
Fox Chase Cancer Center
Philadelphia, Pennsylvania
and
Editor, *Oncology Nursing Forum*

Assistant Editors
Michele Girard Donehower, RN, MSN
Nurse Practitioner
University of Maryland Cancer Center
Baltimore, Maryland

Valerie Lindquist Stalsbroten, RN, MN
Oncology Clinical Nurse Specialist
Anacortes, Washington

Terri B. Ades, RN, BSN, OCN
Coordinator of Nursing Programs
American Cancer Society
Atlanta, Georgia

American Cancer Society
Professional Education Publication

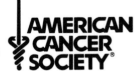

The American Cancer Society, Inc., Atlanta 30329

©1950, 1956, 1963, 1975, 1981, 1991 by the American Cancer Society.
All rights reserved.
Published 1950. Sixth edition 1991
Printed in the United States of America

Library of Congress Cataloging in Publication Data

A cancer source book for nurses / edited by Susan B. Baird; assistant
    editors, Michele Girard Donehower, Valerie Stalsbroten, Terri B. Ades.
        p.   cm. — (Professional education publication)
    Includes bibliographical references.
    Includes index.
    ISBN 0-944235-06-9
    1. Cancer—Nursing.   I. Baird, Susan B.   II. Series.
    (DNLM: 1. Oncologic Nursing. WY 156 C2198)
RC266.C3564 1991
610.73′698—dc20   90-14527
DNLM/DLC   CIP
for Library of Congress

A Cancer Source Book for Nurses
Contents

vii Foreword
   Patricia Greene

ix Contributors

xi Acknowledgments

xi Credits

1 **Unit I. Introduction to Cancer Nursing Care**
   Valerie Lindquist Stalsbroten and Susan B. Baird

9 **Unit II. Cancer as a Disease Process**

10   **Chapter 1. Cancer Incidence and Epidemiology**
      Amy L. Mirand and Joy Miller Knopp
22   **Chapter 2. The Nature of Cancer**
      Beverly Vincent and Amy Mirand
30   **Chapter 3. Cancer Prevention and Risk Reduction**
      Ivana T. Croghan and Margene K. Omoto
40   **Chapter 4. Screening, Detection, and Diagnosis**
      Joy Miller Knopp and Ivana T. Croghan

55 **Unit 3. Treatment Approaches**

56   **Chapter 1. Surgical Oncology**
      Marianne Dietrick-Gallagher and Ella May Brasher
63   **Chapter 2. Radiation Therapy**
      Ryan R. Iwamoto
73   **Chapter 3. Chemotherapy**
      Judy Petersen
83   **Chapter 4. Biological Response Modifiers**
      Mary Ersek
91   **Chapter 5. Bone Marrow Transplantation**
      Louise Schilter and Eileen Rossman

99 **Unit 4. Nursing Management**

100   **Chapter 1. Symptom Management**
      Michele Girard Donehower
111   **Chapter 2. Pain Management**
      Julia Fanslow

121 Chapter 3. Nutritional Support
Karen Barale
132 Chapter 4. Oncologic Emergencies
Brenda Nevidjon
141 Chapter 5. Cancer and Sexuality
Terry Chamorro
150 Chapter 6. Psychosocial Support
Ginette Ferszt and Frances K. Barg
159 Chapter 7. Rehabilitation
Frances K. Barg and Laura Heard

165 Unit 5. Treatment of Specific Neoplasms

166 Chapter 1. Cancers of the Head and Neck
Barbara Albertson
175 Chapter 2. Lung Cancer
Elizabeth J. White
184 Chapter 3. Esophageal and Gastric Cancer
Teresa Coluccio
191 Chapter 4. Colorectal Cancer
Carol Sun Redfield and Nancy Reilly
200 Chapter 5. Cancers of the Pancreas, Hepatobiliary,
and Endocrine Systems
Katherine Talmage Alkire
208 Chapter 6. Urinary Tract Cancers
Julena Lind
216 Chapter 7. Cancer of the Breast
Rebecca Hunter Dorcas
228 Chapter 8. Gynecologic Malignancies
Mary Beth Tombes
242 Chapter 9. Cancers of the Male Genital Organs
Mark Redmond
252 Chapter 10. Cancer of the Central Nervous System
Marybeth Chase
259 Chapter 11. Skin Cancers
Ann Marie Maguire
270 Chapter 12. Cancers of the Bone
Jane Brewer Sloane
276 Chapter 13. Leukemia
Cheryl R. Jedlow
286 Chapter 14. The Lymphomas and Multiple Myeloma
Margie Graff Anderson
296 Chapter 15. Childhood Cancer
Teresa Ely, Denise Giesler, and Ki Moore

309 Unit 6. Resources In Cancer Care
Marilyn Frank-Stromborg and Rhonda Niles

318 Appendices
318 I. Chemotherapeutic Agents
320 II. Hormonal Agents
322 III. American Cancer Society Divisions

325 Glossary
Linda Yoder

339 Index

Italicized words and phrases in the text are
defined in the glossary

FOREWORD

With this edition, *A Cancer Source Book for Nurses* marks its fortieth year of publication. As a textbook, the revisions in this new edition have been purposefully tailored to reflect important changes that have occurred in cancer knowledge and cancer care. It is perhaps an act of Fate, however, that this book is most often referred to as "The Source Book." *Source* is rooted in the Latin *surgere*, to rise, and the presentation and approach of this edition are evidence of the remarkable rise of cancer nursing over the past three decades.

The first issue of *A Cancer Source Book* was written by a physician. The Foreword noted that, "We have not attempted to discuss nursing care techniques, but rather have approached the subject with the conviction that basic knowledge of the facts about cancer is the first step in the control of the disease." That approach was quite consistent with the cancer nursing literature of the time, which typically was written by physicians. In truth, little was known about the nursing care of cancer patients.

This edition of *A Cancer Source Book* addresses the needs of nursing professionals at a time when the specialty of cancer nursing is well developed. Together, in this decade, nurse specialists and nurse generalists are forming a community that is committed to cancer control through primary prevention, early detection, treatment, rehabilitation, and care of persons with advanced disease. Thus, in addition to presenting basic knowledge about the most common cancers and treatments, specific strategies for nursing care of cancer patients have been detailed—by nurse specialists—for nurses in all practice settings.

This revision began as a project of the Nurses' Subcommittee of the Washington Division, Inc, of the American Cancer Society. Valorie Lindquist Stalsbroten, Assistant Editor, worked with volunteers in Washington who developed an outline and began the arduous task of writing the chapters. Later in the project, the work of Washington authors was augmented by contributions from experts around the country. The American Cancer Society is most grateful to the nurses and staff in the Washington Division for their generous and persistent leadership, time, and sharing of talent and knowledge in this effort.

Patricia E. Greene, R.N., M.S.N., F.A.A.N.
Vice President for Nursing
American Cancer Society

CONTRIBUTORS

Barbara E. Albertson, RN, MN
Nurse Practitioner III, Otolaryngology—Head
and Neck Surgery Clinic
University of Washington Medical Center
Seattle, Washington

Katherine Talmage Alkire, RN, MN
Clinical Nurse Specialist—Oncology
St. Lukes Regional Medical Center
Boise, Idaho

Margie Graf Anderson, RN, MN, OCN
Instructor, Associate Degree Nursing
Program
Seattle Central Community College
Seattle, Washington

Susan B. Baird, RN, MPH, MA
Director of Nursing
Fox Chase Cancer Center
Philadelphia, Pennsylvania
and Editor, *Oncology Nursing Forum*

Karen V. Barale, MS, RD, CD
Research Dietitian
Fred Hutchinson Cancer Research Center
Seattle, Washington

Frances K. Barg, MEd
Project Director, School of Nursing
University of Pennsylvania
Philadelphia, Pennsylvania

Ella May Brasher, RNC, OCN
Staff Nurse
Overlake Hospital Medical Center
Bellevue, Washington

Terry Chamorro, RN, MN, CS
Clinical Nurse Specialist, Gynecology
Oncology
Cedars-Sinai Medical Center and Comprehensive Cancer Center
Los Angeles, California

Marybeth Chase, RN, MN
Clinical Nurse Specialist—Neuro Oncology
Childrens Hospital and Medical Center
Seattle, Washington

Teresa Coluccio, RN, MN
Oncology Clinical Nurse Specialist
Providence Medical Center
Seattle, Washington

Ivana T. Croghan, PhD
Assistant to the Chairman for Education
S.U.N.Y. at Buffalo, Department of GYN/OB
Buffalo, New York

Marianne Dietrick-Gallagher, MSN, RN, OCN
Senior Coordinator, Surgical Nursing
Hospital of the University of Pennsylvania
Philadelphia, Pennsylvania

Michele Girard Donehower, RN, MSN
Nurse Practitioner
University of Maryland Cancer Center
Baltimore, Maryland

Rebecca Hunter Dorcas, RN, MN
Director of Oncology and Hospice Services
Visiting Nurse-Home Health Care
Bellingham, Washington

Teresa Ely, RNC, BSN
Staff Nurse, II
University Medical Center
University of Arizona
Tucson, Arizona

Mary Ersek, RN, MN
Doctoral Candidate
University of Washington School of Nursing
Seattle, Washington

Julia Fanslow, RN, EdD, OCN
Oncology Nurse Specialist
St. Joseph Cancer Center
Tacoma, Washington

Ginette G. Ferszt, MSN, RN, CS
Mental Health Nurse Specialist
Private Practice and
University of Pennsylvania School of Nursing
Philadelphia, Pennsylvania

Marilyn Frank-Stromborg, EdD, FAAN
Professor, School of Nursing
Northern Illinois University
DeKalb, Illinois

Denise Giesler, RNC, BSN
University Medical Center
University of Arizona
Tucson, Arizona

Patricia Greene, RN, MSN, FAAN
Vice President for Nursing
American Cancer Society
Atlanta, Georgia

Laura Heard, MS, RN, CRRN
Rehabilitation Clinical Nurse Specialist
Virginia Mason Hospital
Seattle, Washington

Ryan R. Iwamoto, RN, MN, CS
Clinical Nurse Specialist
Division of Radiation Oncology
Virginia Mason Clinic
Seattle, Washington

Cheryl R. Jedlow, RN, BSN
Clinical Nurse Specialist
Fred Hutchinson Cancer Research Center
Seattle, Washington

Joy Miller Knopp, RN, MN, OCN
Oncology Clinical Nurse Specialist
Overlake Hospital Medical Center
Bellevue, Washington

Julena Lind, MN, RN
Executive Director
Center for Health Information, Education &
Research
California Medical Center, and
Adjunct Assistant Professor
Department of Nursing
University of Southern California
Los Angeles, California

Anne Marie Maguire, RN, MN, OCN
Clinical Nurse Specialist
Visiting Nurse Services
Seattle, Washington

Amy L. Mirand, PhD
Epidemiologist/Project Coordinator
Research Institute on Alcoholism
Formerly with
Roswell Park Cancer Center
Buffalo, New York

Ki Moore, RN, DNS
Assistant Professor
College of Nursing
University of Arizona
Tucson, Arizona

Brenda M. Nevidjon, RN, MSN
Oncology Clinical Nurse Specialist
Virginia Mason Medical Center
Seattle, Washington
and Editor, ONS NEWS

Rhonda Niles, RN, MSN, OCN
Doctoral Student in Nursing
University of Washington
Seattle, Washington

Margene K. Omoto, RN, MN
Nurse Educator
Valley Medical Center
Renton, Washington

Judith A. Petersen, RN, MN, OCN
Oncology Clinical Nurse Specialist
Northwest Hospital
Seattle, Washington

Carol Sun Redfield, RN, MN
Oncology Nurse
Northwest Cancer Center
Seattle, Washington

Mark Redmond, RN, MN
Staff Nurse
Virginia Mason Hospital
Seattle, Washington

Nancy J. Reilly, RN, MSN, CURN
GI/GU Clinical Nurse Specialist
Hospital of the University of Pennsylvania
Philadelphia, Pennsylvania

Eileen S. Rossman, RN, BSN
Clinical Nurse Specialist
Fred Hutchinson Cancer Research Center
Seattle, Washington

Louise Schilter-Harms, RN, BSN
Nursing Coordinator, Day Shift
Fred Hutchinson Cancer Research Center
Seattle, Washington

Jane Brewer Sloane, RN, MN
Oncology Clinical Nurse Specialist
Lewisburg, Pennsylvania

Valerie Linquist Stalsbroten, RN, MN
Oncology Clinical Nurse Specialist
Anacortes, Washington

Mary Beth Tombes, RN, MN
Clinical Nurse Specialist
University of Wisconsin Clinical Cancer
Center
Madison, Wisconsin

Beverly J. Vincent, RN, MSN, OCN
Oncology Clinical Nurse Specialist
University of Washington Medical Center
Seattle, Washington

Elizabeth J. White, RN, MN, OCN
Community Hospital Nurse
Seattle Veterans Administration Medical
Center
Seattle, Washington

Linda Yoder, RN, MSN, MBA, OCN
Doctoral Candidate
University of Pennsylvania School of Nursing
Philadelphia, Pennsylvania

Acknowledgements

Many people lent their expertise to this book by contributing content or by reviewing chapters for accuracy and relevancy to practice. Their valuable suggestions and careful reviews added immeasurably to the final text. The time they gave is greatly appreciated.

Nancy Agee*, Kit Bakke, Andrea Barsevick, Ann T. Birkmire, Jennifer Bucholtz, Nilda Bueno*, Savannah Daniels*, Reidun Daeffler*, Susan Dudas, Brenda Eng, Connie Engelking*, Nina Entrekin*, Genevieve V. Foley*, Jayne Fernsler*, Sue Frymark*, Vivian A. Gaits, Elaine Glass*, Dennis Graham, Gloria Haagopian, Karen Heusinkveld, Laura Hilderley*, Pinkie Hutton**, Joanne Iritani, Margaret Irwin, Karen Iseminger*, Joanne Itano*, Ryan Iwamoto* **, Patricia Jassak, Patricia Klopovich, M. K. Tish Knobf, Joy Miller Knopp**, Alice Longman, Margaret Lamb, Elise Lev, Julena Lind, Ester Muscari Lin, Ann McElroy, Bonny Melby**, Marion Morra, Cathleen A. O'Connor, Sarah O'Hara**, Jeanne Pasacreta, Peggy Pierce*, Mark Redmond**, Valeria Lindquist Stalsbroten**, Linda Shegda, Roberta Strohl, Marybeth Tombes**, Marie Whedon, Vicie Whipple**.

*Indicates American Cancer Society National Nursing Advisory Committee member at the time the reviews were done.

**Indicates American Cancer Society Washington Division Nursing Committee member at the time of initial work on this book.

Credits

Copy Editing — Lisa O'Rourke
Art, Design, and Production — Jean Hernandez,
    Anthony J. Jannetti, Inc.
Typing — Exa Murray

UNIT 1

Introduction to Cancer Nursing

Most nurses will encounter patients with cancer at some point in their careers. The extent of cancer as a national health problem necessitates an awareness of the latest advances in research and treatment, regardless of the setting in which nurses practice. Nurses can be involved in every level of cancer control and care. Whether a nurse chooses to specialize in cancer care, provides care to patients with cancer as part of a broad patient mix, or is involved in the cancer care of a family member or neighbor, a vital contribution can be made.

Because the nurse often has closer or more frequent contact with patients and their families than other health care providers, and because this contact usually continues over time, nurses are in a unique position to make a substantial difference in patient care. Nurses work with other health care providers involved in cancer care and can often coordinate care in ways that make the best possible use of resources. This unit explores the many dimensions of cancer nursing and underscores the value of the nurse as a resource in cancer care.

1 AN INTRODUCTION TO CANCER NURSING

Valerie Lindquist Stalsbroten and Susan B. Baird

Perhaps more than any other disease, the diagnosis of cancer is a challenge to nurses. Although nurses have always made substantial and valued contributions to the care of patients with cancer, the emergence of the cancer nursing specialty in the past few decades has drawn attention to both the breadth and depth of these contributions.

Nurses specializing in cancer care can apply those aspects of their nursing knowledge and skill that lend themselves to clinical problem solving, to helping the patient and family along the cancer care continuum. From prevention and detection to rehabilitation and continuing care, cancer nurses work closely with other health care providers to ensure that the best possible care will be available regardless of diagnosis, stage of disease, or geographic location. This book demonstrates the range of activities and concerns that nurses skilled in cancer care bring to the practice setting.

When examining this dynamic field of specialization, several fundamental concepts recur. First, every nurse has a role responsibility in cancer care and can make a valuable contribution. Second, the complexity of the disease provides the nurse with both the opportunity and the challenge for making a difference in patients' and families' lives. Finally, a message of hope pervades these pages—hope for comfort, for quality of life, and for cure.

OPPORTUNITIES FOR NURSES

Every nurse can make a valuable contribution to cancer care. Opportunities have increased because the disease continuum has been expanded and care is now delivered in a variety of settings.

The Disease Continuum

Nurses have traditionally identified themselves with the active, treatment phase of disease. The majority of nurses are employed in acute care settings, working with patients who are newly diagnosed, receiving primary therapy, or being treated for recurrence.

However, increased emphasis on the value of earlier detection for many cancers creates opportunities for nurses to participate in prevention and detection. Because many patients today live longer with their disease than was previously possible, nurses work with patients who have acute disease episodes interspersed with periods of general wellness. Nurses working with patients who are returning to school, work, or family responsibilities have also come to realize the importance of comprehensive rehabilitation plans.

Settings

The number of cancer centers and cancer programs within hospitals is increasing in the United States, making specialized cancer care more available. Cancer outreach programs aimed at rural areas and access to computerized treatment information increase the likelihood that patients will receive modern, multidisciplinary care. Acute care continues to be delivered primarily in hospitals or in ambulatory care programs within hospitals; however, the trend toward shorter hospital stays and outpatient care means that many procedures and treatments traditionally conducted in hospitals are now being performed in ambulatory care settings, office settings, and at home.

For example, cisplatin chemotherapy is a treatment approach that originated as a hospital-based treatment because of the necessity for careful monitoring and hydration. Once information on this regimen accumulated, it became apparent that the regimen could be modified for safe administration in alternative settings. As a result, nurses in these settings are seeing patients with more complex care needs. And, because chemotherapy, and nutritional and hydration products are administered more frequently in the physician's office and at home, nurses in these settings must be familiar with a variety of infusion devices and able to teach patients and families how to use them as well.

Another result of the shift in care practices is an increased demand for skilled oncology nurse clinicians. In addition, nurses who generally have not dealt with patients with cancer may now be involved in their care. Nurses in schools and industrial settings, for example, may be very helpful to patients who are making the transition back to their regular roles as students or workers.

NURSING ROLES IN CANCER CARE

In General Practice

Every nurse should know the signs and symptoms of cancer and why they occur. They should know risk factors for specific cancers, the guidelines for cancer check-ups, and how to perform self-examination techniques. Nurses are often in an advantageous position in their own families and in the community to teach lifestyle changes that can prevent cancer and increase the likelihood of early detection. The American Cancer Society encourages nurses to participate in prevention and early detection activities at the community level.

In addition, nurses in every area of practice should be familiar with general cancer treatment modalities and able to identify both the usual and untoward effects of the disease and its treatment. Nurses should be familiar with the cancer-related resources available at the community, state, and national levels and know how patients can gain access to these services. Coordinating care with other care providers and organizations is a valuable service to patients and families.

Specializing in Cancer Care

Many opportunities exist for the nurse who wants to focus on cancer care. Nurses can work on special units in hospitals or ambulatory care facilities. Some units are organized by treatment modality, such as chemotherapy or radiation clinics; others specialize in a certain type of cancer, such as a gynecological oncology unit. Nurses can also combine their interests and experiences in subspecialties such as pediatric oncology.

Cancer centers with prevention and detection programs frequently employ nurse practitioners for screening and nurse educators for the development of educational programs. The demand for cancer care at home has prompted home care agencies to develop programs and obtain personnel to meet these needs. Nurses with skills that lend themselves to certain cancer populations—such as the enterostomal therapy nurse and the nurse with intravenous therapy skills—will find many opportunities to participate in cancer care.

PREPARATION FOR THE SPECIALTY
Educational Preparation

Continuing education and academic programs can prepare nurses for work in cancer care. The American Cancer Society Divisions and Units, the Oncology Nursing Society, and most cancer centers regularly sponsor continuing education programs to increase nurses' knowledge and provide updates on advances in this rapidly changing field. Cancer organizations and oncology nursing groups have made efforts to increase the cancer content of undergraduate courses so that graduating nurses have a basic knowledge of cancer and have had the opportunity to provide care for this patient population. Programs offering a clinical specialization in oncology at the master's level are available in almost every state. Specialization at the doctoral level is also now available in a limited number of programs. The American Cancer Society and the Oncology Nursing Society (see Unit VI) are good sources of information about current programs and available financial assistance.

Resources

In addition to education programs, many resources are available for the nurse new to the specialty. Cancer nursing textbooks and journals are available in most medical libraries or medical bookstores. Oncology articles appear frequently in nursing journals and in those of other health specialties. The American Cancer Society has both printed and audiovisual materials on many aspects of cancer and cancer care. The Oncology Nursing Society has established standards of care and guidelines for many technical aspects of treatment delivery, such as chemotherapy and infusion management. Unit VI of this book provides information about some of these sources; many others are listed in the bibliographies at the end of each chapter.

Certification

The certification process recognizes the knowledge of skilled clinicians through a testing procedure. The Oncology Nursing Certification Corporation (see Unit VI) offers annual testing opportunities preceding the Oncology Nursing Society Annual Congress and regularly at other sites around the country. A number of groups offer review courses and materials that may be a valuable source of information for nurses preparing for certification as well as those seeking a general update.

Research Opportunities

The greater emphasis throughout the nursing profession on scientifically-based practice has prompted nurses to use research methods to test care approaches and to increase the understanding of many facets of cancer care. Nurses have successfully competed for research funding and have disseminated their findings in publications and presentations. Nursing opportunities are frequently available in medical research as well. Nurses who have a good grasp of cancer, cancer care, and research methods can be valuable members of the research team. They can actively assist in the informed consent process, in providing information to patients, and in data collection.

THE CHALLENGES AND REWARDS OF CANCER CARE

Meeting Support Needs

Whether the nurse has chosen to focus exclusively on cancer care, to deliver cancer care as part of a broader spectrum of responsibilities, or is involved in the care of a friend or family member with cancer, the role is multifaceted and challenging. Because nurses spend considerable amounts of time directly with the patient and family while providing care, they are in an ideal position to provide support in a variety of ways. The patient and family will often express concerns and fears to the nurse, who can, in turn, interpret information, explain what is not clearly understood, and explore alternatives. Nurses can promote cooperation and communication by helping patients and family members develop trust in their care providers and by identifying questions they want to ask the doctor or other provider.

Rapid Changes in Care

The nurse is challenged to keep up with rapid changes in treatment. Nurses will want to have the most current information for planning care, whether it involves prevention and detection, treatment, or side-effect management. Knowing what care options are available and helping patients make the best use of those resources are valuable nursing functions. The nurse can help patients differentiate between standard care approaches, experimental treatment, and unproven methods of treatment. If well-meaning friends and family members suggest unproven treatment methods, nurses can provide current information about these methods and help the patient evaluate them. The American Cancer Society maintains current information about unproven methods.

Community Resources

One major focus in cancer nursing is to identify sources of support and to encourage helpful relationships while helping the patient and family preserve their energy and independence as much as possible. Information about community resources, such as equipment loan closets or transportation, can be particularly useful. Nurses can frequently help coordinate care between settings and providers, a vital function for families with limited resources who are trying to understand competing choices. The nurse can also help families locate the appropriate place to take questions about finances and reimbursement.

The Rewards of Cancer Nursing

Nurses working in cancer care frequently express the satisfaction they feel working in this demanding field. Nurses working in the area of prevention are rewarded when someone makes lifestyle changes or choices that promote health. Participation in screening efforts that detect cancer at an earlier stage, when treatment efforts are the most beneficial, can also be very fulfilling.

The relationships that develop among nurses, patients, and families are very special. Nurses are with them as they make progress and when they face difficulties. When working closely with a person facing life-threatening challenges, the skilled nurse tailors knowledge, experience, creativity, and caring to that individual. Gratification comes from sharing patients' joys, hopes, and sorrows and from recognizing that the care and support given is meaningful and appreciated.

Bibliography

American Nurses' Association and Oncology Nursing Society, (1987). *Standards of oncology nursing practice.* Kansas City, MO: American Nurses' Association.

Longman, A. J. (1990). Cancer nursing education. In S. L. Groenwald, M. H. Frogge, M. Goodman, & C. H. Yarbro (Eds.). *Cancer nursing: Principles and practice.* pp. 1256-1269. Boston: Jones and Bartlett Publishers.

Oncology Nursing Society. (1990). *Standards of advanced practice in oncology nursing.* Pittsburgh, PA: Oncology Nursing Society. Publication No. STAP9001.

Oncology Nursing Society, (1989). *Standards of oncology nursing education: Generalist and advanced practice levels.* Pittsburgh, PA: Oncology Nursing Society.

Oncology Nursing Society. (1989). *Graduate programs in cancer nursing.* Pittsburgh, PA: Oncology Nursing Society, Publication No. FMGP8901.

Oncology Nursing Society and American Cancer Society. (1988). *The master's degree with a specialty in oncology nursing: Role definition and curriculum guide.* Pittsburgh, PA: Oncology Nursing Society, Publication No. JRMD8801.

Hinds, P. (1990). Survey of graduate programs in cancer nursing. *Oncology Nursing Forum,* 17(6), 967-974.

Hinds, P. & Culhane, B. (1990) Cancer Resources in the United States. *Oncology Nursing Forum,* 17(5), 771-774.

UNIT 2

Cancer as a Disease Process

Because growth is an essential part of life, and cancer is a malfunction of the cell growth process, it is not surprising that cancer occurs in all living things. This universal disease develops in all types of plants and animals, has existed since the beginning of recorded history, and crosses boundaries of sex, race, culture, and socioeconomic level. Yet different cancers affect different populations: Some cancers strike the very young, others the very old; some are more prevalent among one gender; some occur in one race but rarely in others. Although the destructive process of cancer is well known, the relationships between the various causes are less well defined and the subject of continuing study.

Preventive measures that could reduce the incidence of some cancers and factors that place certain individuals at risk for other cancers have been identified. Because increased survival is closely linked with early detection in many cancers, nurses play an important role in promoting compliance with guidelines for self-examination, screening, and detection.

The chapters in this unit explain aspects of incidence and epidemiology and review the nature of cancer as a disease process. Content on prevention, risk reduction, screening, detection, and diagnosis will assist nurses in becoming actively involved in helping others recognize the importance of individual awareness and surveillance.

1 CANCER INCIDENCE AND EPIDEMIOLOGY

Amy L. Mirand and Joy Miller Knopp

The term "cancer" refers to a large, commonly encountered group of diseases characterized by the uncontrolled growth and spread of abnormal cells. About 30% of Americans now living will eventually develop cancer, and about 40% of Americans who get cancer this year will be alive 5 years after diagnosis. Survival rates are influenced by the type of cancer, the stage of disease at diagnosis, and the response to treatment. Because nurses work in a wide variety of settings and have contact with various populations, they are very likely to be involved in some way with the care or guidance of people with cancer. Familiarity with cancer incidence and epidemiology is fundamental to understanding prevention and detection, treatment, and continuing care for those with cancer.

BASIC TERMS

To begin to understand the effect of a particular disease in a given population, health care professionals must quantify the occurrence of the disease in that population. There are a number of ways to measure disease frequency. Simple enumeration of the number of cases, however, does not provide enough information to compare the disease experience among different populations.

To acknowledge and allow for differences among populations, the disease frequency is expressed as a rate. A *rate* is a measure of the disease expressed in relation to a unit of the population, along with a specification of time in which the cases are observed. Specifically, a rate has three components: 1. the numerator, the number of persons within the population diagnosed with the disease (cases); 2. the denominator, the population from which the cases are derived; and 3. a specified period during which the population is observed or studied.

The *incidence* of a disease is the number of newly diagnosed cases of disease observed within a given population. Figures 1a and 1b contain projected estimates of cancer incidence and mortality for 1990. The *incidence rate*, a measure of morbidity, is the incidence observed within a specified period of time.

$$\text{Incidence} = \frac{\text{Number of NEW cases observed in the population during the specified time period}}{\text{Number of people at risk of disease in the population during the specified time period}}$$

Incidence rates provide estimates of the risk of developing a disease over a period of time. The statement that the breast cancer incidence rate has increased from 84.7 per 100,000 in 1980 to 104.9 in 1986 illustrates how incidence rates can be compared to demonstrate changes or trends.

In contrast, *prevalence rates* estimate the risk of having a disease at a particular point in time.

$$\text{Prevalence rate} = \frac{\text{Number of EXISTING cases}}{\text{Total population}} \text{ at a point in time}$$

Prevalence rates, which are affected by the relationship between the incidence and the duration of a disease, are useful in evaluating the immediate health care needs of a community. But, when explaining the probability of disease occurrence in a given population, the most applicable measure is incidence.

COLLECTION OF STATISTICS

Tumor registries have been established in many states to collect and record information about the occurrence of cancers within a given population. They are a source of data on local, community, state, and national populations and subsamples.

National cancer incidence rates have been estimated since 1973 by the National Cancer Institute's Surveillance and End Results Program (SEER). The SEER data are actually compiled from data retrieved from 11 population-based cancer registries in the United States. These registries were chosen for their ability to represent a portion of the nation's epidemiologically diverse configuration. The SEER data, derived from about a 10% sample of the national population, appear to provide a representative characterization of national cancer incidence rates. Data on national rates have also been retrieved from several National Cancer Surveys, which also sample a portion of the United States population. The data from these sources have many uses. Table 1 demonstrates how trends

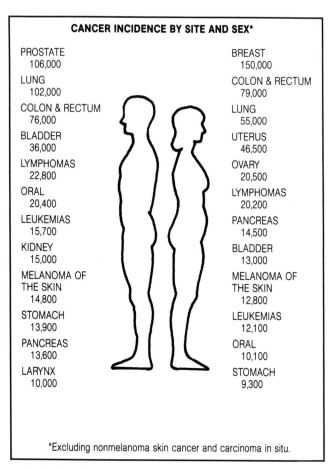

CANCER INCIDENCE BY SITE AND SEX*

PROSTATE 106,000	BREAST 150,000
LUNG 102,000	COLON & RECTUM 79,000
COLON & RECTUM 76,000	LUNG 55,000
BLADDER 36,000	UTERUS 46,500
LYMPHOMAS 22,800	OVARY 20,500
ORAL 20,400	LYMPHOMAS 20,200
LEUKEMIAS 15,700	PANCREAS 14,500
KIDNEY 15,000	BLADDER 13,000
MELANOMA OF THE SKIN 14,800	MELANOMA OF THE SKIN 12,800
STOMACH 13,900	LEUKEMIAS 12,100
PANCREAS 13,600	ORAL 10,100
LARYNX 10,000	STOMACH 9,300

*Excluding nonmelanoma skin cancer and carcinoma in situ.

Figure 1a. Selected cancer sites. Cancer incidence by site and sex—1990 estimates.

Source: From Cancer Facts and Figures—1990, p. 12. Reprinted with permission of The American Cancer Society.

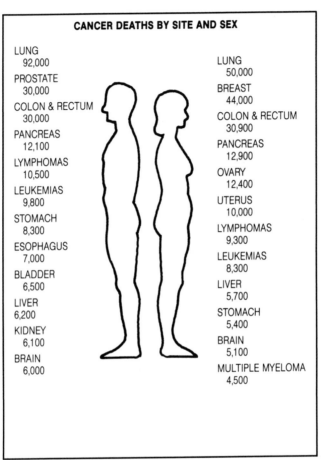

CANCER DEATHS BY SITE AND SEX

LUNG 92,000	LUNG 50,000
PROSTATE 30,000	BREAST 44,000
COLON & RECTUM 30,000	COLON & RECTUM 30,900
PANCREAS 12,100	PANCREAS 12,900
LYMPHOMAS 10,500	OVARY 12,400
LEUKEMIAS 9,800	UTERUS 10,000
STOMACH 8,300	LYMPHOMAS 9,300
ESOPHAGUS 7,000	LEUKEMIAS 8,300
BLADDER 6,500	LIVER 5,700
LIVER 6,200	STOMACH 5,400
KIDNEY 6,100	BRAIN 5,100
BRAIN 6,000	MULTIPLE MYELOMA 4,500

Figure 1b. Selected cancer sites. Cancer deaths by site and sex—1990 estimates.

Source: From *Cancer Facts and Figures—1990*, p. 12. Reprinted with permission of The American Cancer Society.

Table 1. Trends in Survival By Site of Cancer, By Race, Cases Diagnosed in 1960-1963, 1970-1976, 1977-1979, 1980-1985

Site	1960-1963[1] Relative 5-Year Survival Rates (Percent) White	Black	1970-1973[1] Relative 5-Year Survival Rates (Percent) White	Black	1974-1976[2] Relative 5-Year Survival Rates (Percent) White	Black	1977-1979[2] Relative 5-Year Survival Rates (Percent) White	Black	1980-1985[2] Relative 5-Year Survival Rates (Percent) White	Black
All Sites	39	27	43	31	50	39	50	38	51*	38
Oral Cavity	45	—	43	—	55	36	53	36	54	31
Esophagus	4	1	4	4	5	4	6	3	8*	6
Stomach	11	8	13	13	14	16	16	15	16*	19
Colon	43	34	49	37	50	45	52	47	55*	48
Rectum	38	27	45	30	48	41	50	38	53*	39
Liver	2	—	3	—	4	1	3	4	4	2
Pancreas	1	1	2	2	3	2	2	4	3	5
Larynx	53	—	62	—	66	58	68	56	68	53
Lung & Bronchus	8	5	10	7	12	11	13	11	13*	12
Melanoma	60	—	68	—	79	67††	81	37††	81*	66
Breast (Female)	63	46	68	51	75	63	75	62	76*	64
Cervix Uteri	58	47	64	61	69	63	68	61	67	59
Corpus Uteri	73	31	81	44	89	62	87	57	83*	52*
Ovary	32	32	36	32	36	41	37	39	38*	38
Prostate	50	35	63	55	67	58	71	62	73*	63*
Testis	63	—	72	—	78	77*	88	—	91*	91
Urinary Bladder	53	24	61	36	73	47	75	54	78*	56*
Kidney & Renal Pelvis	37	38	46	44	51	50	50	53	52	55
Brain & Nervous System	18	19	20	19	22	28	24	28	24*	30
Thyroid	83	—	86	—	92	88	92	92	93	96
Hodgkin's Disease	40	—	67	—	72	68†	73	73	76*	73
Non-Hodgkin's Lymphomas	31	—	41	—	47	48	48	49	51*	44
Multiple Myeloma	12	—	19	—	24	28	24	32	26*	29
Leukemia	14	—	22	—	34	30	36	30	34	27

[1]Rates are based on End Results Group data from a series of hospital registries and one population-based registry.

[2]Rates are from the SEER program, based on data from population-based registries in Connecticut, New Mexico, Utah, Iowa, Hawaii, Atlanta, Detroit, Seattle-Puget Sound, and San Francisco-Oakland. Rates are based on follow-up of patients through 1986.

*The difference in rates between 1974-1976 and 1980-1985 is statistically significant (p<0.05).

†The standard error of the survival rate is between 5 and 10 percentage points.

††The standard error of the survival rate is greater than 10 percentage points.

—Valid survival rate could not be calculated.

Data Source: Cancer Statistics Branch, National Cancer Institute.

Source: From "Cancer Statistics, 1990," by E. Silverberg, C. C. Boring, & T. S. Squires, 1990, *Ca—A Cancer Journal for Clinicians, 40*(1), p. 9. Reprinted with permission of The American Cancer Society.

in survival can be elucidated through an examination of registry data.

Cancer incidence rates are examined to reveal trends of disease occurrence. Examination of the population data as a whole provides a general picture of disease status. It is clear, however, that subgroups of the general population are at different levels of risk for disease. Therefore, incidence data are often *stratified*, or categorized by the subgroups of interest such as age, race, and sex. The disease experience of one group can then be compared to that of others.

For example, analysis of age-adjusted lung cancer incidence from 1973 to 1986 reveals that the rate for males is declining, while the rate for females is steadily increasing. Further stratification shows that the incidence rate for black males is 50% higher than that for white males. In contrast, the lung cancer incidence rates for black and white females are relatively similar, with the incidence rate for black women only about 6% higher. Other site-specific examples of trends and differences by subgroups are noted in Unit V.

Besides indicating changes in disease trends, incidence rates are monitored for several reasons:

- observed incidence rates can provide estimates of the effectiveness of cancer control programs or provide a rationale for establishing new programs;
- observed patterns of disease occurrence can serve as a basis for generating research hypotheses on reasons for differing disease rates; and
- comparative data from different populations by certain risk factors can provide information leading to the identification of factors associated with the disease.

EPIDEMIOLOGY

Epidemiology is an observational science with two major goals: to identify differences in disease and health distributions among populations; and to investigate the causes or determinants of these differences.

Epidemiology, like any other science, has inherent weaknesses and strengths. One weakness is the fact that the main tools of epidemiologic research are often measures of existing disease in human populations, such as mortality, incidence, and prevalence rates. The people that compose the study group will not benefit from findings that may suggest means to lower disease risks. The main strength of cancer epidemiological studies is that they usually observe a population of human beings in their normal environment. By comparing healthy and ill people in this situation, the risk of disease associated with exposure to or occurrence of identified and measured risk factors can be realistically estimated. Also, if an association between an identified risk factor and increased risk of disease is repeatedly observed, particularly in several populations, it may be possible to suggest preventive measures before actually elucidating the causal mechanisms of the disease. The association between cigarette smoking and an increased risk of lung cancer is an example of an epidemiological study. Cigarette smoking is associated with 83% of lung cancer mortality and 30% of all cancer mortality in the United States. Lung cancer is the single most preventable cause of morbidity and mortality in our country. This causal link between cigarettes and disease was discovered partly through numerous epidemiologic studies.

Several epidemiologic methodologies are available for the study of cancer. The choice of method is dependent on the study objective and the available resources. Some factors to consider are: whether the method can adequately control for the effects of competing or confounding variables that may affect risk estimates, whether the method is specific enough to identify an etiologic agent, and whether the method allows for true inferences of the association between disease and risk factors.

Stratification

The enumeration of cancer cases and deaths is most useful when the data are stratified according to different ages, races, and genders of study population. Analysis of disease by these descriptive variables may provide insight into the factors associated with the development of cancer.

Age: Investigation of disease incidence by age reveals that cancer occurs in all age groups of a population (Figures 2a and 2b). Incidence rates of many types of cancer increase in older age groups. Analysis has also revealed differences in patterns of particular cancers by age. For example, acute lymphocytic leukemia is the most common cancer among children in the United States, but is not common in adults. Conversely, chronic lymphocytic leukemia rarely occurs before age 35.

Data on the occurrence of cancer in different populations must be compared in an age-specific manner: that is, the number of cancer cases in a particular age group of a population must be related to the same age group in another population (Figures 3a and 3b).

A frequently used means of accounting for heterogeneous age distribution is by adjusting the data in reference to the age distribution of a "standard" population. Again, once this is done, the rates of one population can be compared to those of others. This *age-adjustment* of the data eliminates the effect of age when

All Ages	Under 15	15-34	35-54	55-74	75+
All Cancer 250,559	**All Cancer 1,033**	**All Cancer 4,171**	**All Cancer 25,581**	**All Cancer 137,927**	**All Cancer 81,825**
Lung 85,057	Leukemia 383	Leukemia 771	Lung 8,819	Lung 54,050	Lung 21,999
Colon & Rectum 27,469	Brain & CNS 244	Skin 483	Colon & Rectum 2,206	Colon & Rectum 14,532	Prostate 15,888
Prostate 27,262	Non-Hodgkin's Lymphomas 103	Non-Hodgkin's Lymphomas 477	Skin 1,308	Prostate 11,066	Colon & Rectum 10,530
Pancreas 11,403	Bone 46	Brain & CNS 459	Non-Hodgkin's Lymphomas 1,305	Pancreas 6,673	Pancreas 3,571
Leukemia 9,565	Connective Tissue 37	Hodgkin's Disease 300	Brain & CNS 1,251	Stomach 4,445	Bladder 3,376

Source: Vital Statistics of the United States, 1986.

Figure 2b.

All Ages	Under 15	15-34	35-54	55-74	75+
All Cancer 218,817	**All Cancer 798**	**All Cancer 3,548**	**All Cancer 27,210**	**All Cancer 107,681**	**All Cancer 79,556**
Breast 40,539	Leukemia 284	Breast 668	Breast 8,391	Lung 25,153	Colon & Rectum 14,231
Lung 40,465	Brain & CNS 198	Leukemia 472	Lung 4,967	Breast 20,166	Breast 11,308
Colon & Rectum 28,347	Connective Tissue 40	Uterus 368	Colon & Rectum 1,948	Colon & Rectum 11,993	Lung 10,230
Pancreas 12,055	Kidney 36	Brain & CNS 325	Uterus 1,798	Ovary 6,563	Pancreas 5,506
Ovary 11,903	Bone 34	Non-Hodgkin's Lymphomas 215	Ovary 1,688	Pancreas 5,784	Ovary 3,510

Source: Vital Statistics of the United States, 1986.

Figure 2a and 2b. Mortality for the five leading cancer sites for males and for females by age group, United States, 1986.
Source: From "Cancer Statistics, 1990," by E. Silverberg, C. C. Boring, & T. S. Squires, 1990, *Ca— A Cancer Journal for Clinicians, 40*(1), p. 13. Reprinted with permission of The American Cancer Society.

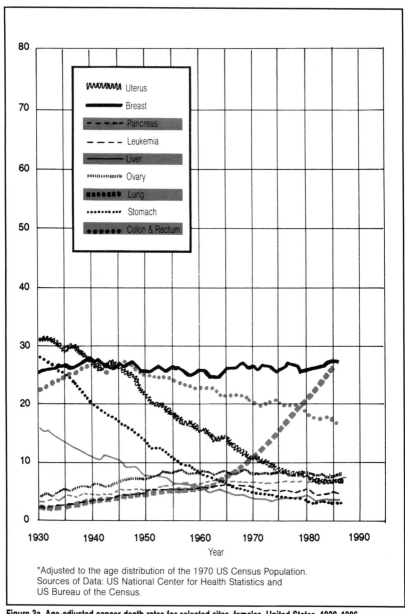

*Adjusted to the age distribution of the 1970 US Census Population.
Sources of Data: US National Center for Health Statistics and
US Bureau of the Census.

Figure 3a. Age-adjusted cancer death rates for selected sites, females, United States, 1930-1986.

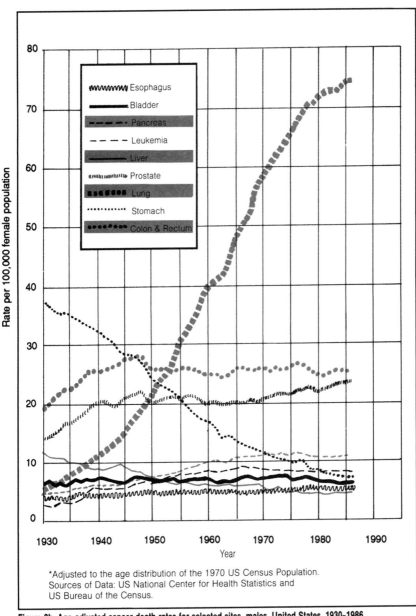

Figure 3b. Age-adjusted cancer death rates for selected sites, males, United States, 1930–1986.
Source: From "Cancer Statistics, 1990," by E. Silverberg, C. C. Boring, & T. S. Squires, 1990, *Ca— A Cancer Journal for Clinicians, 40*(1), p. 16-17. Reprinted with permission of The American Cancer Society.

comparing populations. These methods of stratification and adjustment can also be used in studying other factors.

Gender: Differences in cancer rates by gender are often observed. As with age, analysis of observed differences in rates between males and females may assist in generating hypotheses about factors associated with increased or decreased risk of cancer. The strong positive association between cigarette smoking and the risk of lung cancer provides an example. It had been observed for some time that males faced greater risk of lung cancer than females. Further analysis showed that more males than females smoked cigarettes. However, as cigarette smoking by females became more socially acceptable, females exhibited a concurrent rise in lung cancer cases and deaths. The pattern between exposure (cigarette smoking) and effect (lung cancer) observed in males was thus eventually reproduced in females.

Race: A population is often a heterogeneous group, and each component has unique disease experiences. A breakdown of disease patterns within the United States population by racial/ethnic categories illustrates this fact. For example, black women have a disproportionately higher incidence of cervical cancer than other racial/ethnic groupings. The SEER data show that, since 1973, the incidence rates of cervical cancer for white and black women have declined to a similar extent—3.8% and 4.8%, respectively. However, the actual incidence rate for black women is about two times that for white women. The cervical cancer mortality rates have also declined, about 40% between 1973 and 1986 for both black and white women. But again, the data reveal that black women experience approximately 182% higher mortality for cervical cancer than white women.

Why are there such dramatic differences along racial/ethnic groups? The literature suggests that the differences by race are largely due to differences in lifestyle and culture. Recently the American Cancer Society and other groups have questioned whether race in and of itself influences incidence and survival or whether poverty and ignorance contribute to these differences. Many studies indicate that a disproportionate number of people who develop cancer and die from it are among the socioeconomically disadvantaged—regardless of race. More detailed study of these factors may result in a better comprehension of the etiology of cancer, while providing suggestions for preventive measures.

SUMMARY

The development of a clinically recognized cancer is probably the end result of a multiple-stage process influenced by several factors. By documenting the observed differences in disease distribution, and the factors associated with disease among human populations, cancer epidemiology contributes to the interdisciplinary effort to elucidate the etiology of cancer. It is essential that nurses assisting with cancer control efforts understand cancer incidence and epidemiology and are able to interpret rates and trends to others.

Bibliography
American Cancer Society. (1990). *Cancer facts and figures 1990.* No. 5058-LE. Atlanta: Author.
Freeman, H. P. (1989). Cancer in the socioeconomically disadvantaged. *Ca—A Journal for Clinicians, 39*(5), 266–286.
MacMahon, B., & Pugh, T. F. (Eds.). (1970). *Epidemiology: Principles and methods.* Boston: Little, Brown, & Co.
Schottenfeld, D. & Fraumeni, F. F., Jr. (Eds.). (1982). *Cancer epidemiology and prevention.* Philadelphia, PA: W. B. Saunders Company.
Silverberg, E., Boring, C. C., & Squires, T. S. (1990). Cancer statistics, 1990. *Ca— A Cancer Journal for Clinicians, 40*(1), 9–28.
National Cancer Institute. (1989). *Cancer statistics review 1973-1986, including a report on the status of cancer control, May 1989.* (NIH Publication No. 89-2789). Bethesda, MD: U.S. Department of Health and Human Services, Public Health Service, National Institutes of Health.
Centers for Disease Control, Center for Chronic Disease Prevention and Health Promotion. (1989). *Reducing the health consequences of smoking: 25 years of progress. A report of the surgeon general.* (DHHS Publication No. (CDC) 89-8411). Washington, D.C.: U. S. Department of Health and Human Services, Public Health Service.

2 THE NATURE OF CANCER

Beverly Vincent and Amy Mirand

It is estimated that cancer affects three out of four families in the United States. The disease and, often, its treatment cause substantial mortality and morbidity, prompting intense interest in the exact changes that cells undergo as they became malignant. Scientists are also interested in factors causing clinical disease. Once the course of carcinogenesis and patterns of disease progression are identified, actions can be taken to eliminate or lessen the risk of cancer.

CHARACTERISTICS OF MALIGNANT CELLS

Normal cells reproduce in an orderly, controlled fashion. In some body tissues, such as the epidermis, the bone marrow, and the mucous membranes, new cells are formed regularly in order to compensate for the high rate of cell loss. Other tissues, such as the liver parenchyma or the periosteum of the bone, do not continuously generate new cells but can do so in response to cell loss from injury. Some cells, such as neurons, do not have the ability to reproduce and cannot regenerate even after tissue damage.

Normally, new cells are formed at a controlled rate, keeping the overall number of cells nearly constant. Feedback mechanisms that stimulate or inhibit cell division regulate the growth of normal cells. In contrast, the body's normal regulatory mechanisms are usually unable to control the proliferation of cancer cells once malignant transformation has taken place. Cancer cells also lose the ability to differentiate.

Differentiation is the process by which normal cells undergo physical and structural changes as they develop to form different tissues of the body. Differentiated cells specialize in different physiological functions. For example, in many ways nerve cells look and perform like other cells, yet they are microscopically and functionally different from other cells of the body.

The degree to which malignant cells lose the ability to differentiate varies among tumors. Cancer cells that closely resemble the tissue of origin are called *well-differentiated*, while bizarre tumor cells bearing little similarity to the tissue of origin are termed *undiffer-*

entiated or *anaplastic.* Undifferentiated or anaplastic malignancies are usually more aggressive in their growth and behavior than well-differentiated types.

Although malignant cells frequently lose the function, appearance, and properties associated with the normal cells of the tissue of origin, in some cases they can acquire new cellular functions uncharacteristic of the originating tissue. For example, tumors in non-endocrine tissues sometimes acquire the ability to produce and secrete hormones. This is the case with small-cell lung cancer, which can produce adrenocorticotropic hormone (ACTH) in amounts sufficient to cause Cushing's syndrome.

The term *tumor* is frequently used interchangeably with *cancer,* but the two are not synonymous, because tumor can refer to either *benign* or *malignant growths.* Both benign and malignant tumors result from abnormal cell growth. But unlike malignant cells, benign tumor cells retain their similarity to the tissue of origin, do not invade surrounding tissue, and do not metastasize to distant sites. Benign tumors are generally associated with a more favorable prognosis, unless their presence causes pressure in critical areas such as the brain. Table 1 outlines differences between benign and malignant tumors.

Table 1. Characteristics of Benign and Malignant Neoplasms

Benign	Malignant
Encapsulated	Nonencapsulated
Noninvasive	Invasive
Highly differentiated	Poorly differentiated
Mitoses rare	Mitoses relatively common
Slow growth	Rapid growth
Little or no anaplasia	Anaplastic to varying degrees
No metastases	Metastases

Source: From *Fundamentals of Oncology* (p. 23) by H. C. Pitot, 1981, New York: Marcel Dekker, Inc. Reprinted with permission of the publisher.

CARCINOGENESIS

Carcinogenesis is the process by which a normal cell undergoes malignant transformation. Usually, it is a multistep process involving progressive changes following genetic damage to or alteration of cellular DNA. Figure 1 illustrates the stages of carcinogenesis.

Carcinogens are agents capable of initiating carcinogenesis. Environmental, genetic, and viral factors have been implicated as carcinogens. Table 2 lists the groups of factors that may contribute

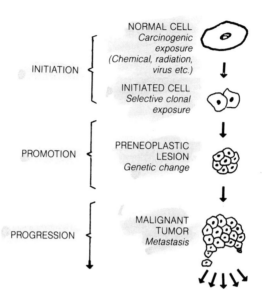

NORMAL CELL
*Carcinogenic
exposure
(Chemical, radiation,
virus etc.)*

INITIATION

INITIATED CELL
*Selective clonal
exposure*

PROMOTION

PRENEOPLASTIC
LESION
Genetic change

PROGRESSION

MALIGNANT
TUMOR
Metastasis

Figure 1. The multistage process of carcinogenesis.
Source: From "Assessment of Carcinogenesis through Epidemiological and Experimental Investigations" by R..T. Senic, 1986, *Seminars in Oncology Nursing* 2(3), p. 155. Reprinted with permission of publisher.

to the development of cancer. Specific risks are discussed in Unit II, Chapter 3.

The early stage of carcinogenesis, initiation, involves an irreversible alteration of the genetic make-up of a cell induced by some agent or factor. Initiation alone does not cause malignant transformation, but a cell thus transformed can pass to its progeny the potential to become cancerous. The initiation of carcinogenesis does not always lead to cancer.

The role of oncogenes in tumor initiation is currently being investigated. *Oncogenes* are pieces of genetic information within the cell that may initiate the cell's transformation from normal to malignant. They are thought to be the abnormal counterparts of *proto-oncogenes*, which in normal cells aid in regulating biological functions such as cell division. Oncogenes may be activated by carcinogens, at which point they alter the regulation of growth in

Table 2. Categories of Known and Suspected Factors in Carcinogenesis

Environmental factors	Chemical carcinogens
	  • hydrocarbons
	    — coal tars
	    — cigarette smoke
	  • industrial factors
	    — asbestos
	  • medications
	    — hormones
	    — cytotoxic drugs
	Dietary Factors
	  • obesity
	  • alcoholism
	Radiation
	  • ultraviolet
	  • ionizing

Genetic (hereditary) factors	
Viruses	Herpes group organisms Hepatitis
Spontaneous mitotic defects Immune deficiency	

the cell. Researchers have also discovered a group of regulatory genes, called *anti-oncogenes*, that have an effect opposite that of oncogenes. When activated, anti-oncogenes can regulate growth and inhibit carcinogenesis.

The second stage of carcinogenesis, promotion, increases the chance for initiated cells to become malignant. The effects of promotion are related to the dose and duration of exposure to the promoting agent; unlike initiation, the effects are reversible. The period of time between exposure to a promoter and the development of a malignancy is referred to as the *latency period*.

Cancer prevention efforts are, potentially, most effective when aimed at avoidance of promoters rather than initiators. The irreversible changes that occur with initiation do not lend themselves to prevention efforts. Avoidance of exposure to promoters, reduction of dose, and reduction of the duration of exposure will lower the probability of malignant expression in initiated cells.

DISEASE PROCESS

Cancers cause morbidity through local growth, metastasis to distant organs, and systemic effects of the disease. Malignant tumors can grow large enough at the primary site to interfere with function of the involved organ or to compress nearby organs and structures. In the abdomen, for example, a tumor mass can cause bowel or ureteral obstruction. Cancer can also spread to adjacent structures and penetrate body cavities by direct extension. For example, ovarian tumors frequently shed cells into the peritoneal cavity, where they grow to cover the surface of abdominal organs.

Malignant tumors differ from benign ones in their ability to *metastasize*, or spread from the primary site to other locations in the body. Metastasis occurs when cells break away from the primary tumor, travel through the body via the blood and/or lymphatic circulation, and become trapped in the capillaries of organs. From there, they infiltrate the organ tissue and grow into new tumor deposits.

Patterns of metastasis differ from cancer to cancer. Cancers tend to metastasize to specific organs or sites in the body, as shown in Figure 2. Clinical symptoms and problems vary according to the organ involved and the extent of disease.

In addition to the local effects of tumor growth, cancer can produce systemic signs and symptoms that are not direct effects of either the tumor or its metastases. These manifestations are collectively referred to as *paraneoplastic syndromes*. Many of these syndromes involve ectopic hormone production by tumor cells or the secretion of biochemically active substances that cause metabolic abnormalities. Paraneoplastic syndromes can also involve the nervous, hematologic, renal, and gastrointestinal systems.

STAGING

Staging is the process of describing the extent of disease at the time of diagnosis in order to aid in treatment planning, predict clinical outcome or prognosis, and compare different treatment approaches. The *TNM classification* proposed by the American Joint Commission on Cancer is the most frequently used system for defining the extent of disease. The *T* refers to the anatomic size of the primary tumor; *N* is the extent of lymph node involvement; and *M* denotes the presence or absence of metastases. This and other staging systems will be referred to in subsequent chapters as they relate to specific types of cancer.

CLASSIFICATION OF TUMORS

Cancers are named according to the site of the primary tumor and the type of tissue involved (*histology*). The three major classifications of normal body tissue are epithelial, connective and muscle, and nerve tissue.

Epithelial tissues cover all external body surfaces and line all internal spaces and cavities. The skin, mucous membranes, gas-

Primary Disease	Common sites of metastasis	Bone	Marrow	Skin	Lung	Liver	Bowel/rectum	Nodes	Spleen	Kidney	Brain	Serosa	Other pelvic organs	Meninges	Adrenal glands
Bladder								X		X			X		
Brain														X	
Breast		X			X	X		X			X			X	
Cervix		X			X	X	X	X		X					
Colon					X	X		X							
Esophagus		X			X	X		X							X
Head/Neck				X	X			X							
Hepatoma		X			X			X							
Kidney		X			X	X		X			X				
Lung		X	X					X		X	X			X	
Melanoma		X		X	X	X		X			X				
Mycosis Fungoides		X	X					X	X						
Ovary					X	X	X	X					X		
Pancreas					X	X	X	X							
Prostate		X			X	X		X							
Sarcoma					X			X							
Stomach		X			X	X		X							
Testes		X			X	X		X							
Thyroid		X			X			X							
Uterus					X									X	

Figure 2. Tumor Type and Metastatic Spread
Source: From *Handbook of Oncology Nursing* (pp. 586–587) by B. L. Johnson and J. Gross, 1985, New York: Delmar Publishers, Inc. Reprinted with permission of publisher.

trointestinal tract, and lining of the bladder are examples of epithelial tissues. The functions of epithelial tissues are to protect, excrete, and absorb. Cancer originating in the epithelial tissue is called a *carcinoma.*

Connective tissue consists of elastic, fibrous, and collagenous tissues, such as bone, cartilage, and fat. The function of such tissue is to connect, support, and protect. Cancers originating in connective tissue and in muscle are called *sarcomas.*

Nerve tissue includes the brain, spinal cord, and nerves. It consists of two types of cells: neurons and glial cells. Tumors arising in nerve tissue do not have a common name, but are named specifically for the type of cell involved. For example, tumors arising from astrocytes, a type of glial cell thought to form the blood-brain barrier, are called *astrocytomas*. Tumors arising in nerve tissue are often benign, but, because of their critical location, are more likely to be harmful than benign tumors in other sites. Table 3 categorizes benign and malignant tumors according to their tissue of origin.

Table 3. Classification of Tumors

Tissue of Origin	Benign Tumor	Malignant Tumor
Epithelial		
surface epithelium	papilloma	carcinoma
epithelial lining of glands or ducts	adenoma	adenocarcinoma
Connective tissue and muscle		
fibrous tissue	fibroma	fibrosarcoma
cartilage	chondroma	chondrosarcoma
bone	osteoma	osteosarcoma
smooth muscle	leiomyoma	leiomyosarcoma
striated muscle	rhabdomyoma	rhabdomyosarcoma
Nerve tissue		
glial		glioma
meninges	meningioma	meningeal sarcoma
retina		retinoblastoma

A tumor's histologic type is determined by the appearance and organization of the cells when examined under a microscope. In many parts of the body, more than one type of tissue may be involved, and cancers of more than one histologic type can develop. Thus, a cancer arising from the glandular tissue of the prostate gland is classified as an "adenocarcinoma" of the prostate, while a tumor arising from the striated muscle in the prostate will be termed "rhabdomyosarcoma" of the prostate. It is important to determine the cancer's histologic type, because this affects decisions about treatment approaches and estimates of prognosis.

CONCLUSION

Each type of cancer expresses characteristics peculiar to itself, but all probably share the same basic nature and process of development. By understanding the process of carcinogenesis and identifying intrinsic and extrinsic factors that affect that process, we may learn how cancer can be prevented and how to effectively treat clinically expressed cancers.

Bibliography

Donehower, M. G. (1985). The behavior of malignancies. In B. L. Johnson & J. Gross (Eds.), *Handbook of oncology nursing* (pp. 1-20). NY: John Wiley and Sons.

Fry, R. J. (1989). Principles of cancer biology: Physical carcinogenesis. In V. DeVita, S. Hellman, & S. Rosenberg (Eds.), *Cancer: Principles and practice of oncology* (3rd edition) (pp. 136-148). Philadelphia: J. B. Lippincott Co.

Groer, M. V. (1987). Risk factors and theories of carcinogenesis. In S. L. Groenwald (Ed.), *Cancer nursing: Principles and practice* (pp. 48-63). Boston: Jones and Bartlett Publishers, Inc.

Liotta, L. A., & Statler-Stevenson, W. G. (1989). Principles of molecular cell biology of cancer: Cancer metastasis. In V. DeVita, S. Hellman, & S. Rosenberg (Eds.), *Cancer: Principles and practice of oncology* (3rd edition) (pp. 98-115). Philadelphia: J. B. Lippincott Co.

Mettlin, C., & Mirand, A. L. (In Press). The causes of cancer. In S. Baird, R. McCorkle, & M. Grant (Eds.), *Cancer nursing: A comprehensive textbook.* Philadelphia, PA.: W. B. Saunders Co.

Pitot, H. C. (1989). Principles of carcinogenesis: Chemical. In V. DeVita, S. Hellman, & S. Rosenberg (Eds.), *Cancer: Principles and practice of oncology* (3rd edition) (pp. 116-135). Philadelphia: J. B. Lippincott Co.

Roberts, A. B., & Senic, R. T. (1986). Assessment of carcinogenesis through epidemiologic and experimental investigations. *Seminars in Oncology Nursing, 2*(3): 154-160.

Sporn, M. B. (1989). Principles of molecular cell biology of cancer: Factors related to cancer biology: Transformation. In V. DeVita, S. Hellman, & S. Rosenberg (Eds.), *Cancer: Principles and practice of oncology* (3rd edition) (pp. 67-80). Philadelphia: J. B. Lippincott Co.

Weinberg, R. A. (1983). Oncogenes (Interview). *Ca—A Journal for Clinicians, 33*(5), 300-306.

3 CANCER PREVENTION AND RISK REDUCTION

Ivana T. Croghan and Margene K. Omoto

Cancer is the second leading cause of death in the United States, exceeded only by cardiovascular disease. In 1990 alone, 1,040,000 individuals are expected to develop cancer and 510,000 will die from it. In other words, one out of three people will have cancer in his or her lifetime; at the current rate, four out of 10 of these individuals will be alive 5 years after diagnosis.

As disease evolves, pathologic changes may become irreversible. Therefore, prevention rather than cure is the focus of cancer control and health maintenance.

LEVELS OF PREVENTION

There are three levels of cancer prevention: primary, secondary, and tertiary.

Primary Prevention

Primary prevention consists of two major types of activities: technological and cognitive. Currently, no known specific technological activity, such as immunization, prevents cancer. Research is increasing in this area, especially in the field of immunology.

Cognitive activities encompass health education, an important nursing responsibility. Nurses can provide health counseling, promote good health habits, and assist the patient to stop or reduce habits hazardous to health, such as smoking or unhealthy eating. Specifically, health education focuses on risk factors suspected to be causally linked with cancer and on minimizing or avoiding exposure to those factors.

For example, if an individual smokes and is therefore at high risk for lung cancer, the nurse can counsel the person on ways to reduce or eliminate this carcinogenic exposure. If the person has a family history of cancer that increases risk, the best services the nurse can provide are cancer education and guidelines for monitoring health status. The nurse can teach the person to recognize the signs of cancer, to follow nutritional guidelines, and to be aware of cancer-causing agents in the environment. The nurse should emphasize the importance of regular health screening and that early diagnosis is directly related to improved prognosis. Nurses can use the information in Table 1 to help identify high-risk patients.

Secondary Prevention

Most known cancer control interventions fall into the category of secondary prevention. The goal of secondary prevention is to prevent morbidity and mortality, so early detection and prompt treatment are the activities emphasized. Secondary prevention measures are extremely important. For example, the American Cancer Society estimates that 42,500 of the cancer deaths that occurred in 1989 could have been avoided through early detection and treatment.

Tertiary Prevention

The third level of cancer prevention is tertiary prevention, defined as the limitation of disability and rehabilitation for patients with cancer. For instance, complications can be prevented by educating patients and monitoring them regularly. Nurses can also contribute significantly to efforts to limit disability by managing symptoms and responding promptly to complications.

CANCER CAUSES AND ASSOCIATION

The causes of cancer are varied, and causative agents are generally subdivided into two categories—those of endogenous (genetic) and those of exogenous (environmental) origin.

According to the American Cancer Society, 80% of all cancers may be associated with environmental exposures and therefore might be prevented if exposure to the causative factors is reduced or avoided. This chapter discusses methods of reducing or eliminating disease occurrence (primary prevention); therefore only exogenous causes will be discussed. Endogenous risk factors will be discussed in the next chapter, on early detection. Tertiary prevention is discussed in Units IV and V.

Many epidemiological studies have demonstrated associations between cancer development and environmental factors. The fact that cancer incidence varies around the world (Table 2) lends support to the idea of modifying an individual's exposure to specific environmental factors to reduce cancer risk. Other epidemiological studies following migrant populations have illustrated that the development of cancer can be influenced by changing environments. For example, when migrants from Japan, an area of low cancer incidence, acquire the lifestyles of Americans, the incidence of breast cancer among them rose to approximate the rate among

Table 1. Risk Factors for Selected Cancer Sites

Cancer Site	High Risk Factors
Lung	Heavy smoker over age 50 Smoked a pack a day for 20 years Started smoking at age 15 or before Smoker working with or near asbestos
Breast	Lump in breast or nipple discharge History of breast cancer in other breast or benign 　breast disease Family history of breast cancer Diet high in fat Nulliparous or first child after age 30 Early menarche or menopause
Colon-Rectum	History of rectal polyps or colonic ademomatosis Family history of rectal polyps Ulcerative colitis or Chron's disease Obesity Increasing age
Uterine-Endometrial	Unusual vaginal bleeding or discharge History of menstrual irregularity Late menopause (after age 55) Nulliparity Infertility, through anovulation Diabetes, high blood pressure, and obesity Age over 50 to 64
Skin	Excessive exposure to sun Fair complexion, burn easily Presence of congenital moles or history of dys- 　plastic nevi or cutaneous melanoma Family history of melanoma
Oral	Heavy smoker and drinker Poor oral hygiene Long term exposure to the sun (lip)
Ovary	History of ovarian cancer among close relatives Nulliparity or delayed age at first pregnancy Age 50 to 59
Prostate	Increasing age Occupations relating to the use of cadmium
Stomach	History of stomach cancer among close relatives Diet heavy in smoked, pickled, or salted foods

Source: From *"Cancer Risk and Assessment"* Cohen, R. F. Frank-Stromborg, M. 1990. In S. L. Groenwald, M. H. Frogge, M. Goodman, & C. H. Yarbro. (Eds.). *Cancer Nursing: Principles and Practice.* Boston, MA: Jones and Bartlett Publishers, Inc. Adapted with permission.

Table 2. Range of Incidence Areas for Common Cancers Among Males (and for Certain Cancers Among Females)

Site of Origin of Cancer	High Incidence Area	Sex	Low Incidence Area
Skin (chiefly non-melanoma)	Australia, Queensland	Male	India, Bombay
Esophagus	Iran (northeast section)	Male	Nigeria
Lung and bronchus	England	Male	Nigeria
Stomach	Japan	Male	Uganda
Cervix uteri	Columbia	Female	Israel, Jewish
Prostate	United States; blacks	Male	Japan
Liver	Mozambique	Male	England
Breast	Canada, British Columbia	Female	Israel, Non-Jewish
Colon	United States; Connecticut	Male	Nigeria
Corpus uteri	United States; California	Female	Japan
Buccal cavity	India; Bombay	Male	Denmark
Rectum	Denmark	Male	Nigeria
Bladder	United States; Connecticut	Male	Japan
Ovary	Denmark	Female	Japan
Nasopharynx	Singapore; Chinese	Male	England
Pancreas	New Zealand; Maori	Male	India, Bombay
Larynx	Brazil; Sao Paulo	Male	Japan
Pharynx	India; Bombay	Male	Denmark
Penis	Parts of Uganda	Male	Israel; Jewish

Source: From *The Causes of Cancer* (p. 1197-1312), by R. Doll & R. Peto, 1981, New York: Oxford University Press. Adapted with permission of publisher.

native United States women. In other studies, when the same community was studied prospectively, it was observed that the incidence of some cancers paralleled lifestyle changes. Two examples are stomach cancer—which decreased in the United States with changes in technology such as refrigeration and in eating habits—and lung cancer, which increased worldwide as cigarette smoking increased.

Risk

Associations between disease and exposure to specific agents or factors are usually quantified in terms of different levels of risks. *Risk* relates the magnitude of effect of a particular factor or characteristic on the outcome being investigated (e.g., mortality rate of a specific cancer). Two types of risk measurement can be calculated: *relative risk* and *attributable risk.*

Relative risk measures the strength of the association between a factor and the outcome. Relative risk of cancer is a ratio of the probability of developing cancer among a group having a characteristic or risk factor to the probability of developing cancer among a similar group without the characteristic or risk factor.

$$\text{Relative Risk} = \cfrac{\left\{\cfrac{\text{Number with cancer in exposed population}}{\text{Number of exposed population}}\right.}{\text{divided by}}$$
$$\left\{\cfrac{\text{Number with cancer in unexposed population}}{\text{Number of unexposed population}}\right.$$

If the relative risk is greater than one, a person with the characteristic or risk factor is more likely to develop cancer than a person without them. If the relative risk is less than one, a person with the characteristic is less likely to develop cancer than the person without the characteristic. If the relative risk is one, the cancer and the characteristic or factor are not associated. The higher the relative risk, the greater evidence of causation. The risk can be expressed numerically or as low or high.

Attributable risk measures the public health effect of a risk factor or characteristic in a population. It is expressed in terms of the proportion of cases in exposed people that can be attributed to the exposure. Attributable risk is the arithmetic difference in cancer rates between the group exposed to the factor and the unexposed group.

$$\text{Attributable Risk} = \left\{\cfrac{\text{Number with cancer in exposed population}}{\text{Number of exposed population}}\right.$$
$$\text{minus}$$
$$\left\{\cfrac{\text{Number with cancer in unexposed population}}{\text{Number of unexposed population}}\right.$$

For example, suppose the mortality rate among heavy smokers subject to low doses of industrial ionizing radiation is 2.7 per 1000 men, and the mortality rate among nonsmokers with the same dose of ionizing radiation is 0.23 per 1000 men. The attributable risk is 2.5, meaning that an additional 2.5 deaths per 1000 men occurred that were attributable to smoking. These excess deaths would have not occurred if the individuals had not smoked heavily.

Researchers continue to uncover various factors that promote cancer and/or predispose individuals to cancer. For example, the causal relationship between cigarettes and the incidence of lung cancer has been proven beyond question. According to the American Cancer Society (ACS), a higher relative risk exists among male smokers than female smokers, but this risk rate might well change as the incidence rises among women due to increased smoking.

Factors Related to Carcinogenesis

Tobacco: Factors associated with increased risk for specific cancers are listed in Table 1. Of all known or suspected carcinogens, cigarette smoking is the primary cause of cancer death in the United States today. Overall, smoking is suspected of being the primary cause of over 83% of all lung cancer cases and of approximately 30% of all cancer deaths. Smokers are at 10 times greater risk of developing cancer than non-smokers. Smoking factors that should be considered are the number of years smoked, the number of cigarettes smoked, and how deeply the smoke is inhaled. Once a person stops smoking, their cancer risk immediately begins to decrease; after 15 years without smoking the risk is equal to that of non-smokers.

Although it has been hypothesized that switching to other forms of tobacco (e.g., cigars or pipe) or even smoking low-tar and low nicotine cigarettes could reduce cancer risks, studies have shown that none of these are healthy alternatives. Cigarette smokers who switch to a pipe or cigars may still maintain the habit of inhaling the smoke and will be running the risk of developing other cancers, such as oral cancer. Smokers who switch to low-tar and low-nicotine cigarettes may smoke more or have a tendency to inhale deeper.

Recently, concern has arisen over the use of "smokeless" tobaccos. Smokeless tobacco (chewing tobacco, snuff) is associated with the development of oral cancers. This relationship is particularly troublesome since smokeless tobacco is popular among adolescent males.

Because there is a strong association between tobacco (in all forms) and cancer of the lung, mouth, tongue, upper airway, bladder, kidney, esophagus, and perhaps pancreas, individuals wishing to ultimately lower their cancer risk should eliminate tobacco completely.

Alcohol: Alcohol is hypothesized to cause 5% of cancer deaths. Excessive consumption of alcohol is associated with cancer of the mouth, pharynx, larynx, and esophagus. It can also indirectly cause liver cancer (i.e., alcohol causes cirrhosis which is, in turn, associated with liver cancer). Alcohol consumption and cigarette smoking together produce a greater risk for esophageal and mouth cancer than either cigarette smoking or alcohol consumption alone. Despite the epidemiological evidence linking alcohol to cancer, the exact carcinogen in alcohol has yet to be determined; however, the American Cancer Society strongly advises a reduction of alcohol consumption.

Occupational Exposure: Occupational exposure to agents such as radiation, ultraviolet rays, asbestos, benzene, and other polycyclic hydrocarbons, chromate, vinyl chloride, nitrosamines, aflatoxins, arsenic, automotive exhaust, and pesticides has been linked to a number of cancers (Table 3). These substances may work alone or in combination with others to cause cancer.

Regulatory agencies, industry, and organized labor have developed a number of policies and regulations to protect the worker. These require companies to provide workers with access to information on all substances to which they are exposed at work. The federal government has also developed health and safety regulations that must be followed to reduce or eliminate cancer in the work force.

Viruses: Viruses have also been linked to a number of cancers. Those identified with specific cancer should be avoided when possible including: the hepatitis B virus (linked to liver cancer in Asia and Africa), the Epstein-Barr virus (associated with nasopharyngeal cancer and Burkitt's Lymphoma), and herpes and papilloma viruses (linked to an increased risk for cervical cancer). The human immunodeficiency viruses type I & II are linked with Acquired Immune Deficiency Syndrome (AIDS), which in turn is associated with Kaposi's sarcoma and lymphoma.

X-rays: High levels of x-rays were used in the past as a form of treatment for many medical conditions (such as cancer, mastitis, acne). Numerous epidemiological studies of the effects of radiation exposure have shown that large doses cause cancer. Although the radiation levels involved in medical procedures have been reduced considerably, patients should be advised to consult their physician and dentist about the use of x-rays. If an x-ray is deemed necessary, the best safeguard is use of an x-ray shield to cover other body parts.

Hormones: A link between large doses of postmenopausal estrogens and endometrial or breast cancer in women has been suggested. Large doses of oral contraceptives were, at one point, associated with cervical and breast cancer. The role of estrogen in cancer remains controversial, so patients considering the use of low-dose estrogens and oral contraceptives should be advised to discuss dosages with a physician.

Ultraviolet rays: Skin cancer is currently on the rise, and excessive exposure to ultraviolet rays (in sunlight) is believed to be the major cause. In the past, skin cancer was easily cured, but the current increase in the incidence of the more intractable melanoma is a cause for concern. Because the strongest ultraviolet rays are emitted from 11:00 a.m. to 3:00 p.m. (10:00 a.m. to 2:00 p.m. daylight

Table 3. Occupational Exposures and Cancer

Cancer sites	Causal Agents	Work or Exposure
Lung	Bichloromethyl ether Chromium Mustard gas	Ion exchange resin producers Ore and pigment manufacturers Poison gas producers
Lung, pleura	Asbestos	Asbestos miners, insulation, shipyard workers
Lung and skin	Arsenic Polycyclic hydrocarbons	Smelter and pesticide workers Mineral oil and tar workers
Lung and nasal Skin Liver	Nickel Ultraviolet light Vinyl chloride Alcohol	Nickel refiners Outdoor workers, fishermen Vinyl chloride workers Brewery workers
Bladder Leukemia Nasal	Aromatic amines Benzene Isopropryl alcohol manufacturers Wood dust	Dye and rubber workers Glue and varnish workers Isopropryl alcohol Furniture workers
Multiple sites	Ionizing radiation	Radium dial painters Uranium miners

Note: Reprinted by permission of The American Cancer Society, Atlanta, GA. From *Cancer Prevention and Detection*, (1986). Costanza, M. E., Li, F. P., Green, H. L., and Patterson, W. B., in B. Cady (Ed.) *Cancer Manual* (7th ed.) (pp. 14–35).

savings time), excessive exposure to sunlight during these hours should be avoided. Individuals with fair skin are at greater risk for developing skin cancer.

To avoid excessive exposure to the sun during the crucial hours, sunscreens should be used. A sunscreen with an SPF (sun protective factor) number above 15 is best. Long sleeves, pants, and a broad-brimmed hat provide added protection.

Foods: Some foods have been suspected to be carcinogens for several years, but more definitive answers are still being sought. To date, many foods have been found to contain carcinogens in the form of additives or as byproducts of storage, cooking, or the host's metabolism.

Findings from studies of cancer and diet are often contradictory or inconclusive. Current research suggests that an increase in dietary fiber may help prevent colon cancer by decreasing the transit time of digested foods in the colon. Foods high in fat content have been associated with an increase in the incidence of colon, prostate, and breast cancers. Current data on the association between fat and breast cancer are inconclusive. Some studies have suggested that obesity (40% or more overweight) is a significant risk factor for colon, breast, endometrial, and prostate cancers. Studies have also shown that salt-cured, smoked, and nitrite-cured foods are risk factors for cancer of the esophagus and stomach. Other studies have suggested that some vitamins may help protect against the development of certain cancers (e.g., lung, larynx, esophagus, and stomach). Nurses should keep abreast of research in these areas and assess study results carefully.

A well-balanced diet is the best dietary means of preventing cancer. The American Cancer Society recommends a diet involving a variety of foods daily, including fruits and vegetables high in vitamins A and C. A diet low in fat is also advisable. Avoid frying foods, limit the use of oils (including butter and margarine), avoid snack foods (e.g., potato chips), and choose low-fat dairy products. Eating foods high in fiber and whole grain—including a number of raw fruits and vegetables, beans, peas, and seeds—is also advisable.

In conclusion, the best cancer prevention tips are:
* Don't smoke or use tobacco in any form (including cigarettes, pipes, cigars, snuff, or chewing tobacco).
* Drink alcohol in moderation (one to two drinks per day).
* Know and follow health and safety rules at your work place.
* Avoid unnecessary x-ray exposure. If the x-ray is necessary, wear a shield to protect other parts of your body.
* Take estrogens only as long as necessary and be sure to discuss dosage with your physician.
* Avoid overexposure to the sun by using sunscreens (an SPF above 15) and wearing protective clothing. Be particularly cautious between 11 a.m. and 3 p.m.
* Eat a diet high in fiber and low in fat (fruits, vegetables, and whole-grain breads and cereals).

Perhaps the most important information nurses can give clients is to adopt a lifetime of good health practices. As part of their primary prevention efforts, nurses can teach other nurses, health professionals, and the public about preventative health practices. Nurses can exert a strong and positive influence on individuals' attitudes and behaviors, helping them to change in ways that will reduce their cancer risk.

Bibliography

American Cancer Society. (1990). *Cancer facts and figures—1990.* Atlanta: Author.

Cohen, R. F. & Frank-Stromborg, M. (1990). Cancer risk and assessment. In S. L. Groenwald, M. H. Frogge, M. Goodman, & C. H. Yarbro (Eds.), *Cancer nursing: Principles and practice* (pp. 103–118). Boston: Jones and Bartlett Publishers.

Costanza, M. E., Li, F. P., Green, H. L., & Patterson, W. B. (1986). Cancer prevention and detection: Strategies for practice. In B. Cady, S. P. Kadish, R. T. Osteen, & P. E. Rosenthal (Eds.), *Cancer manual* (7th ed.) (pp. 14–35). Boston: American Cancer Society.

Derdiarian, A. (1981). Nursing in prevention of cancer. In D. L. Vredevoe, A. Derdiarian, L. P. Sarna, M. Friel, & J. A. G. Shiplacoff (Eds.), *Concepts of oncology nursing* (pp. 270–294). Englewood Cliffs, NJ: Prentice-Hall, Inc.

Fraumeni, Jr., J. F., Hoover, R. N., Devesa, S. S., & Kinlen, L. J. (1989). Epidemiology of cancer. In V. T. DeVita, Jr., S. Hellman, & S. A. Rosenberg (Eds.), *Cancer principles and practice of oncology* (3rd ed.) (pp. 196-235). Philadelphia: J. B. Lippincott.

Hutchison, G. B. (1982). The epidemiologic method. In D. Schottenfeld & J. F. Fraumeni (Eds.), *Cancer epidemiology and prevention* (pp. 3-14). Philadelphia: W. B. Saunders.

National Cancer Institute. (1985). *Cancer rates and risks* (3rd ed.). (NIH Publication No. 85-691). Bethesda, MD: U. S. Department of Health and Human Services.

National Cancer Institute. (1987). *Diet, nutrition, and cancer prevention: The good news.* (NIH Publication No. 27-2878). Bethesda, MD: U.S. Department of Health and Human Services.

Newell, G. R. (1985). Epidemiology of cancer. In V. T. DeVita, Jr., S. Hellman, & S. A. Rosenberg (Eds.), *Cancer principles and practice of oncology* (2nd ed.) (pp. 151-182). Philadelphia: J. B. Lippincott.

Oleske, D., & Groenwald, S. L. (1987). Epidemiology of cancer. In S. L. Groenwald, (Ed.), *Cancer nursing: Principles and practices* (pp. 3-28). Boston: Jones and Bartlett Publishers.

4 SCREENING, DETECTION, AND DIAGNOSIS

Joy Miler Knopp and Ivana T. Croghan

Secondary prevention has become an important part of cancer care in the United States. *Secondary prevention* consists of early screening, detection, and diagnosis of cancer. By detecting cancer at the earliest stage possible, curing it or slowing its progression, preventing complications, and limiting disability, both length and quality of life can be maximized.

Cancer *screening* consists of the prediagnostic procedures used to determine the probability that disease is present. Nurses frequently play an important role in educating the public about screening programs and in conducting screening tests. *Detection* methods, such as mammography and the Papanicolaou (PAP) smear, are used to determine the presence of disease, identify it, and estimate its extent. Nurses' responsibilities may include data gathering, assessment, specimen collection, and further education. *Diagnosis* is the actual confirmation of a specific type of cancer and its location. In addition to fulfilling the above roles, nurses provide support and guidance during these processes.

SCREENING

Cancer screening is an organized effort to assess large numbers of people at risk for disease. Screening involves the use of simple tests or examinations customarily directed at asymptomatic individuals, the vast majority of whom will be free of cancer. The purpose of screening is to detect cancer at an early stage when it is most curable. Some of the most common and life-threatening forms of cancer, such as testicular and cervical cancers, are the most easily treated when detected early.

Three basic principles are applied to screening to assure accuracy and efficacy:

- The test in question must be reasonably accurate, with only a minimum number of missed cases (false negative results) and cancers incorrectly identified (false positives);
- The screening test must be acceptable to the patient—without much discomfort, inconvenience, risk, or expense;

- Early detection through screening must result in a more favorable prognosis than detection at a later stage—in other words, there must be known therapeutic benefit associated with early detection.

The cost-benefit ratios are often favorable for screening for cervical, breast, and colorectal cancers. Cancers for which the screening cost-benefit ratios are unknown, under study, or favorable in very selected circumstances only are lung, prostate, melanoma, head and neck, testes, bladder, stomach, and endometrium.

Effective screening practices should begin with a health history and physical exam. The accuracy and completeness of history-taking and physical examination are essential and lead to a differential diagnosis. Information gathered during history taking includes medical, family, social, occupational, and sexual background. The nurse may also acquire information about exposure to certain cancer-causing agents that place the individual in a high-risk category. The history may lead to detection of vague symptoms that the patient may be unaware of or be denying. Nurses should use an optimistic and empathetic interviewing technique to obtain a history. The physical exam, which includes inspection and palpation, can then follow. Table 1 summarizes The American Cancer Society's recommendations for the early detection of cancer in asymptomatic people. These should be incorporated into the regular physical examinations as appropriate.

According to the American Cancer Society there are seven warning signs that can indicate the presence of cancer (Figure 1). The nurse obtaining a patient's history should obtain information on all these warning signs. Other changes in normal body functions that persist and should be noted are loss of weight, fever, fatigue, and pain. Table 2 summarizes by site the symptoms that should be investigated and the most common detection and diagnostic tests.

The screening process is more than a set of examinations and tests. It is an excellent opportunity for nurses to educate patients about self-examination techniques, stop-smoking programs, and personal and occupational health hazards. Patients can perform self-examination of breasts, testes, skin, and the oral cavity. The American Cancer Society has excellent materials to teach self-examination techniques.

Nurses can receive specialized training in screening techniques such as oral exams, pelvic exams, rectal exams, and breast exams from the American Cancer Society and other organizations. Counseling, especially for high-risk individuals, is an integral part of care (see Unit II, Chapter 3, for risk-related information). Nurses providing

Table 1. Summary of American Cancer Society Recommendations for the Early Detection of Cancer in Asymptomatic People.

Test or Procedure	Population		
	Sex	Age	Frequency
Sigmoidoscopy	M & F	50 and over	Every 3 to 5 years, based on advice of physician.
Stool guaiac Slide test	M & F	Over 50	Every year
Digital rectal examination	M & F	Over 40	Every year
Pap test	F	All women who are, or who have been, sexually active, or have reached age 18, should have an annual Pap test and pelvic examination. After a woman has had three or more consecutive satisfactory normal annual examinations, the Pap test may be performed less frequently at the discretion of her physician.	
Pelvic examination	F		
Endometrial tissue sample	F	At menopause, women at high risk*	At menopause
Breast self-examination	F	20 and over	Every month
Breast physical examination	F	20-40 Over 40	Every 3 years Every year
Mammography	F	35-39 40-49 50 and over	Baseline Every 1-2 years Every year
Chest x-ray			Not recommended
Sputum cytology			Not recommended
Health counseling and cancer checkup**	M & F M & F	Over 20 Over 40	Every 3 years Every year

*History of infertility, obesity, failure to ovulate, abnormal uterine bleeding, or estrogen therapy.
**To include examination for cancers of the thyroid, testicles, prostate, ovaries, lymph nodes, oral region, and skin.

Source: From American Cancer Society Summary of Current Guidelines for the Cancer Related Checkup: Recommendations. No. 3347.0I PE, Rev. 2/89.

screening services can also make an important contribution by educating employers and third party payers about the benefits of screening.

DIAGNOSIS AND STAGING

When cancer is suspected, diagnosis and then staging are performed. Diagnosis confirms a malignancy and determines the cancer type and location. Staging establishes the extent and an-

Change in bowel or bladder habits
A sore that does not heal
Unusual bleeding or discharge
Thickening or lump in breast or elsewhere
Indigestion or difficulty swallowing
Obvious change in wart or mole
Nagging cough or hoarseness

Figure 1. Cancer's seven warning signs.
Source: American Cancer Society

ticipated natural course of the disease; this information is necessary to plan treatment, indicate prognosis, evaluate results, and contribute to cancer research. There are several staging systems, but the most frequently used is the *TNM system*. The letters TNM represent particular characteristics of a tumor: T refers to the primary tumor size, N refers to the degree of local spread to regional lymph nodes, and M indicates presence of distant spread and metastasis.

Another classification system, which uses Roman numerals, is applied to the staging of Hodgkin's disease and other tumors. Stage I, the low end of the scale, usually designates localized disease—encapsulated or well defined—while stage IV, the high end, indicates disseminated disease. More information about the staging of specific cancers and the use of staging in determining treatment is provided in Unit V.

Confirmation of disease diagnosis and stage often requires a synthesis of information obtained from the health history, the physical examination, and radiology, hematology, cytology, histology, and other special studies. The nurse can explain tests, assist in patient preparation, and provide guidance to patients and their families.

Radiologic Examinations

The four types of radiologic examination are conventional radiography with or without contrast media, nuclear medicine, vascular/interventional radiology, and ultrasonography/thermography.

Conventional x-rays focus on specific body parts and project the image of that part onto film. X-rays are frequently used to detect lung and gastrointestinal cancers. A common use of soft-tissue x-ray for detection is mammography. Contrast agents may be used for sites where visualization is difficult, including gastrointestinal tract, gall bladder, liver, and urinary tract. Commonly used contrast agents are iodine and barium.

Table 2. Screening and Detection Recommendations by Cancer Site*

Cancer Site	Signs & Symptoms	Screening/Detection/ Diagnostic Tests
Bladder	- Painless hematuria in the absence of urinary frequency or difficulty voiding - Frequent bladder irritability - Bloody urine or urinary sediment >3-5 red cells per high power field - Marked urgency, dysuria & frequency & a small volume of sterile urine - Interstitial cystitis	- Urine culture - Urinary tract cytology - Washings of bladder - Intravenous urography - Pelvic CT - Cytoscopy evaluation - Biopsy
Breast	- Painless lump or mass - Unilateral serous nipple discharge - Bloody discharge - Dermatitis of nipple/areola - Dimpling of skin in breast - Nipple retraction - Change in contour of breast - Fixation of a mass to the pectoral fascia/ chest wall - Edema & erythema of breast skin - Axillary adenopathy	- Physical breast exam - Mammography - Ultrasound/ Thermography - Percutaneous needle aspiration
Central nervous system	- Increasing intracranial pressure resulting in: headaches, vomiting, lethargy, edema, hemorrhage or infarction, depression - Contralateral homonymous hemianopsia - Epileptic seizures	- Neuroradiographic studies - CT of brain with contrast material - Carotid & vertebral arteriography - MRI - Analysis of cerebrospinal fluid - Endocrine evaluation
Colon/rectum	- Change in bowel habits: obstruction/ diarrhea - Rectal bleeding - Tenesmus - Iron deficiency anemia	- Fecal occult blood test - Digital rectal exam - Air contrast barium enema - CT - Cytoscopy - Colonoscopy - Flexible fiberoptic sigmoidoscopy
Esophagus	- Subtle changes in digestive habits: weight loss, malaise, & anorexia - Dysphagia to solid foods followed by - Dysphagia to liquids - Unexplained "choking" - Gastroesophageal reflux	- Careful physical exam - Radiography (CT) - Fluoroscopy & barium swallow - Endoscopy exam (esophagoscopy with biopsy)

Table 2. Screening and Detection Recommendations by Cancer Site* (Cont.)

Cancer Site	Signs & Symptoms	Screening/Detection/ Diagnostic Tests
Esophagus (continued)	- punch biopsies - brush biopsies - cytology studies of exfoliated cells	
Extrahepatic bile duct	- Jaundice followed by Pruritus - Anorexia & weight loss - Fever - Dyspepsia - Nausea - Vomiting	- Physical Exam (enlarged liver) - Ultrasound - CT - Endoscopic retrograde cholangiopancreatography - Percutaneous trans-hepatic cholangiography by thin-needle
Female genital tract Vulva: Cervical: Endometrial: Ovarian:	- Pruritus vulvae - Postcoital spotting - Postmenopausal bleeding (6 months after menopause) - Enlarged abdomen - Vague digestive disturbance	- GYN exam: Inspection & palpation of superficial lymph nodes (superclavicular, axillary & inguinal areas) - PAP smear - Bimanual palpation - Fractional D & C - Laparoscopy/ laparotomy - CT - Cytology studies - Directed biopsy
Gall bladder	- Acute or chronic cholecystitis - Abdominal pain - Anorexia - Weight loss - Jaundice - Nausea - Vomiting - Occasional fever	- Diagnostic x-rays - Laboratory studies: Liver chemistry Elevated alkaline phosphatase - Laparotomy
Head and neck Oral Cavity: Oropharynx:	- Reddish or whitish patch that persists - Difficulty in chewing, swallowing, or moving tongue or jaws - Firm unilateral lymph nodes in neck - Swelling or ulcer that fails to heal - Ipsilateral referred otalgia - Indurated ulcer - Dysphasia - Local pain - Pain on swallowing - Referred otalgia	- Careful exam of upper aerodigestive tract - Individual indirect mirror exam - Finger palpation - Radiography: Plain films CT Tomographs Orthropantomogram of mandible Barium swallow Laryngogram

Table 2. Screening and Detection Recommendations by Cancer Site* (Cont.)

Cancer Site	Signs & Symptoms	Screening/Detection/ Diagnostic Tests
Head and neck (continued)		
Hypopharynx:	- Dysphasia - Odynophagia - Referred otalgia - Neck mass	Chest X-rays Bone scan Arteriogram - Fiberoptic aerodigestive endoscopy
Larynx:	- Persistent hoarseness - Pain - Referred otalgia - Dyspnea - Stridor	- Biopsy

Nasopharynx:	- Bloody nasal discharge
	- Obstructed nostril
	- Conductive deafness
	- Neurologic problems:
	  atypical facial pain, diplopia, hoarseness,
	  Horner's syndrome
	- Neck mass	

Nose & Sinuses:	- Bloody nasal discharge - Nasal obstruction - Facial pain - Facial swelling - Diplopia	
Parotic & submandibular glands:	- Painless local swelling - Hemifacial paralysis	

Kidney	- Pain
	- Hematuria
	- Palpable abdominal mass
	- Weight loss
	- Polycythemia
	- Fever
	- Erythrocytosis
	- Hepatic dysfunction
	- Seizures
		- Intravenous pyelography
		  & arteriography
		- Ultrasound
		- CT
		- Urography &
		  nephrotomography
		- Radionuclide scan
		- Aspiration
		- Biopsy

Leukemia		

acute leukemia:	- Virus-like syndrome with low grade fever
	- Anemia
	- Fatigue
	- Pallor
	- Thrombocytopenia:
	  oozing gums, epistaxis, petechiae, ecchy-
	  moses, menorrhagia, excessive bleeding af-
	  ter tooth extraction
	- Infections of respiratory, dental, sinus, perirec-
	  tal, & urinary tract with poor response to
	  treatment
		- Fundoscopic exam
		- Laboratory findings of:
		  abnormal white blood
		  cell count
		- Peripheral blood smear
		- Aspiration of bone
		  marrow

Table 2. Screening and Detection Recommendations by Cancer Site* (Cont.)

Cancer Site	Signs & Symptoms	Screening/Detection/ Diagnostic Tests
Leukemia (continued)	- Diffuse adenopathy & - Hepatosplenomegaly - Bone pain - Migratory joint pain accompanied by swelling and tenderness	
Chronic myelogenous leukemia:	- Weight loss despite excellent appetite - Low grade fever - Night sweats - Fatiguability - Splenomegaly (mild sensation of fullness or awareness of actual mass) - Early satiety - Peripheral leg edema - Splenic pain referred to left shoulder - Bone pain - Bleeding problems - Mucous membrane irritation - Infection - Pallor - Adenopathy - Hepatomegaly	- Peripheral blood findings: - Reduced/absent leukocyte alkaline phosphatase (LAP) score -Presence of Philadelphia chromosome (Phi) - Hyperuricemia - Hyperuricosuria
Chronic lymphocytic leukemia:	- Minimal diffuse adenopathy or splenomegaly - Fatigue - Malaise - Occasional fever - Infection - Lymphadenopathy - Night sweats - Weight loss - Uncomfortable neck masses - Enlarged spleen - Anemia - Thrombocytonemia	- Routine blood studies - Bone marrow aspirations
Liver	- Painful hepatomegaly - Liver is tender with nodular enlargement - Splenomegaly - Esophageal varices - Ascites - Jaundice - Gastrointestinal bleeding - Fever - Edema	- Tumor Markers: eg, AFP - Ultrasound - CT with contrast medium - Liver scan - Arteriography - Portal venography - Bone survey - Chest radiography - Needle biopsy
Lung	- Change in pulmonary habits: cough, hoarseness, chest pain, rust-streaked or purulent sputum production, hemoptysis, & dyspnea - Recurrent pneumonitis - Pleural effusion	- Radiography - 3-day sputum cytology

Table 2. Screening and Detection Recommendations by Cancer Site* (Cont.)

Cancer Site	Signs & Symptoms	Screening/Detection/ Diagnostic Tests
Lung (continued)	- Shoulder and arm pain - Paresthesias	
(metastasis to brain):	- Headache - Unsteadiness of gait - Neurologic signs	
(metastasis to liver):	- Weight loss - Jaundice - Anorexia	
(metastasis to skeleton):	- Bony pain - Pathologic fractures	
Lymphoma		
(Hodgkin's Disease):	- Adenopathy in supraclavicular or cervical area - Fever - Night sweats - Weight loss	- Physical exam - CT of abdomen - Radiography of chest - Lymphagiography - Laparotomy

(Non-Hodgkin's Lymphoma):	- Adenopathy
	- Anemia
		- Laboratory findings of
		  -abnormal lymphocytes
		  -leukemia composed of lymphoma cells
		- Bone marrow aspiration
		- Radiographs of chest
		- Bipedal lymphangiography
		- Cytologic exams of any effusions
		- Lung tomography
		- Gallium & bone scans
		- Radiographic exams of gastrointestinal & urinary tract
		- Liver biopsy
		- Laparoscopy
		- Laparotomy & splenectomy

Multiple myeloma	- Anemia
	- Back pain
	- Painful skeletal lesions (osteolytic lesions)
	- Prone to pathologic fractures which result in exacerbations of pain & skeletal instability
	- Hypercalcemia—manifests in weakness, nausea, & altered mental status
	- Renal failure
		- Bone marrow exams
		- Radiographic tests with contrast dyes
		- Laboratory studies:
		  -serum electrophoreses
		  -erythrocyte sediment rate

Pancreas	- Insidious onset of asthenia, anorexia, weight loss, gaseousness & nausea - Dull pain in epigastrium/back - Jaundice - Pruritus	- CT with contrast medium - Ultrasound - Endoscopic retrograde cholangiopancreato-graphy - thin-needle percutaneous biopsy

Table 2. Screening and Detection Recommendations by Cancer Site* (Cont.)

Cancer Site	Signs & Symptoms	Screening/Detection/ Diagnostic Tests
Prostate	- Renal insufficiency & hematuria -weak or interrupted flow of urine -difficulty in starting & stopping urination -need to urinate frequently (esp. at night) -painful burning urination - Blood in urine - Bone pain -Continuous pain in lower back, pelvis or upper thighs	- Digital rectal exam - Blood studies (serum acid phospha- tase & alkaline acid phosphatase) - Radionuclide bone scan - Conventional radiography - Needle biopsy
Sarcoma of bone	- Pain - Presence of mass (initially painless) - Functional deficit - Pathologic fracture	- Physical exam - Bone scan - Chest CT - Full lung planar tomography - Biopsy
Skin/malignant melanoma	- Loss of skin markings - Variegation in pigmentation - Irregular hyperkeratotic areas - Rough area that scabs over, rescabs and fails to heal - Persistent ulcer - Any change in color, size, shape, elevation, surface, surrounding skin, sensation, & consistency	- Complete cutaneous exams - Biopsy
Soft-tissue sarcoma (tumors arising from supportive mesenchymal tissue other than bones)	- Painless mass (esp. in thigh area) - Hard consistency of mass - Peripheral neuralgia - paralysis - ischemia - bowel obstruction - weight loss - fever - general malaise - episodic hypoglycemia	- Physical exam - Radiographic studies: CT Angiography - Biopsy - Radioisotope studies
Stomach	- Complaints of indigestion & epigastric distress - Loss of appetite - Weight loss or anorexia - Dysphagia - Mass in abdomen - Colonic obstruction - Ulcer-type pain - Iron deficiency anemia	- Radiographic studies - Endoscopic exam - Gastroscopy with muc- osal biopsies - Abrasion balloon cytology - Flexible fiberoptic gastroscope
Testis	- Painless scrotal mass that does not illuminate - Orchitis - Infarction	- Physical exam (palpation) - Transillumination of in- trascrotal lesions - Abdominal exam

Table 2. Screening and Detection Recommendations by Cancer Site* (Cont.)

Cancer Site	Signs & Symptoms	Screening/Detection/ Diagnostic Tests

Testis (continued)	- A feeling of heaviness
	- At times trauma
	- A change in pre-existing hydrocele
	- An attack resembling epididymitis
	  (it does not respond to medical treatment
	  within 14 days)
	- Spermatocele
	- Hydrocele
	- Fatigue
	- Pallor (from Anemia)
	- Cough
	- Hemoptysis
		- Radiography of chest
		  Abdominopelvic Computed Tomographic
		  scanning
		- Hematologic survey
		  (RIA):
		  Chorionic gonadotropin
		  Alpha-feto protein
		  Lactic hydroglucose
		- Lymphangiography

Thyroid	- Mass in neck or cervical lymph node
	- Existing goiter may suddenly enlarge
	- Hoarseness
		- Careful palpation of the
		  thyroid gland
		- Have patient swallow
		  small quantities of water, while palpating
		  gland
		- Indirect mirror
		  laryngoscopy

Ureters	- Hematuria - Pain from obstruction	- Urine exam - Cytology - Excretory urography - Cystoscopy - Retrograde ureterography - Pyelography

*Childhood Cancers are not included.
Composite information found in: Rubin, P. (Ed.). (1983). *Clinical Oncology: A Multi-disciplinary Approach.* New York: American Cancer Society. (1986). *Cancer Manual (7th Ed.).* Boston: American Cancer Society, pp 478. (1990). *Cancer Facts and Figures—1990* (No. 5008-LE) Atlanta.

Computerized axial tomography (CAT or CT) is a radiologic technique that inspects a selected cross section of the body at a focal point. This technique provides visualization of inaccessible structures—such as those in the peritoneal area—and permits more precise estimation of tumor size, shape, and location than conventional x-rays. Low concentrations of contrast agents may be used to enhance a CT scan.

Magnetic resonance imaging (MRI) is a technique that uses conventional x-rays but provides superior contrast of soft tissues and allows visualization of multiple planes, including regions where bones hamper visualization by x-ray or CT scans. Standard MRI scans do not require iodine-based contrast media and are especially useful for studying the central nervous system.

Nuclear medicine refers to the use of a radioactive substance (*radionuclide*) administered orally or intravenously, which enables a physician to visualize practically every organ of the body. The most frequently investigated organ sites are the liver, spleen, bones, urinary tract, lungs, heart, thyroid, and brain.

Contrast studies provide information about vessel structure and condition by using a dye contrast. They are often useful in locating tumors. There are three types of contrast studies.

- Arteriography involves the injection of a contrast medium into an appropriate artery. It is used to localize a mass, identify relationships to adjacent organs, and gain information about the vascular supply of the tumor.
- Venography is the evaluation of the venous pathway and is helpful in studying mediastinal masses and retroperitoneal tumors.
- Lymphangiography, which is useful for staging, employs a contrast medium injected into a small lymph vessel of the foot to outline the lymph nodes of the groin and pelvis. It is used mainly to evaluate retroperitoneal nodes in patients with lymphoma, testicular cancer, or gynecologic cancer.

Ultrasound and thermography are two additional types of radiologic tests. *Ultrasound* uses high-frequency sound waves instead of x-rays to locate deep tumors. *Thermography* measures localized areas of elevated skin temperature, a phenomenon that occurs over inflammatory or malignant lesions.

Hematology

Abnormal findings from lab studies routinely performed as part of the physical examination (e.g., hemoglobin, blood sugar, uric acid studies) indicate the need for further work-up. Blood studies are also used to confirm metastasis from the primary disease site.

Biochemical tumor markers are the most specific and sensitive of the approaches available for detecting and monitoring the presence and/or quantity of tumor. Most tumor markers are immunologic products, including: oncofetal antigens (*carcinoembryonic antigen* or CEA); protein or hormonal products such as *human chorionic gonadotropin* (HCG) and *adrenocorticotropic hormone* (ACTH); enzymes such as acid and alkaline phosphatases; or metabolic substances such as polyamines or plasma proteins (ferratins and cereplasma B_2 immunoglobulin, for example). Thus far, these markers have been used clinically to monitor the effects of therapy on the tumor burden and to detect recurrent disease after initial therapy. Although these tests seem promising as diagnostic tools, their accuracy and efficacy have not yet been confirmed.

Cytology and Histology

In cytologic studies, exfoliative cells and material removed from various organs by scrapings, brushings, and thin-needle aspiration biopsy are analyzed. These help to determine the number of involved cells, cell types, and whether the mass is malignant or premalignant.

Cytologic smears are routinely used to test the female genital tract (e.g., *PAP smear*), the mouth, and nipple discharge. Other specimens, obtained from the amniotic fluid and pleural effusions, require special collection techniques.

Materials submitted for tissue examination may be classified according to their histologic or cellular characteristics. Broder's classification, a basic method for tumor categorization, is based on the degree of cell differentiation. The higher the grade number, the less differentiated cells are, and the poorer the prognosis. Grade I tumors have many well-differentiated cells, while grade IV tumors have few well-differentiated cells.

Cytologic smears showing evidence of a malignancy are followed by a biopsy to provide a comprehensive picture of the malignancy. The biopsy shows the histologic pattern and the relationship of the cancer to the surrounding tissue.

Biopsies can provide definitive diagnoses, an evaluation of tumor grade, depth of invasion, detection of *in-situ* lesions and premalignant changes, and information on other tumor properties needed for treatment planning. Surgical biopsy approaches include: excisional biopsy, incisional biopsy, and needle aspiration. Biopsies are performed under local or general anesthesia, depending on the degree of invasiveness; they are frequently performed on an outpatient basis.

Excisional biopsy, usually performed on discrete tumors 2 to 3 cm in diameter, removes the entire suspected tumor. *Incisional biopsy* is performed on tumors larger than 3 cm in diameter and on tumors for which local excision would prohibit definitive surgical resection later. *Needle biopsy,* in which core tissue samples are obtained through a small needle or syringe inserted into the tissue mass, is usually simple to perform, creates little disturbance in surrounding tissue, and is relatively inexpensive. Internal organs may be biopsied during endoscopic procedures such as cytoscopy, bronchoscopy, and sigmoidoscopy.

Two forms of biopsy specimens are used for evaluation: frozen sections and fixed tissue samples. Frozen sections are obtained when the patient is on the operating table. Tissue samples are hardened by freezing, allowing a pathologic diagnosis to be made within 10 to 15 minutes. The results can be reported at once to the surgical team, so they can perform the appropriate surgical procedures. Fixed tissue specimens are placed in a fixative solution immediately after removal. The tissue is then processed and embedded in paraffin, cut, and stained. Pathological reports using this procedure require at least 24 hours; usually the patient receives the results several days later.

SUMMARY

Secondary preventive efforts, such as screening and early detection, coupled with vastly improved diagnostic and staging techniques, provide a very real and potent weapon against diseases that only 20 years ago were considered incurable. Nurses need to understand the technical aspects of screening and detection procedures in order to create an atmosphere of openness and trust that will encourage the patient's participation in the screening, diagnosis, and treatment of cancer. Information on specific early detection methods may be obtained from local units of the American Cancer Society. The possibility of a cancer diagnosis can have a devastating psychological and physiological impact on a person. By preparing the patient for testing, assisting with procedures, and understanding the implications of test results, nurses fulfill vital caregiving, teaching, and supportive roles.

Bibliography

American Cancer Society. (1990). *Cancer facts and figures—1990*. (Report No. 89-45M-No.5008-LE) Atlanta, Georgia: Author.

Costanza, M. E., Lit, F. P., Green, J. L., & Patterson, W. B. (1986). Cancer prevention and detection: Strategies for practice. In B. Cady (Ed.) *Cancer Manual* (7th ed.) (pp. 14–35). Boston: American Cancer Society.

du Toit, J. P. (1985). The role of the nurse in the early detection of cervical carcinoma in a developing country. *Cancer Nursing, 8*(2), 121–127.

Faulkenberry, J. E. (1983). Cancer prevention and detection programmed instruction: Risk assessment. *Cancer Nursing, 6*(1), 59–64.

Holleb, A. I. (1986). *The American Cancer Society cancer book*. New York: Doubleday & Co.

Nevidjon, B. (1986). Cancer prevention and early detection: Reported activities of nurses. *Oncology Nursing Forum, 13*(4), 76–80.

Rosevelt, J. Frankel, H. (1984). Colorectal cancer screening by nurse practitioners using 60-cm flexible fiberoptic sigmoidoscope. *Digestive Diseases and Sciences, 29*(2), 161–163.

White, L. N. (1986). Cancer prevention and detection: From twenty to sixty-five years of age. *Oncology Nursing Forum, 13*(2), 59–64.

White, E. N., & Faulkenberry, J. E. (1985). Screening by nurse clinicians in cancer prevention and detection. *Current Problems in Cancer, 9*(4), 1–42.

UNIT 3

Treatment Approaches

Cancer treatment approaches can have three aims depending on the histologic nature of the tumor, stage of disease, and presence or absence of metastasis: cure, control, or palliation. For many years three basic treatment approaches have been used, either alone or in combination: surgery, radiation therapy, and chemotherapy. Research efforts have focused on evaluating different treatment combinations, dosages, and schedules. Treatment approaches are constantly being modified to increase their effectiveness and to minimize side effects and toxicities.

Two newer treatment modalities have received increased attention: biologic response modification and bone marrow transplantation. Research has focused on their efficacy against specific cancers at different stages, on their use with other treatment approaches, and on the sequencing of these approaches. The chapters in this unit discuss the principles, use, and general nursing considerations of each treatment approach, providing readers with an appreciation of the complexity of modern cancer treatment.

1 SURGICAL ONCOLOGY

Marianne Dietrick-Gallagher and Ella May Brasher

Surgery is the oldest form of cancer therapy and remains one of the most important treatment components for solid tumors. Surgery alone can be curative in patients with localized disease, but because approximately 70% of patients have evidence of micrometastases at diagnosis, combining surgery with other treatment modalities is usually necessary to achieve higher response rates.

Continuing advances in cancer surgery have improved patient outcomes and permitted more complex operative procedures. These include:

- improved technical ability to perform complex, radical surgeries, as well as greater understanding about the appropriate applications of radical surgery;
- the use of radiolabeled monoclonal antibodies to facilitate excision of the entire tumor;
- the use of antibiotic therapy to reduce morbidity secondary to infection;
- advanced technology in surgical intensive care units resulting in increased survival after radical surgical procedures; and
- new techniques and improved prosthetics to decrease disability and disfigurement caused by radical surgery.

Knowledge of the natural history of cancer—especially of the patterns of metastases—provides a more scientific basis for the selection and combination of treatment modalities. For example, the Halstead radical mastectomy was the treatment of choice for breast cancer in 1890 and remained the primary treatment well into the 1960s. Today, information about how breast cancer progresses and the knowledge that it is often a systemic disease at the time of presentation have changed the surgical approach to this disease. Breast cancer surgery has become less radical and is frequently followed by radiation or chemotherapy.

PRINCIPLES OF CANCER SURGERY

A number of principles guide the surgical oncologist in the treatment of malignancy.

- Slow-growing cancers are the most amenable to surgical treatment.
- The initial surgery for malignancy is more successful than a secondary operation for recurrence. This is the guiding principle behind many radical surgeries.
- A margin of normal tissue must be excised to assure an adequate resection.
- Clinical *staging* to determine the extent of the disease should be completed before definitive surgery.
- Removal of the tumor with adjacent lymph nodes is preferable to simple tumor excision (if no serious disfigurement would result).
- The patient must find the potential impairment resulting from surgery acceptable.
- Reconstruction and rehabilitation are essential components of cancer surgery and postoperative care.

TYPES OF CANCER SURGERY

Surgical procedures for malignancies may be divided into the following categories: diagnostic, staging, definitive (curative), preventative, reconstructive, palliative, and supportive. Surgical procedures are also used in the management of some oncologic emergencies.

Diagnostic

Tissue biopsy is essential to confirm the diagnosis and identify the specific type of cancer (*histology*). Each histologic disease type responds differently to treatment; this is a factor in planning surgical and adjuvant therapy.

Several biopsy techniques are used to confirm diagnosis. These include: aspiration biopsy, needle biopsy, excisional biopsy, and incisional biopsy (See Table 1). The approach used depends on the type of tumor suspected, its size, location, and characteristics of growth. Patients will need to be taught to care for the biopsy site and to report any complications, such as bleeding or signs of infection.

In addition to confirming the histologic diagnosis of the primary cancer, biopsy techniques are also used to diagnose opportunistic infections in immunosuppressed patients.

Staging

Staging surgeries are performed to determine the extent of disease. The information obtained helps the oncologist select the surgical procedure and additional therapy most appropriate for that

Table 1. Biopsy Procedures Used in the Diagnosis of Cancer

Type	Definition	Note
Aspiration	Aspiration of cells and tissue fragments through a needle that has been guided into suspected malignant tissue.	Cytologic analysis can provide a tentative diagnosis. Since the tumor can be missed, only a positive test is diagnostically significant.
Needle	Obtaining a core of tissue through a specially designed needle introduced into suspected malignant tissue.	Sufficient for the diagnosis of most tumors. Differentiating benign and reparative lesions from malignancies is often difficult with soft tissue and bony sarcomas. Since the tumor can be missed, only a positive test is diagnostically significant.
Incisional	Removal of a small wedge of tissue from a larger tumor mass.	Preferred method for diagnosing soft tissue and bony sarcomas.
Excisional	Excision of the entire suspected tumor tissue	Procedure of choice for small, accessible tumors when they can be done without compromising the ultimate surgical procedure.

Source: From "Principles of Surgical Oncology" by S. A. Rosenberg, 1985, pp. 220-221. In V. T. DeVita, S. Hellman, & S. A. Rosenberg, (Eds.), *Cancer: Principles and Practice of Oncology.* Philadelphia: J. B. Lippincott Co. Adapted by permission of publisher.

stage of disease. Exploratory surgery is commonly used to stage disease in patients with lymphomas or ovarian cancers. During staging operations, abdominal organs are exposed and palpated for gross evidence of disease. Multiple biopsies are taken from the peritoneal cavity.

In cases of metastatic disease, where surgery alone would not be curative and other treatment modalities will be used, staging surgery can help caregivers determine the exact extent of disease. Preparations may also be made for further treatment or observation; for example, radio-opaque clips for tumor delineation may be placed during staging surgery. This tailoring spares the patient the morbidity associated with more radical or unnecessary procedures that may be beneficial at certain stages but not at others.

Definitive

The goal of definitive surgery is to excise as much of the tumor as possible. During a curative surgery the entire tumor, associated lymphatics, and a margin of surrounding tissue are removed as one specimen. This decreases the possibility of seeding normal tissue with cancer cells. Surgery can be curative for early-stage cervical, breast, skin, and vulvar cancers, among others. Ultimately, the selection of the appropriate surgical procedure considers the size of the tumor, its anatomic extent, and the patient's physiological status.

When patients have large or unresectable tumors, cytoreductive or *debulking* surgery may be performed. Reducing the tumor mass in certain cancers can increase the effectiveness of subsequent radiation or chemotherapy, both of which are most effective against small numbers of cancer cells. For example, cytoreductive surgery has proven beneficial for ovarian cancer and Burkitt's lymphoma. This approach to treatment will be beneficial only in cancers where other treatment modalities are effective in controlling residual disease.

Surgery may also be useful to manage metastatic disease. When metastasis is confined to solitary lesions or a few nodules—as it may be to the lung, brain, or liver—surgical removal of those specific areas is frequently of value.

Two other surgical techniques are used in select clinical situations. Cryosurgery, in which malignant cells are destroyed by the application of liquid nitrogen, may be used for cancers of the oral cavity, skin, and prostate. Laser surgery is another procedure used for local excisions of laryngeal cancers and in the treatment of cervical dysplasias. It is also being used to treat other diseases, such as breast cancer, because it results in less bleeding and scarring. Both laser and cryosurgery cause only minor complications and can be done on an outpatient basis.

Preventative

Surgery plays a limited role in the prevention of malignancy. Surgical intervention may be indicated for a patient with a strong family history of cancer, an underlying condition, or congenital predisposition that increases the risk of developing cancer. For example, colectomy may be recommended for a patient with ulcerative colitis or a history of familial polyposis who has a increased risk of developing colon cancer. Occasionally, prophylactic subcutaneous mastectomies are considered for women with a very strong family history of breast cancer and previous fibrocystic disease. Because cryptorchidism is associated with the development of testicular cancer, orchiopexy before age 6 is advised for males with this condition. The protective effect of orchiopexy diminishes with increasing age. Before any prophylactic surgery, patients should be informed of the statistical risks of developing malignancy as well as the risks and benefits of prophylactic surgery.

Reconstructive

Reconstructive surgery is becoming more common to repair anatomic defects and improve function and cosmetic appearance following radical surgery. Reconstructive techniques that can minimize deformity and improve the quality of life include: breast reconstruction after mastectomy, restoration of acceptable appearance and function after head and neck surgery, the use of artificial joints after surgery for sarcoma, and the use of penile implants after urological organ surgery.

Palliative

Surgery can be effective in relieving symptoms in more advanced stages of cancer. For example, when pain cannot be controlled through pharmacologic or behavioral interventions, the nerve pathways may be interrupted surgically (see Unit IV, Chapter 2). Surgery is also indicated in patients with obstructions related to local expansion of the tumor. Common sites of obstruction are the bowel in colorectal and ovarian cancer, biliary obstruction in hepatobiliary tumors, and urinary tract obstruction from cancers of the cervix, ovary, bladder, prostate, or rectum.

Supportive Care

Several surgical interventions are useful in the supportive care of oncology patients. Venous access devices (see Unit III, Chapter 3) may be surgically inserted for administration of chemotherapy or parenteral nutrition, and for blood drawing. Ventricular reservoirs permit direct delivery of chemotherapy to the cerebrospinal fluid. Gastrostomy and jejunostomy tubes are often placed in patients with gastrointestinal malignancies to provide enteral nutrition.

SURGERY FOR ONCOLOGIC EMERGENCIES

Surgical interventions are frequently required for the management of oncologic emergencies (see Unit IV, Chapter 4). The effects of both the primary tumor and of the treatments can cause such emergencies. Exsanguinating hemorrhage, perforation, obstructive disease, and inflammatory lesions may occur, posing a major threat to the patient whose status may already be compromised by neutropenia and thrombocytopenia.

NURSING CONSIDERATIONS

Some patients with cancer may be at greater risk of postoperative complications such as bleeding and infection. This heightened risk results from the underlying disease process and/or side effects of previous therapy. Nurses must assess patients carefully to identify potential problems early in their course. Figure 1 highlights the most important nursing care considerations.

Patients and their families are always anxious about surgery. When the reason for surgery is cancer, another dimension is added:

- Maintenance of basic physiological functions
- Protection of operative sites
- Accurate monitoring, interpretation, and documentation of pertinent observations about changes in condition
- Prevention of infection through aseptic management of surgical sites
- Maintenance of respiratory function
- Passive exercises and assistance with early ambulation
- Management of pain with analgesics
- Physical and psychosocial rehabilitation
- Preparation of patients for radiation or chemotherapy where required.

Figure 1. Important postoperative considerations

Source: From "Cancer Treatment" by S. M. Hubbard, 1985, p. 26. In B. Johnson & J. Gross (Eds.),*Handbook of Oncology Nursing.* New York: Delmar Publishers, Inc. Adapted with permission of the publisher.

uncertainty about long-term survival and subsequent treatments. In addition to general pre- and postoperative considerations, nursing care should focus on patient education, emotional support, and successful rehabilitation.

Preoperative teaching should include a discussion of the extent of the planned surgery and of any expected functional limitations. Nurses should repeat and reinforce information when possible, because anxiety may decrease patients' abilities to understand and retain information. Careful planning to ensure continuity of care is paramount in most care settings, where patients are discharged from the hospital sooner than was standard in the past. Communication with the office nurse and home health nurse may ease the transition from hospital to home.

Beyond the immediate pre- and postoperative instructions, educational efforts should focus on information about other treatments, such as radiation or chemotherapy. Patients and/or family members at a high risk for a specific malignancy should also be instructed on appropriate health-promoting behaviors such as breast self-examination.

The nurse may also need to address patient and family adjustment to the long-term effects of both surgery and cancer during the postoperative period. American Cancer Society support groups such as Reach to Recovery, Lost Chord, or community-based support groups such as United Ostomy (see Unit VI) may help patients deal with body image and sexuality issues related to their surgery. Contact with disease-free, well-adjusted, rehabilitated volunteers from these groups may help reduce fears and contribute to a sense of well being and self esteem.

Bibliography

Frogge, M., & Goodman, M. (1987). Surgical therapy. In S. Groenwald (Ed.), *Cancer nursing: Principles and practice* (pp. 312-320). Boston: Jones and Bartlett Publishers.

Hubbard, S. M. (1985). Cancer treatment In B. L. Johnson & J. Gross (Eds.), *Handbook of oncology nursing* (pp 21-27). New York: John Wiley & Sons.

Patterson, W. (1984). Principles of surgical oncology. In P. Rubin (Ed.), *Clinical oncology: A multidisciplinary approach* (pp. 30-40). New York: American Cancer Society.

Pilch, Y. (1984). *Surgical oncology.* New York: McGraw-Hill Book Company.

Szopa, T. (1987). Surgery. In C. Ziegfeld (Ed.), *Core curriculum for oncology nursing* (pp. 199-207). Philadelphia: W.B. Saunders.

Rosenberg, S. A. (1989). Principles of surgical oncology. In V. T. DeVita, S. Hellman, & S. A. Rosenberg (Eds.), *Cancer: Principles and practice of oncology* (pp. 236-246). Philadelphia: J. B. Lippincott Company.

2 RADIATION THERAPY

Ryan R. Iwamoto

Radiation therapy is one of the major treatment modalities for cancer. Approximately 60% of all people with cancer will be treated with radiation therapy sometime during the course of their disease. Its effectiveness as a treatment for cancer was first reported in the late 1800s. Advances in equipment technology, combined with the science of radiobiology, have led to today's highly sophisticated treatment centers. Radiation therapy can now be delivered with maximum therapeutic benefits, minimizing toxicity and sparing healthy tissues.

BIOLOGIC EFFECTS OF RADIATION

Radiation therapy uses high-energy ionizing radiation to kill cancer cells. It is considered a local therapy because cancer cells are destroyed only in the anatomic area being treated. The radiation causes the breakage of one or both strands of the DNA molecule inside the cells, thereby preventing their ability to grow and divide. While cells in all phases of the cell cycle can be damaged by radiation, the lethal effect of radiation may not be apparent until after one or more cell divisions have occurred. Although normal cells can also be affected by ionizing radiation, they are usually better able to repair the DNA damage.

PRINCIPLES OF TREATMENT

The dose of radiation administered is determined by a number of factors, including the radiosensitivity of the tumor, the normal tissue tolerance, and the volume of tissue to be irradiated. The *Gray*, the Systeme Internationale Unit, has now replaced the "rad" (radiation absorbed dose) as the accepted term for radiation dosage. One Gray (Gy) = 100 rads; therefore, 1 cGY = 1 rad.

A radiosensitive tumor is one that can be eradicated by a dose of radiation and is well tolerated by the surrounding normal tissues (Table 1). The sensitivity of tumor cells to the effects of radiation is also dependent on the presence of oxygen. Killing hypoxic cells

Table 1. Relative Radiosensitivity of Various Tumors and Tissues

Tumors or Tissues	Relative Radiosensitivity
Lymphoma, leukemia, seminoma, dysgerminoma	High
Squamous cell cancer of the oropharyngeal, glottis, bladder, skin, and cervical epithelia; adenocarcinomas of the alimentary tract	Fairly high
Vascular and connective tissue elements of all tumors; secondary neurovascularization, astrocytomas	Medium
Salivary gland tumors, hepatoma, renal cancer, pancreatic cancer, chondrosarcoma, osteogenic sarcoma	Fairly low
Rhabdomyosarcoma, leiomyosarcoma, and ganglioneurofibrosarcoma	Low

Source: From "Principles of Radiation Oncology and Cancer Radiotherapy" by P. Rubin, 1983 p. 60. In P. Rubin, (Ed.), *Clinical Oncology for Medical Students and Physicians,* Atlanta: American Cancer Society. Reprinted with permission of the publisher.

requires 2 to 3 times the dose of radiation required to achieve the same therapeutic effect in well-oxygenated cells. Hypoxic cells occur when tumor growth exceeds the blood supply and the central core of the tumor becomes necrotic. New strategies are being developed to increase the radiosensitivity of these hypoxic, resistant cells with chemicals that mimic the presence of oxygen or with hyperthermia (the use of heat).

The dose of radiation that can be delivered to a tumor is also limited by the radiation tolerance of the adjacent normal tissues. This limit is the point at which normal tissues are irreparably damaged. The maximum dose of radiation that can be administered to parts of the body varies with the tissue involved.

Because administration of the tumor-lethal dose of radiation in a single treatment would result in unacceptable toxicity or even death, the total prescribed dose of radiation is usually divided into several smaller doses or *fractions.* Treatments are usually given on a daily basis, 5 days per week for an average of 25 to 30 treatments. With fractionation, a *tumoricidal* dose can be delivered while minimizing the damage to normal tissues. In addition, gradual shrinkage of the tumor during treatment brings hypoxic cells closer to the vascular supply, where they become oxygenated and more susceptible to the effects of radiation.

For some tumors, a "boost" or "reduced field" of radiation is administered to complete the course of therapy. These treatments are delivered to limited areas within the treatment field that are at greatest risk for recurrence. In this way, the tumor can be treated with a higher dose than the normal surrounding tissues would tolerate or need. The "boost" may be administered externally or internally.

USES OF RADIATION THERAPY FOR THE TREATMENT OF CANCER

Primary Therapy

Radiation therapy is a primary therapy for basal cell carcinomas of the skin, early-stage laryngeal cancers and other head and neck cancers, early stage Hodgkin's disease, non-Hodgkin's lymphomas, early stage breast cancer following lumpectomy, certain lung cancers, seminomas, carcinomas of the cervix, prostate cancers, bladder cancers, thyroid cancers, certain pediatric tumors, and certain brain tumors.

Radiation and surgery, both of which are local therapies, may achieve comparable responses and cure rates in some diseases; however, radiation may offer some treatment advantages to certain patients. In some cases, the functional and cosmetic outcomes of radiation therapy are superior to the results that can be achieved surgically. Also, some individuals may be unable to undergo surgery due to pre-existing medical conditions, thus making radiation therapy the better treatment choice.

Combined Modality Therapy

Radiation therapy may be used in addition to other primary treatment modalities. Postoperative radiation therapy is frequently used to decrease the risk of local recurrence following surgery for breast, lung, high-risk rectal cancers, and brain tumors. Preoperative radiation is used to shrink the size of a tumor so that a less radical or disfiguring surgical procedure is possible.

Radiation therapy and chemotherapy are frequently combined to increase tumor destruction. Certain chemotherapeutic agents increase the radiosensitivity of cancer cells. However, combination approaches may exacerbate known side effects of these therapies. For example, when cyclophosphamide, which damages bladder mucosa, is administered to someone receiving pelvic radiation, an increase in cystitis is noted.

Tumors cells appear to be especially sensitive to heat. Hyper-thermia is used in some treatment centers in conjunction with radiation therapy to potentiate the effects of iradiation.

Prophylaxis

Radiation therapy may also be used to prophylactically treat tissues or organs before disease is clinically evident. The central nervous system is frequently treated with radiation to prevent relapse of certain forms of leukemia in the brain.

Palliative Therapy

Radiation therapy may be used to palliate the symptoms of metastases in patients with widespread disease. Pain, bleeding, compression of vital structures such as the brain, ulcerating skin lesions, and metastases in weight-bearing bones that are susceptible to fracture can be managed with palliative radiation.

Oncologic Emergencies

Radiation therapy is also used in the management of spinal cord compression and superior vena cava syndrome. Refer to Unit IV, Chapter 4 for a discussion of these complications.

ADMINISTRATION OF RADIATION THERAPY

Radiation treatments can be administered externally or internally, depending on the type and extent of the tumor. X-rays, radioactive elements, and radioactive isotopes are most often used.

External Beam Radiation

External radiation treatments are administered with machines that deliver high-energy radiation. These machines vary according to the amount and type (eletromagnetic or particulate) of energy produced. The kind of machine used will differ depending on the type and extent of the tumor. The Cobalt-60 was the first meg-avoltage machine, and is still used in many institutions. Linear accelerators, which use high-energy x-ray beams, are now the most commonly used machines. Technological advances have permitted the development of machines with increased energy, which allow for more precise treatments of deeply seated tumors with less damage to superficial tissues.

Simulation and Treatment Planning

The purpose of treatment planning is to determine the best way to deliver the radiation treatment and to limit the radiation dose to normal tissues. An x-ray machine called a simulator is used to visualize and define the exact treatment area. Customized shielding devices (*blocks*) may be created to protect healthy tissue from the radiation beam. Temporary dye or permanent tattoos about the size of a small freckle may be used to mark reference points on the skin so that the exact same area is treated each day. In order to deliver treatments precisely, immobilization devices may be used to support and assist the patient in maintaining an exact position during treatment.

Internal Radiation

Internal radiation, or *brachytherapy*, is the use of radioactive isotopes for either temporary or permanent implants. Methods of delivering brachytherapy include intracavitary or interstitial placement of sources, instillation of colloidal solutions, and parenteral or oral administration. Sealed sources are those encapsulated in a metal seed, wire, tube, or needle. Unsealed radioactive sources are prepared in suspension or solution.

Encapsulated radioactive elements are placed in body cavities or inserted directly into tissues with suitable applicators. The applicator is usually placed into the body cavity or tissue surgically or using fluoroscopy. The applicators, usually plastic or metal tubes, may be sutured into or near the tumor. Later, when the patient returns to the hospital room, the radioactive isotope is placed into the applicator. This "after loading" technique is used to reduce the radiation exposure to hospital personnel. These implants provide radiation to a limited area while minimizing normal exposure. Radioactive implants are used in the treatment of cancers of the tongue, lip, breast, vagina, cervix, endometrium, rectum, bladder, and brain.

Encapsulated sources may also be left within the patient as permanent implants. "Seeding" with small beads of radioactive material is an approach that can be used for the treatment of localized prostate cancers, and localized but inoperable lung cancers. The patient's body attenuates, or blocks, most of the radiation so radiation precautions are usually not required. Radioactive isotopes can also be given orally, parenterally, or instilled into intrapleural or peritoneal spaces. Thyroid cancer, for example, is frequently treated with oral administration of radioactive iodine (^{131}I). The period of greatest radioactivity for ^{131}I is 8 days.

**Table 2. The Immediate and Delayed Response
of Tissues to Radiation Exposure**

Site of Radiation Exposure	Acute Response to Radiation	Subacute Response to Radiation	Late Response to Radiation
Skin	Denuding of the epidermal layer. Redness, edema, itching, dryness, and weeping may occur. Begins in 1–6 weeks and recovers 2–3 weeks after the exposure to radiation ends.	Fibrosis, atrophy, telangiectasis and a tan appearance. ⟶	
Epithelial lining of the gastrointestinal tract: Oral cavity	Dryness, redness, edema, denuding, ulceration, pain, necrosis, taste alerations, anorexia.	Fibrosis, telangiectasis, taste alterations. ⟶	
Esophagus	Denuding and sloughing of epithelial cells, necrosis, ulceration, pain, anorexia.	Fibrosis. ⟶	
Stomach	Sloughing of epithelial cells, nausea, vomiting.	Infarction, fibrosis, necrosis.	Ulceration, obstruction
Intestines	Sloughing of intestinal villi, diarrhea.	Infarction, fibrosis, necrosis.	Ulceration, obstruction
Epithelial lining of the genitourinary tract: Kidneys		Vascular occlusion leading to radiation nephritis, renal shut-down. ⟶	
Bladder	Cystitis, ulceration.	Fibrosis, contracted bladder. ⟶	
Bone marrow:	Depression of the white blood cels (neutrophils), platelets, and red blood cells. Complete recovery of the neutrophils and platelets in 2–6 weeks.	Anemia. ⟶	
Hair Follicle	Hair loss.	Permanent hair loss. ⟶	

(Continued)

Site of Radiation Exposure	Acute Response to Radiation	Subacute Response to Radiation	Late Response to Radiation
Respiratory system	Pneumonitis; significant if 25% of the lung tissue is involved, fatal if 75% of the lung tissue is involved.	Fibrosis.	→
Cardiovascular system	Rare myocarditis or pericarditis.	Fibrosis.	→
Central nervous system: Brain and Spinal cord	Inflammation and edema.	Vascular obliteration leading to infarction and occlusion.	→
Peripheral nerves	Inflammation and edema.		
Eyes		Lenticular opacities.	**Cataracts.**
Bones and cartilage: Child		Arrest of growth, shortening of bone.	→
Adult	No response. ———————————————————————→		
Gonads: Sperm:	Radioresistant, will remain for 90-120 days.		
Mature sperm	Some possibility of mutation.		
Spermatogonia	100-300 cGy, temporary ————————————→ sterility with possible mutations. 300-600 cGy, permanent sterility.		Normal levels with 100-300 cGy
	——————————————————————————————————→		
Ovary:	All oocytes are present; 600-1000 cGy, permanent sterility.————————————————————————→		

SPECIAL NOTE: The fetus is very sensitive to radiation. Pregnant women or those women who suspect they may be pregnant must avoid all possible exposure to sources of radiation. The most radiosensitive period for the fetus is during the period of organ development which is 2-12 weeks post-conception. Congenital abnormalities have been detected at doses of 5 cGy with radiation-induced abortion occurring at 500 cGy. The development of cancer, especially leukemia and thyroid cancer, as well as the central nervous system disorders of microencephaly and mental retardation, are the defects most often reported when the fetus is exposed to a source of radiation.

Source: From *Care of the Client Receiving External Radiation Therapy.* (pp 53-54) by J.M. Yasko, 1982, Reston, VA: Reston Publishing Co. Inc. Reprinted with permission of Appleton Lange, Norwalk, CT.

NURSING CONSIDERATIONS

Many patients are frightened by the concept of radiation, making assessment of the patient's knowledge all the more important. Nurses can provide information about the use of radiation therapy in the treatment of cancer, the process of treatment planning, the treatment schedule, and the self-care activities the patient can perform to control treatment side effects.

With internal irradiation, patients may require special radiation precautions based on the principle of time, distance, and shielding. Health care personnel should limit the amount of time spent in close proximity to the patient, minimize the time spent in the room, and use lead shielding as appropriate.

Patients receiving internal irradiation via either sealed or unsealed sources are generally physically isolated from other patients and staff members in a private room. People under 18 years old and pregnant women are not permitted in the room. With sealed sources, body fluids and materials from the patient are not radioactive. Special precautions are not needed when handling bodily fluids and materials from the patient. Bed rest may be required to prevent dislodging the radioactive source. Once the implant is removed and returned to the lead-lined container, the patient is no longer radioactive.

In patients treated with unsealed radioactive isotopes, secretions may be contaminated with radioactive material. Health care personnel should wear gloves when handling these secretions, and when possible, disposable items (e.g., eating utensils, urinals) should be used. Non-disposable items (equipment, linens, etc.) should be placed in plastic bags and left in the patient's room to be checked for radioactivity and removed when permissible. These patients may be discharged from the hospital when it is determined that the total body retention of the isotope is at a safe level.

Side effects occur as normal tissues within the treatment area are damaged by the radiation. Skin toxicity, fatigue, and anorexia can occur with treatment to any site, while other toxicities are seen when specific areas of the body are treated (Table 2). The severity of side effects depends on many factors, including volume of tissue treated, total dose, daily dose (fractionation) of therapy, method of treatment, and certain individual factors. Acute radiation reactions, such as skin reactions, occur during the course of therapy and generally resolve 2 to 4 weeks following the completion of therapy. However, delayed side effects may occur many months or years after treatment and may persist on a long-term basis.

Nursing care for side effects involves assessment and intervention to prevent or minimize the occurrence of the side effects and to

1. Assess skin within the treatment area for erythema, pain, and dry or moist desquamation (peeling of the skin).
2. Markings on skin for treatment purposes must not be removed unless otherwise instructed.
3. Wash the treated area only with tepid water and a soft wash cloth.
4. Within the treatment area *avoid* the use of soaps, deodorants, powders, perfumes, cosmetics, heavily scented lotions, and skin preparations.
5. Avoid wearing tight-fitting clothing over treatment area.
6. Wear cotton clothing close to the skin.
7. Items that produce extreme temperatures such as hot water bottles, electric heating pads and hot and cold packs must not be applied to the treatment area.
8. Protect the treatment area from the sun, wind, and cold. Utilize protective clothing. Following treatment, if sun exposure to the treatment area is unavoidable, use a SPF #15 sun screening agent. Increased skin sensitivity within the treatment area may be a permanent outcome of irradiation.
9. If dry desquamation occurs, a moisturizing lotion may be prescribed.

Figure 1. Guidelines for skin care during external radiation therapy.

provide relief of symptoms that do occur. A discussion of the nursing management of the more common problems can be found in Unit IV, Chapter 1. General guidelines for skin care during radiation therapy are summarized in Figure 1. Individual radiation therapy departments may have additional or special instructions regarding symptom management and nursing care of patients receiving radiation therapy.

Bibliography

Bucholtz, J. (1987). Radiation therapy. In: C. R. Ziegfeld (Ed.), *Core curriculum for oncology nursing* (pp. 207-224). Philadelphia: W. B. Saunders.

Godwin, C., Bucholtz, J., & Wall, S. (1985). Hidden hazards on the job: radiation. *Nursing Life,* (Nov./Dec.), 43-47.

Hassey, K. (1985). Demystifying care of patients with radioactive implants. *American Journal of Nursing, 85,* 788-792.

Hassey, K., Hilderley, L. (Eds.). (1990). *Nursing perspectives in radiation oncology.* Albany, NY: Delmar Publications, Inc.

Hilderley, L., Hassey, K. & Dudjak, L. (1988). *Nursing management of the patient receiving radiation therapy.* From the Fifth National Conference on Cancer Nursing, American Cancer Society. Publ. No. 3480.04-PE.

Hilderley, L. (1987). Radiotherapy. In: S. Groenwald (Ed.), *Cancer nursing principles and practice,* pp. 320-347. Boston/Monterey: Jones & Bartlett Publishing, Inc.

Hilderley, L. (1983). Skin care in radiation therapy: A review of the literature. *Oncology Nursing Forum,* 10(1), 51-56.

McNally, J., Campbell-Stair, J., & Summerville, E. (Eds.). (1985). *Guidelines for cancer nursing practice.* Orlando, FL: Grune & Stratton, Inc.

Rubin, P. (Ed.). (1983). *Clinical oncology for medical students and physicians* (Ed. 6). Rochester, NY: American Cancer Society.

3 CHEMOTHERAPY

Judy Petersen

Chemotherapy, or the use of chemical agents to destroy cancer cells, is a mainstay in the treatment of malignancies. Its possible therapeutic role was discovered when the bone marrow suppressive effects of nitrogen mustard gas were noted during World War I. Since that time, the search for drugs with anticancer activity has continued, and the goal of treatment with chemotherapy has evolved from palliation to cure (Table 1). A major advantage of chemotherapy is its applicability to the treatment of widespread or metastatic disease, because surgery and radiation therapy are limited to the treatment of localized disease. Today, approximately 50 anticancer drugs and hormones are commercially available in the United States.

CHEMOTHERAPEUTIC AGENTS

Almost all currently available chemotherapeutic agents kill neoplastic cells by affecting DNA synthesis or function, but the drugs vary in their mechanism of activity within the cell cycle (Figure 1). Cell cycle specific (CCS) drugs exert their action only when cells are in a specific phase of the cell cycle (i.e., S phase, M phase). Cell cycle nonspecific (CCNS) drugs affect dividing and resting cells in all phases of the cell cycle.

The major categories of chemotherapeutic agents are alkylating agents, antimetabolites, plant alkaloids, antitumor antibiotics, and steroid hormones; these are grouped according to their effects on the cell cycle and cell chemistry. The mechanisms of action of several of these drugs are illustrated in Figure 2.

Alkylating agents (CCNS) act by directly attacking DNA, causing breaks in and cross linking of the DNA strands. Alkyating agents may be used in the treatment of chronic leukemias, Hodgkin's disease, lymphomas, and certain carcinomas of the lung, breast, prostate, and ovary. Cyclophosphamide is an example of a commonly used alkylating agent.

Antimetabolites (CCS) block cell development by interfering with metabolic processes, usually DNA synthesis. They compete with normal substances for incorporation in the cell, and once ingested

Table 1. Tumors Responsive to Chemotherapy

Tumors Potentially Curable by Chemotherapy

Choriocarcinoma	Acute myelogenous leukemia
Acute lymphocytic leukemia in children and adults	Wilms' tumor
	Burkitt's lymphoma
Hodgkin's disease	Embryonal rhabdomyosarcoma
Diffuse large-cell lymphoma	Ewing's sarcoma
Lymphoblastic lymphoma (in children and adults)	Peripheral neuroepithelioma
	Neuroblastoma
Follicular mixed lymphoma	Small-cell cancer of the lung
Testicular carcinoma	Ovarian cancer

Tumors Potentially Curable by Adjuvant Chemotherapy

Breast cancer	Soft tissue sarcoma
Osteogenic sarcoma	Colorectal cancer

Tumors Potentially Responsive in Advanced Stages
But Not Yet Curable by Chemotherapy

Bladder cancer	Endometrial cancer
Chronic myelogenous leukemia	Adrenal cortical carcinoma
Chronic lymphocytic leukemia	Medulloblastoma
Hairy cell leukemia	Polycythemia rubra vera
Multiple myeloma	Prostatic cancer
Follicular small-cleaved cell lymphoma	Glioblastoma multiforme
Cervical carcinoma	Insulinoma
Soft tissue sarcomas	Breast cancer
Head and neck cancer	Carcinoid tumors

Tumors Poorly Responsive in Advanced Stages to Chemotherapy

Osteogenic sarcoma	Colorectal cancer
Pancreatic cancer	Non-small cell lung cancer
Renal cancer	Melanoma
Thyroid cancer	Hepatocellular carcinoma
Carcinoma of the vulva or penis	

Source: From "Principles of Cancer Chemotherapy" by V.T.DeVita, 1989, p. 297. V. T. DeVita, S. Hellman, and S. A. Rosenberg, (Eds.), *Cancer: Principles and Practice of Oncology*, Philadelphia: J. B. Lippincott and Co. Adapted with permission of the publisher.

they halt normal development and reproduction. All drugs in this category are cell cycle specific, affecting the cell during the "S" phase. Examples of commonly used antimetabolites include 5-fluorouracil and methotrexate. Antimetabolites may be used in the treatment of acute and chronic leukemias, choriocarcinoma, and some tumors of the gastrointestinal tract, breast, and ovary.

Nitrosoureas (CCNS) act similarly to akylating agents and also inhibit enzymatic changes necessary for DNA repair. These agents cross the blood-brain barrier and are used to treat brain tumors, lymphomas, multiple myeloma, and malignant melanoma. Carmustine (BCNU) and lomustine (CCNU) are the major drugs in this category.

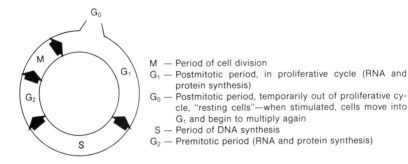

M — Period of cell division
G_1 — Postmitotic period, in proliferative cycle (RNA and protein synthesis)
G_0 — Postmitotic period, temporarily out of proliferative cycle, "resting cells"—when stimulated, cells move into G_1 and begin to multiply again
S — Period of DNA synthesis
G_2 — Premitotic period (RNA and protein synthesis)

Figure 1. The cell cycle.

Antitumor antibiotics are a diverse group of compounds; most are considered to be CCNS. In general, they act by binding with DNA and preventing RNA synthesis. The most commonly used drugs in this group are doxorubicin, mitomycin-C, and bleomycin. These agents are widely used in the treatment of a variety of malignancies.

Plant (vinca) alkaloids (CCS) are naturally occurring substances that block cell division by inhibiting spindle formation during mitosis. Vincristine, vinblastine, and VP-16, commonly used agents in this group, are used in the treatment of acute lymphoblastic leukemia, Hodgkin's and non-Hodgkin's lymphomas, neuroblastoma, Wilms' tumor, and cancers of the lung, breast, and testes.

Steroidal hormones useful in treating some types of tumors include adrenocorticosteroids, estrogens, antiestrogens, progesterones, and androgens. Although their specific mechanism of action is not clear, steroid hormones modify the growth of certain hormone-dependent cancers.

In addition, other **miscellaneous antineoplastic** drugs exist whose mechanisms of action do not permit broad categorization. All agents and their major toxicities are listed in Appendices I and II.

PRINCIPLES OF TREATMENT

An understanding of the normal cell cycle and the behavior of malignant cells is necessary in order to comprehend how chemotherapy destroys cancer cells (see Unit II, Chapter 3).

The ultimate goal of chemotherapy is the destruction of all malignant cells. Chemotherapy is selective for cancer cells over most normal host cells. Malignant cells are more susceptible to

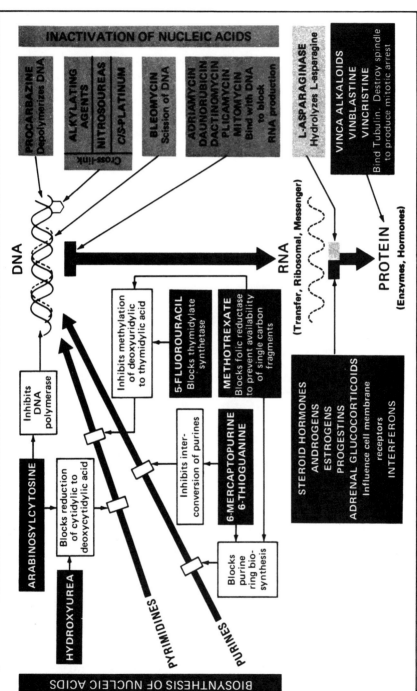

Figure 2. Mechanism of action of anticancer drugs.

Source: From "Cancer Chemotherapeutic Agents;" by I. H. Krakoff, 1987, *CA-A Cancer Journal for Clinicians, 37,* pp. 93–105. Reprinted with permission of the American Cancer Society.

Table 2. MOPP, A Combination Chemotherapy Regimen for Treatment of Hodgkin's Disease

Drug	Cell Cycle	Route	Days	Major Toxicity
M = Mechlorethamine (Mustargen, nitrogen mustard)	CCNS	IV	1 and 8	Myelosuppression, nausea and vomiting
O = Oncovin® (vincristine)	CCS-M Phase	IV	1 and 8	Neurotoxicity, alopecia
P = Procarbazine (matulane)	CCNS	Orally	1 thru 14	Myelosuppression, neurotoxicity
P = Prednisone	CCNS	Orally	1 thru 14	Hyperglycemia, osteoporosis, immunosuppression

CCS = cell cycle specific, CCNS = cell cycle non-specific
Source: From *Cancer Chemotherapy: A Reference Guide* (pp. 82-83) by L. Tenenbaum, 1989. Philadelphia: W. B. Saunders Co. Adapted with permission of the publisher.

the effects of these agents not only because they reproduce more rapidly than most normal cells, but because the proportion of tumor cells dividing at any one time (growth fraction) is higher than that in normal tissue counterparts. Although the growth fraction of host tissues does not approach that of a tumor, the rapid dividing rate of certain normal cells increases their sensitivity to chemotherapy. Because of the toxicity of chemotherapeutic agents to these normal tissues, the maximum single dose that can be safely administered to patients may be less than is required to achieve complete eradication of all cancer cells.

Several strategies may be used to maximize the cytotoxic effect of chemotherapy. Chemotherapy is generally given intermittently over an extended period to progressively lower the number of tumor cells to the point where the body's own immune responses can control further tumor growth.

Combination Chemotherapy

Chemotherapy agents that differ in both their cell cycle specificity and their toxicities are frequently combined to achieve maximum tumor effect with minimal toxicity. Table 2 outlines MOPP, one of the combination regimens commonly used for treatment of Hodgkin's disease. Because tumor cells have different biological characteristics (heterogeneity), combining drugs may more effectively eradicate cancer cells resistant to a single agent.

Adjuvant Chemotherapy

This treatment may be administered when no objective evidence of cancer can be found but when certain prognostic factors (e.g., metastasis to lymph nodes) predict a high probability of residual microscopic disease and an increased risk of systemic recurrence. Use of chemotherapy at an earlier stage of tumor growth may preclude the development of resistance to chemotherapy often observed in large or metastatic cancers.

Combined Modality Therapy

Chemotherapy may also be used in combination with other treatment modalities, such as radiation or surgery. Local and systemic therapies are combined to obtain a greater response rate than could be achieved with a single treatment modality.

Hormonal Manipulation

Because the growth of certain tumors is partially dependent on hormones, the hormonal environment may be manipulated in patients with endocrine-related cancers. Hormone therapies are not cytotoxic, and therefore not curative; their purpose is prevention of cell division and of further growth of hormone-dependent tumors. Their use is frequently reserved for the management of patients with locally advanced or metastatic disease. Available hormonal agents are listed in Appendix II.

INVESTIGATIONAL THERAPY

The identification and development of effective new anticancer drugs is an on-going process. Following rigorous testing in laboratory animals and experimental model systems, chemotherapeutic agents with demonstrated antitumor activity are evaluated in clinical trials. In Phase I trials, the initial phase of clinical investigation, a new treatment is evaluated in cancer patients for the first time. The purpose of these studies is to determine the associated toxicity, maximum tolerated dose, and optimal schedule or mode of delivery of a new therapy. Phase II trials test a new therapy (using the dose, method of administration, and schedule defined in Phase I) in patients with a variety of tumors to determine whether there is objective antitumor activity. In Phase III trials, new therapies that exhibited activity in Phase II are compared to the standard or best available therapy for each type of tumor tested.

Participation in a clinical trial is one treatment option frequently offered to patients at some point during therapy. The continued progress of cancer treatment depends upon the participation of adequate numbers of patients in such studies. Nurses can help patients understand the purpose of clinical trials and what participation will entail. Nurses can also assess the patient's understanding of the clinical trial and can help patients formulate questions they may want to ask physicians in order to make an informed choice. A very useful booklet for this purpose is *What are Clinical Trials All About?* (Available free by calling 1-800-4-CANCER, NIH Publication No. 85-2706, 1984).

CHEMOTHERAPY ADMINISTRATION

Although studies of the potential health hazards of the preparation and administration of antineoplastic agents have been inconclusive, health care personnel involved in these activities should be aware of the possible risks in handling chemotherapeutic agents and of the recommendations developed for their safe handling. The main routes of cytotoxic drug exposure for health care personnel are inhalation, absorption, and ingestion during drug preparation, administration, or disposal of contaminated materials. The Occupational, Safety and Health Administration (OSHA), the Oncology Nursing Society, and other groups have developed guidelines for the safe handling of chemotherapeutic agents to guide practice and to minimize the chances of accidental exposure. Hospitals and other practice settings have incorporated these guidelines when developing specific drug administration policies and procedures. Nurses administering chemotherapy, assisting in its administration, or otherwise coming in contact with supplies used in administration, must be familiar with the operating guidelines at their institutions and assist in the practice of safe handling techniques.

Nurses should be familiar with the agent(s) to be administered (dosage, route of administration, toxicity). Individual chemotherapy doses are usually based upon body surface area (m^2), calculated from the person's height and weight. The sequence of chemotherapy administration may be critical to its effectiveness. Careful adherence to written chemotherapy orders can prevent errors in scheduling or method of administration.

The most common routes of administration for chemotherapy are oral, intravenous, and intramuscular. More recently, other methods have been used to increase the local concentration of chemotherapy at the tumor site (intracavitary, intraperitoneal, intrathecal, intrapleural, intravesical, topical, and intra-arterial).

Because many chemotherapeutic agents are toxic to organs, several points in the patient's laboratory data should be checked before chemotherapy administration: white blood cell count, hemoglobin/hematocrit, platelet count, renal function tests, liver function tests, and assessment for specific drug toxicities (e.g., doxorubicin-induced congestive heart failure). Abnormalities in these values may require dose modifications or the delay of therapy. Additionally,

Table 3. Patient Assessment Criteria for a VAD

<table>
<tr><td colspan="2" align="center">CRITERIA

Frequency of Venous Access
Longevity of Treatment
Mode of Administration
Venous Integrity
Patient Preference</td></tr>
<tr><td>LOW PRIORITY</td><td>HIGH PRIORITY</td></tr>
<tr><td>Infrequent venous access
Short-term therapy
Intermittent single injections
Non-vesicant/non-irritating drugs
No previous IV therapy
Both extremities available

Venous access with 2 or fewer
   venipunctures
Patient does not prefer VAD</td><td>Frequent venous access
Long-term indefinite treatment period
Continuous infusion chemotherapy
Home infusion of chemotherapy
Vesicant/irritating drugs
Venous thrombosis/sclerosis due to
   previous IV therapy
Venous access limited to one
   extremity
Prior tissue damage due to extra-
   vasation
Multiple (> 2) venipunctures to secure
   venous access
Patient prefers VAD</td></tr>
</table>

Source: From "Venous Access Devices: An Overview" by M. S. Goodman and R. Wickham, 1984, *Oncology Nursing Form 11*(5), p. 17. Reprinted with permission of the publisher.

other pretreatment actions, such as hydration or administration of antiemetics, may be ordered to minimize side effects. Institution-specific chemotherapy administration guidelines should be available to guide the nurse in preparing patients, administering agents, and monitoring patient response.

Successful intravenous drug administration is dependent upon careful vein selection and venipuncture. Patients with poor peripheral venous access may ultimately require placement of a venous access device. These devices can provide long-term venous access for administration of chemotherapeutic agents, blood products, antibiotics, hyperalimentation, and blood drawing. A wide variety of venous access devices, implantable ports, and infusion pumps is available. Factors considered in choosing equipment include frequency of access, longevity of treatment, mode of administration, venous integrity, and patient preference. Patient assessment criteria are summarized in Table 3.

Leakage of chemotherapy from the vein into the surrounding tissues during infusion (*extravasation*) is a potential problem when administering vesicants, or drugs that can cause tissue damage or necrosis if infiltrated. Careful vein selection and monitoring of

1. Stop the infusion immediately and notify the physician.
2. Attempt to aspirate drug through existing needle with a tuberculin syringe (greater suction ability).
3. Check institutional guidelines regarding administration of antidote, if indicated.
4. Remove needle.
5. Apply ice (or heat if vinca alkaloids) per institutional guidelines.
6. Document interventions and response.

Figure 3. Guidelines for the treatment of extravasation.

the infusion site for blood return are crucial to preventing extravasation. If extravasation should occur, general guidelines for its management are listed in Figure 3. Institutional guidelines for extravasation management vary and should be checked before administering chemotherapy.

Patients should be provided with verbal and written information regarding chemotherapy and its potential side effects. In many cases, their understanding and cooperation are needed to prevent or minimize toxicity. In addition, many patients will receive chemotherapy as part of a clinical trial. In such cases it is vitally important that patients clearly understand the nature and risks of the trial to assure that consent is truly informed. Nurses should be familiar with the informed consent process and the regimen planned in order to assist patients with their decision-making.

SIDE EFFECTS

Normal tissues with rapid doubling times are sensitive to the toxic effects of chemotherapeutic drugs. These tissues include bone marrow, hair follicles, gastrointestinal epithelium, and reproductive cells. *Myelosuppression*, the suppression or inhibition of the bone marrow, occurs as a side effect of many chemotherapeutic agents. The *nadir*, or time that the blood count reaches its lowest point after chemotherapy administration, varies with each drug (usually somewhere between 7 and 14 days). Calculating the occurrence of the nadir is important in predicting, monitoring, and responding to myelosuppression. Alopecia, nausea and vomiting, mucositis, and sterility are commonly observed side effects when tissues with rapid doubling times are damaged. The pathophysiology and management of these toxicities are discussed in Unit IV, Chapter

1, and the major toxicities of all chemotherapeutic agents are listed in Appendix I. Issues arising from the effects of cancer treatment on fertility are addressed in Unit IV, Chapter 5.

Chemotherapeutic agents are also associated with a variety of organ system toxicities that can result in cardiac, pulmonary, hepatic, renal, and neurological impairment. In general, these effects are observed after prolonged administration of chemotherapeutic agents and may be permanent or irreversible. Knowledge of the offending agents and careful monitoring of organ function permits early recognition of toxicity. Reducing the dosage or discontinuing the toxic antineoplastic agent may prevent further deterioration of organ system function.

Bibliography

Brager, B., & Yasko, J. (1984). *Care of the client receiving chemotherapy.* Reston, VA: Reston Publishing Co.

DeVita, V., Hellman, S., & Rosenberg, S. (Eds.). (1989). *Cancer: Principles and practices of oncoLogy* (3rd ed.). Philadelphia: J.B. Lippincott Co.

Fischer, D. S. & Knobf, M. K. (1989). *The cancer chemotherapy handbook* (3rd ed.). Chicago: Year Book Medical Publishers.

Goodman, M. S., & Wickham, R. (1984). Venous access devices: An overview. *Oncology Nursing Forum, 11*(5), 16-23.

Gullo, S. M. (1988). Safe handling of antineoplastic drugs: Translating the recommendations into practice. *Oncology Nursing Forum, 15*(5), 595-601.

Hughes, C. (1986). Giving cancer drugs IV, some guidelines. *American Journal of Nursing, 86*(1), 34-38.

Johnson, B, L., & Gross, J. (1985). *Handbook of oncology nursing.* New York: John Wiley & Sons.

Oncology Nursing Society. (1988). *Cancer chemotherapy guidelines. Modules I through V.* Pittsburgh, PA.

Oncology Nursig Society. (1989). *Access device guidelines, recommendations for nursing education and practice. Module I, Catheters; Module 2, Access Device Guidelines.*

Preston, F. A., & Wilfinger, C. (1988). *Memory bank for chemotherapy.* Baltimore: Williams and Wilkins.

Tenebaum, L. (1989). *Cancer chemotherapy: A reference guide.* Philadelphia: W. B. Saunders.

4 BIOLOGICAL RESPONSE MODIFIERS

Mary Ersek

INTRODUCTION

Biologic response modifiers (BRMs) constitute the fourth cancer treatment modality. These agents modify the relationship between tumor and host by strengthening the host's biologic response to tumor cells.

BRMs can be divided into three major categories according to mechanism of action:

1) agents that restore, augment, or modulate the host's normal immunological mechanisms;

2) agents that have direct antitumor effects; and

3) agents that have other biologic effects, such as interference with a tumor cell's ability to metastasize or survive after metastasis, promotion of cell differentiation, or interference with neoplastic transformation in cells.

Scientists began studying BRMs for cancer therapy in the 1960s, labeling the treatment modality "immunotherapy." After promising results in animal studies, researchers initiated many large-scale clinical trials to stimulate cancer patients' immune systems using the bacterial agents *Bacillus Calmette-Guerin* (BCG) and *Corynebacterium parvum (C. parvum)*. The results of these trials were discouraging, so the research into immunotherapy as a possible modality for cancer treatment lost momentum.

Recent technological advances have prompted a renewed interest in BRMs, and today biologic response modification, or biotherapy, is an important area in cancer research and treatment.

OVERVIEW OF THE IMMUNE SYSTEM

The body's immune system is a coordinated combination of nonspecific and specific responses to foreign substances (e.g. microbes and certain other toxins, called *antigens*).

Both physical injury and the presence of antigens can invoke nonspecific host defenses. These defenses include physical barriers and chemical factors, such as the skin and mucous membranes, acidic gastric secretions, and normal intestinal flora. The inflammatory response is another nonspecific host defense that serves to control the growth of microorganisms and prevent systemic infection.

Specific immune responses are elicited by the presence of an antigen. These reactions are characterized by a memory: that is, following the initial exposure to an antigen, specific portions of the immune system produce memory cells that allow a more vigorous response to subsequent exposures to the same antigen. These specific memory responses are generally divided into *humoral* and *cell-mediated* immunity.

Humoral immunity refers to immunity conferred by B-lymphocyte cells produced in the lymph system. These lymphocytes, also called *B cells*, produce plasma cells, which in turn produce antibodies (Figure 1). Antibodies are small proteins that can deactivate antigens by a variety of mechanisms, usually by binding with them. Antibody-antigen interaction is specific: Only one type of antibody can interact and neutralize a specific type of antigen. This interaction then activates the complement cascade, a system of proteins that "complements" antibody activity by destroying bacteria and helping the body rid itself of antibody/antigen complexes.

Cell-mediated immunity refers to immunity conferred by the mutation of T-lymphocytes, which is thought to occur in the thymus gland. These lymphocytes, also called *T cells*, directly or indirectly destroy viruses, malignant cells, cells infected with intracellular organisms, and cells of grafted organs. Different types of T cells have different immune functions: *cytotoxic* T cells directly destroy antigens; helper T cells activate the humoral immune system and cytotoxic T cells; and suppressor T cells inhibit antibody production and other immune responses.

Other cells that are important in the immune response are *macrophages* and *natural killer* (NK) *cells*. Macrophages are white blood cells with a number of important functions. They bind to an antigen and "present" the antigen to undifferentiated cells (precursor cells); these, in turn, become activated and produce mature lymphocytes. Without this macrophage processing, the T and B cells could not respond to some types of antigen. NK cells are cytotoxic to tumor cells and virus-infected cells.

Many cells in the immune system produce chemicals that aid in regulating the immune response. These substances are referred to as mediators and broadly referred to as *cytokines*. Scientists are currently studying many cytokines to determine their effect on the immune system. Table 1 lists several cytokines and their mechanisms of action.

TYPES OF BRM THERAPY

A brief review of BRM agents currently being evaluated follows.

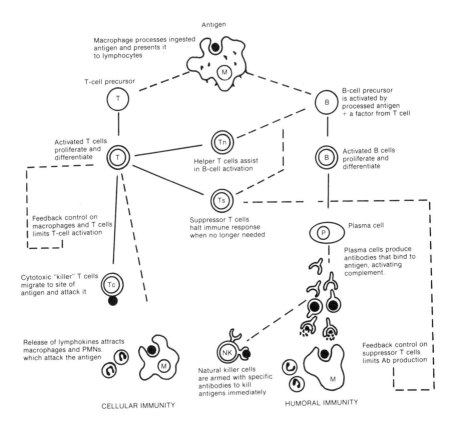

Figure 1. Overview of cell cooperation in the immune response. Solid lines show cell differentiation. Dashed lines show cells' effects.
Source: From *Medical-Surgical Nursing: A Psychophysiologic Approach* (p. 94) by J. Luckmann and K. Sorensen, 1987, Philadelphia: W. B. Saunders Company. Adapted with permission of publisher.

For additional information, the reader is referred to the bibliography at the end of the chapter.

Monoclonal Antibodies

The use of monoclonal antibodies (MoAbs) involves the development of specific antibodies directed against antigens located on the surface of tumor cells. Samples of the patient's tumor cells are taken and processed to reveal specific antibodies to the tumor-associated antigens. In order for this approach to work, a sufficient quantity of antigens unique to the tumor cells must be present. In addition, the tumor antigens must be sufficiently different from

Table 1. Cytokines Used as Biological Response Modifiers

Mediator	Source	Mechanisms of Action*
Interleukin-1 (IL-1)	Macrophages	Promotes proliferation of T lymphocytes Stimulates production of IL-2
Interleukin-2 (T-cell growth factor, IL-2)	T lymphocytes	Promotes proliferation of several types of T cells and LAK cells Increases NK cell activity
Colony stimulating factor (CSF)	T lymphocytes	Stimulates bone marrow cells to differentiate
Gamma interferon (γ INF)	T cells B cells Macrophages	Same as for gamma interferon
Tumor necrosis factor (TNF)	Macrophages	Cytotoxic to tumor cells Stimulates IL-1 Stimulates CSF synthesis

*Not all mechanisms of action for each cytokine are listed. Moreover, some are probable mechanisms which have not actually been identified yet in humans.

antigens elaborated by normal cells to provoke an antibody response.

The antibodies can be used alone to kill cancer cells or as carriers of other substances used for either therapeutic or diagnostic purposes. For example, chemotherapeutic agents can be attached to monoclonal antibodies to deliver high concentrations of these toxic substances directly to the tumor cells. In theory, this approach is less toxic and more effective than conventional chemotherapy because the delivery of harmful agents to normal tissues is decreased.

Monoclonal antibodies can also be used diagnostically. They carry radioactive substances to cancer cells, thus pinpointing the location of metastases previously undetected by other methods.

Despite these uses, monoclonal antibody treatments have limitations. Because monoclonal antibodies are made using mouse antibodies, they are, themselves, foreign proteins that often trigger an immune response; thus, they can be neutralized before any therapeutic effect occurs. In addition, monoclonals may lack specificity for tumor antigens. Tumor cell antigens may not be different enough from those on normal cells to ensure only cancer cell destruction; studies have revealed that most monoclonal antibodies interact with antigens on both normal and cancer cells. Technological developments may resolve these issues in the future.

In the clinical setting, therapeutic monoclonal antibodies are usually given over 4 to 6 hours by continuous intravenous infusion. Because of the risk of serious allergic reactions, patients are premedicated with acetaminophen and an antihistamine and monitored closely. Emergency drugs are kept at the bedside. Side effects of monoclonal antibodies include dyspnea and mild wheezing, fever, chills, headache, rash, nausea, vomiting, tachycardia, and allergic reactions.

Research studies are currently underway using monoclonals for a variety of diseases, including T cell lymphoma, chronic and acute lymphocytic leukemia, melanoma, colorectal cancer, and neuroblastoma.

Interferons

Interferons (IFNs) are small proteins that inhibit viral replication and promote the cellular (T-cell) immune response. Interferon use for cancer treatment was limited until the late 1970s, when technological advances enabled production of large amounts of IFN.

There are currently three major types of IFNs: alpha (α), beta (β), and gamma (γ). Each type has similar but distinctive capabilities for altering biological responses. Although results of clinical studies have failed to fulfill the high expectations that the medical community initially had about IFNs, promising results have been obtained.

Alpha-IFN was the first BRM approved by the Food and Drug Administration (FDA) in 1986. It is currently indicated for use in the treatment of hairy cell leukemia and AIDS-associated Kaposi's sarcoma. It has also demonstrated therapeutic effectiveness against hematologic diseases such as low-grade non-Hodgkin's lymphoma, cutaneous T-cell lymphoma, multiple myeloma, and chronic myelogenous leukemia. In addition to alpha interferon's use in hematologic diseases, clinical reports indicated a therapeutic response when used in the treatment of viral hepatitis.

Interferons produce side effects of varying frequency and intensity depending on dose, schedule, route of administration, and type of IFN. One of the most common side effects of IFN therapy is a flu-like syndrome. Symptoms include fever, chills, tachycardia, muscle aches, malaise, fatigue, and headaches. This reaction is extremely common during a patient's first exposure to IFN, but usually decreases in intensity with continued daily therapy.

Other common side effects of IFN include decreased white blood cell count, anemia (with prolonged therapy), and decreased platelets. Gastrointestinal symptoms such as loss of appetite, nausea, vomiting, and diarrhea may also be present. Central nervous system toxicities range from mild confusion and sleepiness to seizures. Acute kidney failure is rare but can occur. Loss of hair may also be a problem.

Interferon can be administered by intravenous bolus or infusion, or intramuscular, subcutaneous, or intrathecal injection. It can also be given intranasally. Redness and irritation at the injection site may occur. Since IFN is often administered on an outpatient basis, it is essential that the patient and family are taught the technique of administration and how to manage side effects.

Interleukin-2

Interleukin-2 (IL-2) is a substance produced by lymphocytes. In addition to being an essential factor for the growth of T cells, IL-2 augments various T-cell functions and enhances NK cell function. IL-2 also activates *lymphokine-activated killer* (LAK) *cells*, which are a type of killer T cell produced when lymphocytes are incubated with IL-2. LAK cells destroy tumor cells and improve the recovery of immune function in certain immunodeficiency states. To date, patients with renal cell cancer, melanoma, and non-Hodgkin's lymphoma have responded to IL-2 therapy.

The most severe toxicities result from IL-2's ability to increase capillary permeability, which causes hypotension, ascites, generalized body edema, and pulmonary edema.

Chills and fever also frequently occur within a few hours after IL-2 administration. Headache, malaise, and other flu-like symptoms are also common. Gastrointestinal effects include nausea, vomiting, loss of appetite, diarrhea, and mucositis. Some liver dysfunction is common during therapy but resolves once treatment is stopped. Central nervous system toxicity is manifested by lethargy, confusion, disorientation and hallucinations, anxiety, and sometimes depression. Although the effect of IL-2 on the kidneys is generally mild, renal failure can result if severe hypotension occurs. Hypotension, anemia, and a decrease in platelets are more likely with higher, cumulative doses. Skin changes include redness, rash, pruritus, and occasionally skin desquamation.

Although many research studies with IL-2 require intensive supportive care in acute care settings, other current treatment regimens can be given on an outpatient basis. Patient education in these situations is especially important because patients must be alert to potential side effects that should be reported immediately.

Colony Stimulating Factors

Colony stimulating factors (CSFs) are growth factors which mediate the proliferation, maturation, regulation, and activation of granulocytes, macrophages, lymphocytes, monocytes, erythrocytes, and platelets. Four types of CSFs have been produced synthetically and are in various stages of clinical trials. Generally, CSFs have been named for the major cell lineage they affect: Granulocyte-macrophage CSF (GM-CSF) affects both granulocyte and macrophage lineage; granulocyte CSF (G-CSF) targets only granulocytes; pleuripoietin IL-3, or multi-CSF affects early cell lineage; and macrophage CSF (M-CSF) targets macrophage production. Erythropoietin (EPO®), which targets erythrocyte production, was approved by the FDA in 1989 for use in anemia caused by end-stage renal disease. Current clinical trials are assessing its effectiveness in treating anemia related to cancer and its therapies.

GM-CSF and G-CSF have been administered by intravenous bolus, subcutaneously by daily injection, or by continuous intravenous infusion. G-CSF therapy has been associated with only minimal toxicity, mainly bone pain. GM-CSF produces more systemic toxicities, including fatigue, fever, muscle aches, anorexia, rash, and diarrhea. Blood levels of alkaline phosphatase and aminotransferases may also be increased.

Medical use of these growth factors is an important step in understanding and manipulating the immune system. Future studies will test their efficacy in the treatment of congenital hematologic diseases and their ability to reduce neutropenia during cancer treatment, thus allowing patients to receive higher doses of chemotherapy without myelosuppression.

Tumor Necrosis Factor

Tumor necrosis factor (TNF) is a substance naturally secreted by macrophages. When activated by endotoxins, the macrophages release TNF, which then binds to receptors on cell membranes. Once bound to the cell membrane, TNF initiates cellular activity and is possibly cytotoxic to that cell.

TNF is in the early phases of clinical trials and has not yet demonstrated therapeutic effectiveness against malignant diseases. Side effects of TNF are similar to those experienced with interferon therapy, including a flu-like syndrome and soreness at the injection site. Fever and chills are generally mild and disappear with subsequent doses of TNF.

NURSING CONSIDERATIONS

With the exception of alpha interferon, most BRMs are currently being evaluated in Phase I/II clinical trials. (For descriptions of the phases of clinical trials see Unit III, Chapter 3.) Most patients eligible for Phase I and II clinical trials have advanced disease or disease unresponsive to standard therapy. These patients may feel a sense of desperation and believe that a new therapy will bring a cure or at least a reprieve.

It is difficult but absolutely essential to give accurate, realistic information about investigational agents and participation in clinical trials. Patients must fulfill strict eligibility criteria before entry into clinical trials; not every advanced cancer patient will be eligible. Nurses must counsel patients that the new therapy is not a panacea, and there are many known and unknown risks of participation. For these reasons, informed consent is obtained before the trial begins to ensure that patients understand and agree to the proposed treatment. Frequent and consistent information must be provided to patients and families to support their needs once a clinical trial begins.

Nurses caring for patients receiving BRMs must be knowledgeable about this modality in order to administer investigational agents safely, evaluate treatment-related toxicities, and inform patients and their families about self-care strategies. Current information on the status of BRM therapies is available through the Cancer Information System (refer to Unit 6).

Bibliography

Foon, K. A. (1988). Advances in immunotherapy of cancer: Monoclonal antibodies and interferon. *Seminars in Oncology Nursing, 4*(2), 112-119.

Gallucci, B. B. (1987). The immune system and cancer. *Oncology Nursing Forum, 14*(6, Supplement), 3-12.

Gallucci, B. B., & Rokosky, J. S. (1986a). Immune responses. In M. L. Patrick, S. L. Woods, R. F. Craven, J. S. Rokosky & P. M. Bruno (Eds.), *Medical-surgical nursing: Pathophysiological concepts* (pp. 186-202). Philadelphia: J.B. Lippincott & Co.

Hahn, M. B., & Jassak, P. F. (1988). Nursing management of patients receiving interferon. *Seminars in Oncology Nursing, 4*(2), 95-101.

Haeuber, D., & Di Julio, J. E. (1989). Hemopoietic colony stimulating factors. An overview. *Oncology Nursing Forum, 16*(2), 247-255.

Mitchell, M. S., & Bertram, J. H. (1985). Immunology and biomodulation of cancer. In P. Calabresi, P. S. Schein, & S. A. Rosenberg (Eds.), *Medical oncology: Basic principles and clinical management of cancer* (pp. 363-389). New York: MacMillan Publishing Company.

Moldower, N. P., & Figlin, R. A. (1988). Tumor necrosis factor: Current clinical status and implications for nursing management. *Seminars in Oncology Nursing, 4*(2), 120-125.

Oldham, R. K. (1984). Biologicals and biological response modifiers: Fourth modality of cancer treatment. *Cancer Treatment Reports, 68*(1), 221-232.

Simpson, S., Seipp, C. A., & Rosenberg, S. A. (1988). The current status and future applications of interleukin-2 and adoptive immunotherapy in cancer treatment. *Seminars in Oncology Nursing, 4*(2), 132-141.

5 BONE MARROW TRANSPLANTATION

Louise Schilter and Eileen Rossman

Bone marrow transplantation (BMT) was attempted in the early 1950s with very disappointing results. All patients treated were in late stages of their disease and relapsed following transplant. By the late 1970s, with improvements in supportive care such as modern antibiotics and parenteral nutrition, and advances in basic sciences such as tissue typing, BMTs were performed more successfully. Today, BMT is no longer considered a last resort for the treatment of certain diseases. Over 10,000 transplants have been performed worldwide and more than 200 marrow transplant centers exist.

POTENTIAL INDICATIONS

BMT is used for cancers that are responsive to high doses of chemotherapy or radiation therapy. These high doses kill cancer cells but are also toxic to bone marrow. Because BMT provides a method for "rescuing" patients from bone marrow damage, higher doses of chemotherapy and/or radiation therapy can be given. Diseases of bone marrow are treated with BMT because the donor marrow replaces deficient hematopoietic elements by reconstituting the population of stem cells in the bone marrow cavities. Malignancies that may be treated with BMT are listed in Table 1.

SOURCES OF BONE MARROW

Marrow for transplantation is obtained from three sources: an identical twin (syngeneic), an HLA-matched sibling or unrelated donor (allogeneic), or the patient's own stored bone marrow (autologous). In allogeneic and syngeneic transplants, the person's abnormal or diseased marrow is replaced with healthy marrow from a donor. With autologous transplants, bone marrow is taken from the patient before a treatment is started that will be lethal to the marrow for reinfusion following marrow ablative therapy. In some hematologic malignancies, the transplant may be done during remission.

As with any organ transplant, the problem of organ or tissue rejection is a major consideration. In allogeneic transplants, human-leukocyte antigens (HLA), found on all nucleated circulating and

Table 1. Malignant Diseases. Potential Indications for Bone Marrow Transplantation

Acute myelogenous leukemia
Acute lymphocytic leukemia
Chronic myelogenous leukemia
Chronic lymphocytic leukemia*
Myelodysplastic syndromes
Preleukemia
Multiple Myeloma*
Non-Hodgkin's lymphoma
Hodgkin's disease
Responsive solid tumors*
  Neuroblastoma*
  Testicular cancer*
  Small-cell lung cancer*
  Breast cancer*
  Other sensitive solid tumors*

*Diseases currently under investigation or with the potential to be treated with bone marrow transplantation.
Source: From "Bone Marrow Transplantation," by G. B. Vogelsang, 1989, *Mediguide to Oncology 9*, p. 1. Adapted with permission of DellaCorte publications.

tissue cells, are involved in the immune response to foreign tissue. When the donor marrow regenerates and begins to produce white blood cells, those white blood cells will recognize the recipient's tissues as foreign and begin to attack these tissues. For this reason, HLA typing for antigen compatibility between the donor and the recipient is conducted. Marrow from a donor whose HLA type matches that of the transplant recipient is more likely to successfully engraft, and the patient will experience fewer complications.

The ideal donor for a BMT is an identical twin, because the donor and the recipient are genetically identical for all transplantation antigens. Siblings of a prospective patient have a 25% chance of being perfect matches (Figure 1). Approximately 60% of patients lack a suitably matched sibling donor. For this reason, bone marrow donor registries have been established to match more HLA-identical people. The odds are 1 in approximately 100,000 that any two unrelated individuals will be HLA-matched. As the number of donor registries increases throughout the United States, the chances of finding a matched donor for every patient who needs one also increase.

PSYCHOSOCIAL CONSIDERATIONS

The BMT procedure involves a major emotional and economic commitment from patients and their families. Because there are not many major transplant centers, patients and some family

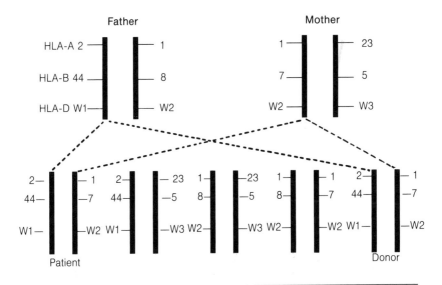

Figure 1. Diagrammatic representation of the inheritance of the human leukocyte antigen (HLA) region of chromosome 6 in a family. The patient and the sibling donor have inherited the same two HLA haplotypes and thus are HLA genotypically identical.
Source: Reprinted by permission of the American Cancer Society, from E. D. Thomas, Bone marrow transplantation" *Ca-A Cancer Journal for Clinicians, 37*(1987):293.

members may have to temporarily move to the location where the transplant will be performed. They must depend on unfamiliar medical and nursing staff in a new city for their support during a particularly stressful time. Most transplant centers sponsor support groups and offer counseling to patients and their families.

The costs of BMT are high. Inpatient hospital expenses range from $100,000 to $200,000. Although these costs may be reimbursed by insurance carriers, many patients have exhausted their benefits by the time a BMT is recommended. When BMT is performed in a state other than the patient's residence, insurance difficulties are frequent. The patient's community may be a major source of economic assistance through locally organized fundraising.

TRANSPLANT PROCESS

Preparative Regimen

Cancer patients preparing for BMT must first undergo a *conditioning* or *preparative* regimen that involves high doses of chemotherapy and/or radiation therapy. These regimens aim to eradicate the existing marrow so that the patient is essentially

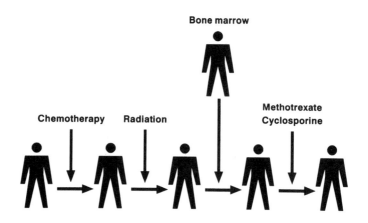

Bone marrow

Methotrexate
Cyclosporine

Chemotherapy   Radiation

Figure 2. A typical schema of an allogeneic bone marrow transplant in patients with leukemia.
Source: From "The management of acute leukemias," 1989, *Clinical Advances in Oncology Nursing, 1,* p. 1. Reprinted with permission of Wyeth-Ayerst Laboratories.

incapable of mounting an immune response to, and ultimately rejecting, the donor marrow. In cancers involving the bone marrow, the regimen also eradicates residual malignant cells. In cancers not involving the bone marrow, the patient may also receive additional chemotherapy or radiation therapy specific to that type of malignancy. The preparative regimen varies depending on the disease being treated. The typical sequencing of the preparative regimen, the BMT, and immunosuppressive regimen is shown in Figure 2.

Bone Marrow Harvest

Bone marrow harvest is a commonly used phrase referring to the collection of bone marrow for transplantation. For syngeneic and allogeneic transplants, the bone marrow donor is admitted to the hospital to donate marrow. With the donor under general or spinal anesthesia in the operating room, the marrow is aspirated from the anterior and posterior iliac crests with a needle and syringe (Figure 3). Between 1-5% of the total bone marrow is removed, an amount not large enough to cause anemia. Following the harvest, the donor may have some soreness and hip discomfort that disappear within a day or two. Donors are often discharged the day after surgery.

Autologous transplant candidates go through the same harvesting or collecting procedure. Harvested bone marrow is then filtered to remove bone particles and fat, and heparinized to prevent clotting. Following this, the bone marrow may be *purged* or treated to destroy any residual malignant cells and then frozen for reinfusion.

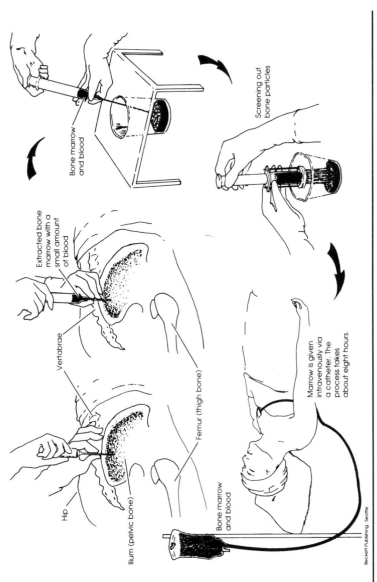

Bone marrow and blood

Screening out bone particles

Extracted bone marrow with a small amount of blood

Vertebrae

Femur (thigh bone)

Hip

Ilium (pelvic bone)

Bone marrow and blood

Marrow is given intravenously via a catheter. The process takes about eight hours.

Beckett Publishing, Seattle

Figure 3. Bone marrow aspiration and reinfusion process in an allogeneic transplant. In an autologous transplant, the marrow is defrosted and manually "pushed" into a central line. The DMSO preservation is cytotoxic.

Source: From *Patient Information Handbook, 1988,* Seattle, WA: Becker Publishing. Reprinted with permission of publisher.

If the bone marrow is not to be purged, it will be refrigerated or cryopreserved for reinfusion. The projected number of days to reinfusion dictates the storage method.

Marrow Infusion

Autologous BMT patients receive their preparative regimen and other disease treatment after the bone marrow harvest to avoid marrow-ablative drug effects. The marrow for these patients is not reinfused until the preparative drugs have cleared the patient's system. Allogeneic and syngeneic BMT patients can receive the preparative regimen and disease treatment before the harvest of the donor marrow because the donor marrow is obviously not exposed to the drugs.

The marrow is infused into the patient intravenously over 2 to 6 hours while the patient is being monitored for any problems associated with infusing such a large amount of fluid. The new marrow enters the general circulation, migrates to the bone marrow cavities, and begins to produce cells within 2 to 4 weeks.

COMPLICATIONS

Patients undergoing BMT experience a variety of complications. Some are specific to BMT, such as graft-versus-host disease and veno-occlusive disease. Other complications are commonly seen secondary to radiation or chemotherapy but may be more intense following BMT.

Graft-versus-host disease: *Graft-versus-host disease* (GVHD) occurs in approximately 50% of allogeneic transplant patients. GVHD involves an immunologic response of the immunocompetent cells produced by the donor marrow (graft) to the recipient's (host) tissue. Even though the white blood cells produced are HLA matched to the host tissue, the lymphocytes in the donor marrow recognize the recipient as foreign and attack the patient's gastrointestinal tract, skin, and liver. Since GVHD occurs despite HLA-matching, there are probably other unknown antigens that are involved in this response. GVHD generally occurs at the time of bone marrow recovery (acute GVHD) but can occur as a very late complication, from 6 months to 1½ years post BMT (chronic GVHD). Patients who receive partially HLA-matched marrow and older patients are at a higher risk of developing GVHD.

Treatment for GVHD has improved; however, patient response is variable. Of the 50% of patients who develop GVHD, 30% experience a fairly severe form, with 20% of these having life-threatening cases. Patients receiving allogeneic transplants may be given prophylactic immunosuppressive treatment with methotrexate and/or cyclosporine or steroids to prevent GVHD (Figure 2).

Veno-occlusive disease: The high-dose preparative regimen for bone marrow transplant seems to predispose the patient to veno-occlusive disease (VOD), a condition in which deposits of fibrin in the small venules of the liver obstruct blood flow. This complication occurs more frequently with patients who have pre-existing liver abnormalities. Veno-occlusive disease is rarely seen outside the BMT population. Symptoms include weight gain, ascites, right upper quadrant pain, elevated bilirubin and liver enzymes, and, in extreme situations, encephalopathy. One-third of all BMT patients develop significant VOD. There is no treatment other than supportive care.

Bleeding: Bleeding can occur during the first few weeks following transplant because of the thrombocytopenia associated with high-dose preparative regimens. Patients are supported with platelet transfusions from community donors and/or family members. The most common sites of bleeding include the nose, mouth, gastrointestinal tract, urinary tract, and site of any invasive procedure.

Infection: Because the new bone marrow takes considerable time to mature and begin to function, patients are susceptible to unusual and potentially life-threatening bacterial, fungal, and viral infections during their prolonged period of immunodeficiency. Pneumonia is the leading cause of death in the first 3 months following BMT. Viral pneumonias account for over 50% of all pneumonias in BMT patients and for 13% of all transplant deaths.

Renal insufficiency: Renal insufficiency can result from damage induced by chemotherapy and other nephrotoxic medications—e.g., antibiotics, immunosuppressive drugs—or from potentiation of pre-existing renal insufficiency caused by this rigorous treatment. Management of a patient with renal problems is a challenge; when encountered in association with VOD, this complication can result in high mortality.

Gastrointestinal effects: Patients generally experience a variety of gastrointestinal toxicities related to the preparative regimen. Severe mucositis involving the oropharynx and esophagus is frequently observed. This disruption in the integrity of the mucosa further predisposes the patient to infectious complications, including viral (e.g., *herpes simplex*), bacterial, and fungal infections.

Patients frequently develop nausea, vomiting, and diarrhea in reaction to the high doses of chemotherapy and radiation used in the preparative regimen. Because the patient experiencing these toxicities will probably not get adequate nutrition, assessment is done periodically to identify problems and to initiate appropriate nutritional support.

Long-term effects: Fatigue, sterility, and cataracts are frequently observed long-term effects of treatment. Other late complications that can occur include delayed onset of GVHD, impaired growth and development associated with the preparative regimen, late infectious proccesses, and the possibility of relapse or second malignancy.

PATIENT DISCHARGE

The average hospital stay for a BMT patient is 35 to 40 days, but can be longer if complications arise. Before release from the hospital, the patient must be free of infection, afebrile, and off antibiotics; have a granulocyte count greater then 500; and be able to maintain an adequate nutritional intake. Once discharged, the patient must be monitored regularly and be observed closely for GVHD (if an allogeneic BMT recipient), infections, adequate caloric intake, and function of the engrafted bone marrow. BMT patients generally stay in the hospital area for approximately 100 days.

A patient's long-term prognosis depends on many factors: the type of disease, the degree of HLA matching, whether the patient is in remission or relapse at the time of transplant, prior organ damage, previous exposure to chemotherapy, and the patient's age. In recent years significant advances have been made in BMT techniques, and many transplant teams are investigating and implementing new techniques to improve results. BMT has progressed from an investigational treatment modality to a standard treatment for several diseases.

Bibliography

Ballard, B., & Ford, R. (1988). Acute complications after bone marrow transplantation. *Seminars in Oncology, 4*(1), 15-24.

Corcoran-Buchsel, P. (1986). Long-term complications of allogeneic bone marrow transplantation: Nursing implications. *Oncology Nursing Forum, 13*(6), 61-70.

Haberman, M. R. (1988). Psychosocial aspects of bone marrow transplantation. *Seminars in Oncology Nursing, 4*(1), 55-59.

Klemm, P. (1985). Cyclosporin-A: Use in preventing graft-versus-host disease. *Oncology Nursing Forum, 12*(5), 25-31.

Margolies, C. P. (1983). *Understanding leukemia* (pp. 108-119). New York: Scribner's Sons.

Nims, J., & Strom, S. (1988). Late complications of bone marrow transplant recipients: Nursing care issues. *Seminars in Oncology, 4*(1), 47-54.

Schryber, S., Lacasse, S. R., & Barton-Burke, M. (1987). Autologous bone marrow transplantation. *Oncology Nursing Forum, 14*(4), 74-80.

Thomas, E. D. (1987). Bone marrow transplantation. *CA-A Cancer Journal for Clinicians, 37*(5), 291-301.

UNIT 4

Nursing Management

In many ways, nursing care during cancer therapy is similar to that involved in the treatment of other diseases. However, there are important differences that attest to the tremendous need for skilled nursing intervention.

Initiation of treatment is usually immediate, sometimes precluding extensive patient preparation. The patient often enters treatment in a debilitated state as a result of tumor growth, disease recurrence, or secondary problems such as anemia or infection. In addition, the patient and family are most often fearful, anxious, and experiencing disruption of their usual routines. Treatment approaches may be aggressive, multimodal, conducted for extended periods, and accompanied by side effects and toxicities.

Nursing research and expert clinical practice have contributed to the definition of common problems and to the development of care approaches. Some problems may be prevented, minimized, or controlled through prudent assessment and intervention. Patient and family teaching are important aspects of nursing management in cancer care. Increased survival of patients with cancer has prompted intensified interest in rehabilitation and quality of life issues. The chapters in this unit highlight common concerns throughout the disease continuum.

1 SYMPTOM MANAGEMENT

Michele Girard Donehower

A growing malignancy or the local or systemic effects of cancer treatment can affect virtually all body systems. A variety of symptoms can result, depending on the location of the tumor and the specific toxicities of treatment. Nurses caring for patients with cancer need to be aware of the more common symptoms associated with the disease or its treatment, because those that are particularly distressful can lead to morbidity, affect compliance with treatment regimens, and affect overall quality of life. Nursing interventions focus on the prevention, early detection, and management of these complications. Nurses have demonstrated increasing autonomy in symptom management. It is an area of patient care that provides opportunities to be creative and to make a significant difference in patients' quality of life.

BONE MARROW DYSFUNCTION

Bone marrow dysfunction can be caused by primary or metastatic disease involving the bone marrow or by myelosuppressive therapy. The normal production of hematopoietic cells is impaired, resulting in granulocytopenia, thrombocytopenia, and anemia.

Granulocytopenia (a decrease in white blood cells) increases susceptibility to infection and is a common cause of morbidity and mortality in the cancer patient. Both exogenous microorganisms and normal endogenous flora can be pathogenic in these immunosuppressed patients. Nearly 80% of infections in patients with cancer originate in the lower respiratory tract, perianal area, pharynx, genitourinary tract, or skin. Health care professionals frequently initiate infection control measures in patients with granulocyte counts of less than $1000/mm^3$ (Table 1). Handwashing is the single most important intervention to reduce risk of exogenous infection.

Thrombocytopenia (a decrease in platelets) can result in bleeding or hemorrhage when the platelet count falls below $50,000/mm^3$, and platelet transfusions may be required. Spontaneous hemorrhage can occur with platelet counts of less than $20,000/mm^3$. Administration of platelet transfusions to keep the platelet count above $20,000/mm^3$, thereby reducing bleeding risk, is standard protocol in many treatment settings. Patients must participate in measures to prevent bleeding and learn to recognize when to report it (Table 1).

Anemia (a decrease in red blood cells) results in general fatigue, headache, dizziness, shortness of breath, and other symptoms. Because the body is able to compensate for a gradual decline in red blood cells, patients with treatment- or disease-related anemia may not become symptomatic until the hematocrit falls below 30%. These cases are routinely managed with transfusions of red blood cells and interventions to control the associated symptoms (Table 1).

Nurses should educate patients about the signs and symptoms of granulocytopenia, thrombocytopenia, and anemia. Patients should also be informed of the potential for bleeding and increased susceptibility to infection associated with low platelet and white blood cell counts. Infection prevention should be stressed.

NAUSEA AND VOMITING

Nausea and vomiting are most commonly seen in patients receiving chemotherapy, biologic response modifiers, or radiation therapy involving the gastrointestinal tract. However, a variety of other phenomena related to tumor growth and metastasis, organ dysfunction, and metabolic abnormalities may cause these symptoms.

Patients receiving chemotherapy frequently experience nausea and vomiting, due to either the direct irritation of the gastrointestinal tract or a central nervous system effect on the area of the brain that controls vomiting. Patients sometimes experience symptoms before chemotherapy administration—a conditioned response known as anticipatory nausea and vomiting. Its exact mechanism is unknown, and management is difficult. Premedicating patients with antiemetics before chemotherapy is one of the most effective ways to deal with this problem.

Localized damage to the epithelial lining of the esophagus, stomach, and intestines, and accumulation of toxic waste products of cell destruction are the probable causes of nausea and vomiting in patients receiving radiation.

The management of treatment-related nausea and vomiting has improved due to an increased variety of antiemetics with different mechanisms of action. Antiemetics are also being combined in new ways to achieve maximal control of nausea and vomiting. The choice of a single agent or combination regimen is determined by the chemotherapeutic agents administered and by the patient's response to the antiemetic. Table 2 lists the more frequently used antiemetics.

Table 1. Bone Marrow Suppression

Clinical Manifestations	Interventions
	Granulocytopenia
Fever (may be masked in patients receiving steroids)	• Avoid exposure to:
	— potential sources of infection
Usual signs & symptoms of inflammation may be absent or diminished (redness, heat, pus formation, edema, pain) due to lack of white blood cells.	— persons with transmissible diseases
	— all sources of stagnant water (humidifiers, water pitchers, etc.)
	— dust, sprays, etc.
	— contaminated medical equipment
	— dogs, cats, birds, and other animals
	— fresh fruit and vegetables, cut flowers
Changes in usual respiratory pattern	Change room air filters between patients or monthly
— Dyspnea (with or without productive cough)	Wash hands meticulously when caring for patient
— Sore throat	• Ensure good daily personal hygiene for patients
Changes in usual urinary patterns	• Inspect skin daily for signs of infection
Perirectal discomfort	• Cleanse oral cavity after each meal and at bedtime
	• Restrict patients with WBC <1000/mm³ to private room
	• Avoid injury to skin and oral and rectal mucosa
	Avoid use of indwelling urinary catheters
	Provide site care to all venous catheters qd & prn
	• Avoid deodorants (block secretions of sebaceous glands)
	Administer newly ordered antibiotics as soon as possible
	• Keep antibiotics on schedule
	• Report fever (>100°F) to physician
	Thrombocytopenia
Bleeding gums	• Avoid activities with potential for physical injury
Petechiae, ecchymoses	— Sports, recreational activities
Frank bleeding from body	— Shaving with razor
— mouth, vagina, rectum, urethra, nose	— Cutting finger or toe nails
	• Avoid medicines that alter platelet function and normal coagulation (e.g. ASA, heparin)
Prolonged bleeding from venipuncture sites, cuts	Minimize number of invasive procedures—apply pressure to procedure site for 5–10 min.
	Check all urine, stool, and emesis for blood
	Avoid IM injections
	• Gently cleanse oral cavity with soft toothbrush. Do not use dental floss for platelets <100,000
	• Avoid constipation
	— promote hydration
	— increase mobility
	— administer stool softeners

Table 1. **Bone Marrow Suppression (Continued)**

Clinical Manifestations	Interventions
	• Avoid sneezing (if possible) and forcefully blowing nose • Encourage use of water-based lubricant before sexual intercourse • Use precautions to prevent falls • Avoid rectal manipulation with enemas, suppositories, thermometer • Report a headache, especially frontal, to physician • Inspect skin for new signs of bleeding or bruising Transfuse with platelets as ordered
	Anemia
Fatigue, weakness Shortness of breath Headache Dizziness, syncope, tachycardia, postural hypotension	• Allow for periods of rest between daily activities • Assure adequate sleep at night • Instruct patient to rise slowly from lying or sitting position • Provide adequate nutritional intake Administer O_2 and analgesics for headache as ordered Transfuse with RBCs as ordered

• Indicates interventions that patients should know and perform as they are able in the hospital and at home.

Patients with treatment-related symptoms receive antiemetics before treatment and on a scheduled, around-the-clock basis for 24 to 72 hours following treatment, often in high dosages and in combinations. By administering antiemetics around the clock instead of as needed (PRN), better prevention and control of emesis can be achieved.

Important nursing interventions include educating patients about antiemetic scheduling and side effects, administering antiemetics, and evaluating the patient's response to the antiemetic regimen.

Other behavioral interventions, such as relaxation training, distraction, and guided visual imagery, have been employed to manage nausea and vomiting with varying degrees of success.

BOWEL DYSFUNCTION

Oncology patients frequently exhibit alterations in bowel function such as diarrhea, constipation, and bowel obstruction.

Common causes of diarrhea include: chemotherapy, radiation therapy, antibiotics, graft-versus-host disease, bowel resection, food intolerance, hyperosmolar dietary supplements, tube feedings, in-

Table 2. Commonly Used Antiemetic Drugs

Antiemetic	Sites of action	Route	Dose
PHENOTHIAZINES	Vomiting center (TVC)		
chlorpromazine		IV/IM, PO, rectal	10-50 mg
prochlorperazine		IV/IM, PO, rectal	10-50 mg
promethazine		IV/IM, PO, rectal	12.5-25 mg
BUTYROPHENONES	Chemoreceptor trigger zone (CTZ)		
haloperidol		IV/IM, PO	1-4 mg
droperidol		IV/IM	1.25-2.5 mg
CANNABINOIDS	Higher CNS structures*		
tetrahydrocannabinol		PO	2.5-10 mg
nabilone		PO	1-2 mg
ANTIHISTAMINES	TVC, higher CNS structures*		
diphenhydramine		IV/IM, PO	25-50 mg
CORTICOSTEROIDS	Unknown		
dexamethasone	?periphery**	IM/IV, PO	8-20 mg 10-40 mg
BENZODIAZEPINES	Higher CNS structures*		
lorazepam		IV/IM, PO	0.5-3 mg
METACLOPROMIDE	CTZ periphery**	IV, PO	1-2 mg/kg
TRIMETHOBENZAMIDE	CTZ	IM, PO, rectal	200-250 mg

*higher CNS structure = brain stem and cortical structures
**periphery = GI tract and other viscera (heart, testes)
Source: From PDQ (Physicians Data Query) (1990). Information file, Supportive Care Submanuscript, National Cancer Institute, Bethesda, MD.

flammation of the bowel, fecal impaction, and anxiety. Bloody diarrhea may be indicative of drug toxicity. Clinical effects of diarrhea may include fluid and electrolyte loss, fecal incontinence, and the development of severe perianal irritation. Treatment depends on the etiology, but may include: antidiarrheal and narcotic agents (Lomotil®, Imodium®, codeine, tincture of opium), aluminum-containing antacids (Amphogel®, Basalgel®), bulk-forming agents (Metamucil®), the avoidance of high dietary fiber and other bowel stimulants, and the restriction of oral intake to rest the bowel.

Constipation can result from impairment of peristaltic activity by neurotoxic chemotherapy, narcotic analgesics, immobility, changes in eating habits, dehydration, hypercalcemia, and neurogenic phenomena secondary to metastatic disease (e.g., spinal cord compression). Constipation can be managed by preventive techniques, including the elimination of causative factors, or by judicious use of stool softeners. Patients at risk for constipation should be started on a prophylactic bowel regimen that includes a high fiber diet, increased fluid intake, bulk-forming agents, and stool softeners. Further drug administration may have to be delayed until the underlying problem is resolved.

Bowel obstruction most frequently occurs in patients with advanced abdominal malignancies, ovarian cancer, or adhesions caused by prior surgery or radiation therapy to the abdomen. Patients who have received neurotoxic chemotherapy often experience this problem as well. Obstruction secondary to advanced cancer can be insidious in onset and produce only intermittent symptoms. Abdominal pain, nausea, and vomiting are common symptoms. Initially, patients may be treated conservatively with nasogastric suction and restriction of all oral intake; some may require surgical intervention to relieve the obstruction.

MUCOSITIS

Cytotoxic chemotherapy and radiation can damage the epithelial cells lining the gastrointestinal tract. Although toxicity can affect all mucosal surfaces from the mouth to the anus, the majority of symptomatic complaints are related to inflammation of the oral mucosa, or mucositis. Almost 40% of patients receiving chemotherapy experience mucositis. In addition, all patients receiving head and neck irradiation will experience this problem to some degree. Symptoms usually begin 5 days to 2 weeks after therapy starts, so preventive oral care should start as soon as therapy does. When selecting interventions such as rinses or coating agents, the available solution, application techniques, and application frequencies should be considered. Medications designed to prevent infection (i.e., antifungals, antivirals) and to minimize pain (Table 3) are added to the basic regimen.

ALOPECIA

Treatment-induced *alopecia* (hair loss) can be a devastating physical and emotional event for the cancer patient. Hair loss is primarily seen in patients receiving certain chemotherapeutic agents, although patients receiving cranial irradiation will experience this problem as well. Alopecia results from the cytotoxic treatment's disruption of the mitotic activity of the hair follicle, which weakens the shaft and causes the hair to break. Scalp hair is primarily affected, although loss of pubic, axillary, and facial hair may also

Table 3. Commonly Used Agents for Oral Application in Mucositis

Indication	Product	Administration	Nursing implications
Cleansing: for tenacious mucus	Hydrogen peroxide	One quarter strength with normal saline. Swish, gargle, and expectorate.	Rinse oral cavity with warm water or saline. Remove mucus with swabs if necessary. Both hydrogen peroxide and sodium bicarbonate may have unpleasant taste. May be flavored with oil of wintergreen as mouthwash.
	Sodium bicarbonate solution	1 teaspoon in 8 oz. water. Swish, swallow, and expectorate.	
Pain and discomfort: local anesthetic for oral/pharyngeal/ esophageal pain	Benzocaine 20%	Apply directly to painful area or wish and swallow.	Comes in a tube for spot application.
	Dyclonine hydrochloride (Dyclone®) 0.5%	15 min before meal; 5–10 ml swish for 2 min, gargle, and discard.	Avoid serving hot food to patients receiving local anesthetics because sensitivity to temperature is diminished.
		Swab on to painful sites prn, using an applicator. 5–10 ml swish and swallow. Onset: 10 min Duration: 1 hr or more.	Contraindicated in patients with compromised swallowing function. Decreases gag reflex.
	Lidocaine (Xylocaine®) viscous 2%	10–15 ml swish and swallow/ discard q 3 hr prn. Duration: 20 min.	Note the longer duration of dyclonine hydrochloride as compared to lidocaine. Note systemic effects of lidocaine in larger doses (cardiovascular depression, CNS depression, or excitation).

Table 3. Commonly Used Agents for Oral Application in Mucositis (Continued)

Indication	Product	Administration	Nursing implications
	Vitamin E capsule	Puncture capsule with a sterile needle and apply contents directly to painful lesions.	Recommended by oncology nurses as promoting healing and reducing pain. No research results available.
5-FU-related stomatitis	Allopurinol mouthwash	5-10 ml, 4 times a day (300 mg/15 ml solution)	Observe for allergic reactions.
Painful oral mucosa: antihistamine to soothe.	Diphenhydramine hydrochloride	5-10 ml swish for 2 min, gargle and discard/swallow prn.	Note that drug also is used to treat motion sickness, allergic reactions (except asthma), extrapyramidal reactions. It may cause sedation, dizziness, and hypotension, especially in older patients.
	Kaolin	Mix 10 ml with pain reliever (above) to coat mucosa and keep pain reliever in place.	
Dry mouth and throat; decreased saliva	Zilastin® remineralizing solution	Apply with swab to affected areas before meals and at bedtime. Duration: 2-4 hrs. As prescribed by producer/pharmacy.	Contains tannic acid and alcohol. Stings initially but results in a white film that protects the area while eating. Speeds healing.
	Artificial salivas (e.g., saliva substitute)	Swish 5-15 ml prn in a clean oral cavity; swallow or discard or apply on painful areas with a swab.	Commercial salivas consist of sorbitol, carboxymethyl cellulose, and a flavoring agent and have no known side effects. Dispenser bottles allow patient to squirt a small amount directly into mouth.

Source: Adapted from *Handbook of Oncology Nursing* (pp. 270-271) by B. L. Johnson and J. Gross, 1985, New York: Delmar Publishers, Inc., and from *Guidelines for Cancer Nursing Practice* (p. 179) by J. C. McNally, J. C. Stair, and E. T. Somerville, 1985, Orlando: Grune & Stratton. Adapted with permission of publisher.

occur. Hair loss usually begins 2 to 3 weeks after the initial treatment, and regrowth occurs within 8 weeks of cessation of therapy. In patients receiving cranial radiation doses >4500 rads, alopecia may be permanent.

When alopecia is anticipated, nurses should prepare patients for the possibility of hair loss and discuss with them the option of purchasing a wig before therapy. Patients vary in their response to hair loss and altered body image. Nurses can assist patients in understanding their feelings and in using a variety of head coverings. The American Cancer Society's program, *Look Good, Feel Better*, is an example of specific assistance available to patients with alopecia.

Scalp tourniquets and scalp hypothermia have been used with limited success in selected chemotherapy patients. These techniques decrease blood supply to the superficial scalp vessels by external compression or by vasoconstriction due to cooling, this, in turn, decreases the amount of toxic chemotherapy that reaches the hair follicles. Malignant cells sequestered in the scalp may be inadequately treated when these interventions are employed, so health care professionals should exercise caution in the use of these interventions for patients with hematologic malignancies or at risk for malignant infiltrates in the scalp.

DYSPNEA

Patients with lung cancer or disease metastatic to the lung frequently develop pulmonary obstructions and restrictions that can cause dyspnea. Factors that cause these problems include: lymphatic spread of tumor, pleural effusion or scarring, loss of functional lung tissue following surgical resection, fibrotic changes due to radiation and pulmonary toxic chemotherapy, pericardial effusion or tamponade, congestive heart failure, anemia, infection, and vascular changes in pulmonary blood supply.

Medical interventions focus on the treatment of the underlying malignancy with chemotherapy, radiation therapy, or surgery. Patients with recurrent pleural effusions will require thoracentesis and possibly instillation of sclerosing agents to prevent reaccumulation of fluid. Antibiotics, diuretics, bronchodilators, steroids, and low-dose narcotics may also be used to alleviate dyspnea. Nurses can also use general measures, such as teaching breathing and relaxation techniques, providing emotional support, positioning to facilitate ventilation, controlling room temperature, and administering oxygen therapy when indicated.

Table 4. Factors Contributing to Fatigue in Cancer Patients

Physiological	Psychological	Situational
Accumulation of toxic waste products secondary to radiation, chemotherapy, or the tumor	Anxiety	Sensory deprivation due to disturbance of sleep pattern
	Depression	
	Anticipatory nausea and vomiting	Immobility
Hypermetabolic state associated with active tumor growth, infection, fever, or surgery	Grief	Crisis
		Problems with relationships
Competition between tumor and the body for nutrients		Drugs—antibiotics, antidepressants, alcohol, nicotine, antianxiety agents, long-acting sleeping agents, analgesics, medications, caffeine
Inadequate intake of nutrients secondary to anorexia, nausea, vomiting, gastric obstruction		Sleep deprivation
Chronic pain		Diagnostic tests
Impairment of aerobic energy metabolism secondary to dyspnea and anemia due to various causes		Loss

Source: From "Fatigue in the Cancer Patient: A Conceptual Approach to a Clinical Problem" by J. Aistairs, 1987, *Oncology Nursing Forum, 14*(6), p 26. Reprinted with permission of Oncology Nursing Society.

PRURITUS

Although pruritus does not occur as frequently as the other symptoms discussed here, it can cause discomfort and impair the integrity of the skin, reducing its effectiveness as a protective barrier. Pruritus can be a secondary symptom of an underlying malignancy, and has been reported primarily in patients with Hodgkin's disease. This symptom may also be a clinical manifestation of a local hypersensitivity reaction to chemotherapy, radiation therapy, antibiotics, or opiates.

Nursing management aims to eliminate stimuli that produce itching and to control the tendency to scratch. Commonly used interventions include: cleansing and moisturizing the skin, avoiding application of irritating lotions and creams, and administering antihistamines and corticosteroids, if indicated. Cool compresses and distraction are other techniques frequently used.

FATIGUE

In oncology patients, fatigue can be a chronic problem resulting from a combination of physical, psychological, and situational factors. Fatigue is frequently one of the presenting signs of malignant disease. Although the exact mechanism of fatigue in this population is unknown, a variety of factors are thought to contribute to its development (Table 4).

Lack of knowledge about fatigue mechanisms has hindered scientific development of appropriate interventions. Treatable physical causes, such as anemia or nutritional deficits, are corrected whenever possible. Working with health professionals, patients can develop an activity/rest program based on assessment of their fatigue patterns that allows them to use their energy most effectively. To promote the patient's adaptation and adjustment to a potentially chronic condition, nurses can evaluate home care needs and recommend support services.

Bibliography

Aistairs, J. (1987). Fatigue in the cancer patient: A conceptual approach to a clinical problem. *Oncology Nursing Forum, 14*(6), 25-30.

Carlson, A. (1985). Infection prophylaxis in the patient with cancer. *Oncology Nursing Forum, 12*(3), 56-64.

Daeffler, R. (1980-81). Oral hygiene measures for patients with cancer [a series of articles]. *Cancer Nursing, 3*, 347-356; *3*, 429-432; *4*, 29-35.

Dangel, R. B. (1986). Pruritus and cancer. *Oncology Nursing Forum, 13*(1), 17-21.

Foote, M., Sexton, D. L., & Pawlik, L. (1986). Dyspnea: A distressing sensation in lung cancer. *Oncology Nursing Forum, 13*(5), 25-31.

Johnson, B. L. & Gross, J. (Eds.). (1985). *Handbook of oncology nursing.* New York and Bethany, CT: John Wiley & Sons and Fleschner Publishing Co.

Nerenz, D. R., Leventhal, H., & Love, R. R. (1982). Factors contributing to emotional distress during cancer chemotherapy. *Cancer, 50*, 1020-1027.

Peterson, D. E., & Sonis, S. T. (1982). Oral complications of cancer chemotherapy: Present status and future studies. *Cancer Treatment Reports, 66*, 1251-1256.

Portenoy, R. (1989). Constipation in the cancer patient: Causes and management. *Medical Clinics of North America, 20*, 801-807.

Triozzi, P. L., & Laszlo, J. (1987). Optimum management of nausea and vomiting in cancer chemotherapy. *Drugs, 34*, 136-149.

Yasko, J. M. (1982). *Care of the client receiving external radiation therapy.* Reston, VA: Reston Publishing Co., Inc.

Yasko, J. M. (1983). *Guidelines for cancer care: Symptom management.* Reston, VA: Reston Publishing Co., Inc.

2 PAIN

Julia Fanslow

INCIDENCE

Approximately 50-80% of patients with advanced cancer experience pain during the course of their disease. The majority of these patients will not obtain satisfactory relief. This fact constitutes a major problem, because unrelieved pain can significantly diminish the patient's quality of life. Among the factors that may contribute to inadequate pain management are the overriding fear of addiction, health care professionals' lack of knowledge about pain medication and new pharmacologic interventions, and lack of confidence in the efficacy of behavioral techniques.

Cancer pain can be acute or chronic. Acute pain generally results from tissue damage and is of limited duration. The physiologic effects (e.g., tachycardia) observed result from stimulation of the autonomic nervous system. Once the cause of the pain has been identified, it can be successfully treated and often completely eradicated. Chronic pain, on the other hand, is persistent, usually greater than 3 months in duration. Because the pathology or cause of the pain cannot be altered, the nervous system eventually adapts and ceases to be hyperactive; the pain may then manifest itself as depression, anxiety, and insomnia.

CAUSES

The severity and prevalence of pain that cancer patients experience depends on many factors, including the site and stage of disease and the location of metastases. Cancer-related pain can result from the disease process or cancer therapy. The most common causes of pain from direct tumor involvement are metastatic bone disease, nerve compression or infiltration, and hollow viscus (e.g., bowel) involvement resulting in obstruction. All of the major treatment modalities may also cause pain syndromes; these are listed in Table 1. Additionally, patients may have pre-existing chronic pain that is not associated with either the disease or its treatment.

Pain affects each person differently, depending upon factors such as age, sex, personality, perception, pain threshold, and past experiences with pain. Psychological factors such as fear, worries, or

Table 1. Sources of Pain Associated with Cancer Treatment

I. Diagnostic procedures
- Lumbar punctures
- Blood samples
- Angiography
- Endoscopy
- Biopsies

II. Surgery
- Acute postoperative pain
- Chronic postoperative pain
  - Mastectomy
  - Radical neck resection
  - Lymphedema
  - Thoracotomy
  - Phantom-limb

III. Chemotherapy
- Acute
  - Gastrointestinal distress
  - Mucositis
  - Myalgia
  - Joint pain
  - Cardiomyopathy
  - Pancreatitis
  - Extravasation
  - Peripheral neuropathy
- Chronic
  - Peripheral neuropathy
  - Steroid pseudorheumatism
  - Aseptic osteonecrosis

IV. Radiation
- Acute
  - Skin burn
  - Gastrointestinal cramping
  - Proctitis
  - Mucositis
  - Itching
- Chronic
  - Osteonecrosis
  - Fibrosis
  - Keratitis
  - Demyelination
  - Pneumonitis
  - Bowel ulceration or obstruction
  - Myelopathy

V. Other Treatments and Treatment Complications

Source: From "Painful Complications of Cancer Diagnosis and Therapy" by C. R. Chapman, J. Kornell, and K. L. Syrjala, 1987. p. 48. In D. McGuire & C. Yarbro (Eds.), *Cancer Pain Management.* Orlando: Grune & Stratton, Adapted with permission of publisher.

knowledge of impending death can also influence the effect of pain. Insomnia, fatigue, and anxiety can lower the pain threshold, while rest, sleep, and diversion can raise it.

PAIN ASSESSMENT

An accurate assessment of the patient's pain experience provides a basis for an evaluation of various pain management techniques. A comprehensive assessment includes information about the following dimensions of pain: location, intensity, factors influencing its occurrence, observed behaviors during pain, psychosocial variables (i.e., attitudes, situational factors), effects of pain, effects of therapy, and patterns of coping. A variety of pain assessment tools have been developed, ranging from simple self-reports about pain intensity to detailed descriptive information (Figure 1). Assessment of chronic pain may be enhanced through the patient's use of a pain diary, in which descriptions of the characteristics of the pain and the effectiveness of management techniques can be recorded. Individual institutions may use a variety of pain assessment tools.

PAIN MANAGEMENT

The goal of pain management is not only relief from pain, but the maintenance of the patient's normal quality of life. All methods of pain management attempt to either control the cause of the pain or alter the patient's perception of it. Currently available methods of managing cancer-related pain are listed in Table 2.

Although pain management techniques are many and varied, therapeutic approaches can be classified as either pharmacologic or nonpharmacologic. Pharmacologic pain control involves the use of analgesics, as well as other medications that either potentiate the analgesics' effects or modify the patient's mood or pain perception. Nonpharmacologic approaches include behavioral techniques, radiation, surgery, neurological and neurosurgical interventions, and traditional nursing measures to promote comfort and evaluate the effectiveness of therapy. Because of the complex nature of cancer-related pain, successful management usually involves combining techniques.

Cancer pain management in the elderly calls for special considerations. Aging patients are at an increased risk for drug reactions, because drug absorption, distribution, metabolism, and elimination change with age, disease status, and medication interactions.

Pharmacologic Management

Health care personnel must aggressively manage acute pain in the cancer patient with medication to return the patient to a pain-

Date _____

Patient's Name _____ Age _____ Room _____

Diagnosis _____ Physician _____

Nurse _____

I. Location: (Patient or nurse mark drawing.)

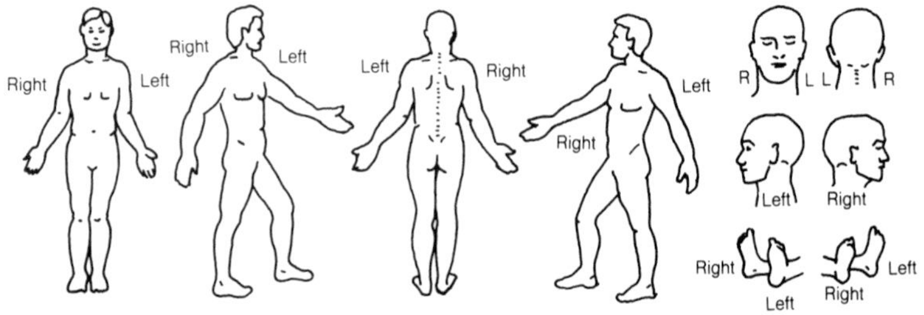

II. Intensity: (Patient rates the pain.) Scale used _____

Present _____

Worst pain gets_____

Best pain gets _____

Acceptable level of pain_____

III. Quality: (Use patient's own words, e.g., prick, ache, burn, throb, pull, sharp.) _____

IV. Onset, duration, variations, rhythms:_____

V. Manner of expressing pain: _____

_____

_____

VI. What relieves the pain? _____

_____

_____

VII. What causes or increases the pain? _____

VIII. Effects of pain: (Note decreased function, decreased quality of life.)

Accompanying symptoms (e.g., nausea) _____

Sleep _____

Appetite _____

Physical activity _____

Relationship with others (e.g., irritability)_____

Emotions (e.g., anger, suicidal, crying) _____

Concentration_____

Other _____

IX. Other comments: _____

X. Plan: _____

Figure 1. An Initial Pain Assessment Tool.
Source: From *Pain: Clinical Manual for Nursing Practice* (p. 21) by M. McCaffery and A. Beebe, 1989, St. Louis, MO: C. V. Mosby. Reprinted with permission of publisher.

Table 2. Existing Methods of Alleviating Cancer-Related Pain

I. Primary Control Methods
  • Therapy directed toward control of the disease process itself
    — Surgery
    — Radiation therapy
    — Chemotherapy (cytotoxic & hormonal agents)
  • Therapy directed toward a specific, disease-related (reversible pathophysiologic) event
    — Infection with antibiotics
    — Inflammation with anti-inflammatory drugs
    — Gout with antihyperuricemic agents
II. Symptomatic Control Methods
  • Systemic analgesics
    — Interference with specific chemical substances involved in pain perception peripherally (anti-inflammatory/antipyretic agents)
    — Interference with conduction of pain away from affected site (local anesthetics)
    — Interference with central nervous system perception of pain and the development of affective responses (narcotic analgesics)
    — Interference with anxiety, tension, or depression (sedative/hypnotics, phenothiazines, tricyclic antidepressants)
  • Surgical procedures on the spinal cord and brain
  • Behavioral techniques

Source: From "Pharmacologic Management of Cancer Pain" by R. Catalano, 1987, p. 155. In D. McGuire & C. Yarbro (Eds.), *Cancer Pain Management.* Orlando: Grune & Stratton. Adapted with permission of publisher.

free state as quickly as possible. Once the pain is relieved, the pain medication is decreased to the lowest dosage or mildest analgesic that will maintain the pain-free state. When the pain cycle is broken, patients can be sustained on minimal amounts of pain medication.

Chronic pain, however, requires very different medication management. For example, a patient with chronic pain is usually started on a non-narcotic analgesic and moves to a narcotic as more effective pain control is needed.

The World Health Organization (1987) states that "analgesic drugs are the mainstay of cancer pain management" and advocates a three-step "analgesic ladder" for decision making. Step one includes use of a non-opioid drug with or without an adjuvant drug (e.g. acetaminophen ± amitriptyline). If pain persists or increases pain management moves to step two, a weak opioid plus a non-opioid, with or without an adjuvant drug (e.g. acetaminophen, codeine, ± carbamazepine). If pain persists or increases, pain management moves to step three, a strong opioid, with or without a non-opioid, with or without an adjuvant drug (e.g. morphine, ± acetaminophen, ± dexamethasone).

Non-narcotic agents are best used for mild cancer pain. This category includes aspirin, acetaminophen, and non-steroidal anti-inflammatory drugs (NSAIDs). Non-narcotic agents may also be used to potentiate the effect of narcotic analgesics in patients with severe pain. However, these agents have a ceiling effect: that is, increasing the dosage beyond a certain point doesn't produce additional pain relief.

Narcotic analgesics (opioids) are used for the treatment of moderate to severe cancer pain. They are categorized as either narcotic agonist or narcotic agonist-antagonist drugs. One theory or model explaining the actions and effects of the opioids, the Multiple Opioid Receptor Theory, proposes that narcotic agonist drugs, such as morphine and codeine, bind with specific opiate receptor sites. There are three kinds of receptor sites, or portions of the nerve cell to which a drug can bind: the *mu* receptor associated with analgesia and respiratory depression; the *kappa* receptor with sedative effects; and the *sigma* receptor with psychomimetic effects.

Although the Multiple Opioid Receptor Theory is still evolving and does not yet completely explain narcotic analgesia, nurses should understand that pure narcotic agonists, such as morphine and codeine, are thought to occupy the *mu* receptor without antagonizing activity at the other receptor sites. Narcotic agonists-antagonists occupy the *kappa* receptor for pain relief while also antagonizing the effects of pure agonists at the *mu* receptor. The three available agonist-antagonists are butorphanol, nalbuphine, and pentazocine. Citations in the bibliography at the end of this chapter are sources of further information. Nurses will find the McCaffery and Beebe book a particularly good resource on the Multiple Opioid Receptor Theory.

Adjuvant analgesic drugs are also used to treat cancer pain. This group includes amphetamines, anticonvulsant agents, phenothiazines, tricyclic antidepressants, steroids, antihistamines, and levodopa. Although their exact mechanisms of action for pain relief are not well understood, these drugs relieve pain when used alone or in combination with other non-narcotics or narcotics.

Pain medication may be given by the following routes: orally, rectally, subcutaneously, intramuscularly, intravenously, intrathecally, and epidurally. Conditions such as thrombocytopenia, neutropenia, and duration of a medication's effect must be taken into account when selecting the route. The peak of a drug's effect is largely dependent on the route of administration. Oral medications usually peak in 2 hours, intramuscular drugs in 1 hour, and intravenous drugs in 15 to 30 minutes. Duration of effect varies widely and should be carefully considered.

The schedule for administering analgesics appears to be an important factor in their effectiveness. Research shows that around-the-clock (ATC) rather than as needed (PRN) administration of analgesics is more effective in the control of chronic pain. In many cases, doses of analgesics may be decreased with ATC scheduling because the pain intensity is consistently less.

Nurses are responsible for knowing the pharmacology of the drugs being given and the expected effects on the patient (Table 3). Using information obtained from pain assessments, nurses also collaborate with physicians to select the most effective medication and route of administration for each patient.

Patients with cancer may be undermedicated for their pain because health care personnel fear that patients will become addicted to narcotics. Although the possibility of becoming psychologically dependent on narcotics may exist for some patients, cancer patients usually develop a tolerance to the effects of opioids rather than an addiction. *Addiction* and *tolerance* are not synonymous terms. Tolerance to narcotics can occur at anytime and requires increasing doses to produce the same level of analgesia. Patients also develop tolerance to the serious side effects of narcotics (e.g., sedation, respiratory depression) at the same rate as tolerance to analgesia, so they can accept larger doses of narcotics without overdosing. In contrast, psychological dependence involves the preoccupation with obtaining and using drugs for non-medical purposes, and can arise in the absence of tolerance.

New Methods of Analgesic Delivery

Like insulin, pain medications can now be administered on a continuous basis into subcutaneous tissue through a small-gauge butterfly needle taped in place.

Patient-controlled analgesia (PCA), also known as demand or self-administered analgesia, now allows patients to manage their pain by allowing them to self-administer their pain medication. Pain medication is delivered through a PCA device similar to an intravenous infusion pump. When patients experience pain, they press a button on the PCA pump, and a preset volume or dose of medication is delivered. The role of this approach in the overall management of cancer related pain is currently being explored.

Narcotics can also be continuously infused epidurally and intrathecally with the placement of an indwelling intrathecal catheter. This technique is associated with fewer central nervous system effects than systematic administration of narcotics. The major problem observed with intraspinal delivery of narcotics is respiratory depression.

Table 3. Duration of Effect of Commonly Used Pain Medication

Medication	Route	Onset	Peak (Hours)	Dose (Mg)	Duration (Hours)
Aspirin	PO	1 hr.	2	600	3
Acetaminophen					
Tylenol®, Datril®,	PO	1 hr.	2	600	3
Tempra®, Nebs®	Rectal	30 min.	1-2	600	3
Codeine	PO	35-45 min.	1-2	200	4
	IM	10-30 min.	30-60 min.	130	
	SC	10-30 min.	30-60 min.		
Hydromorphone HCL					
Dilaudid®	PO	30 min.	30-90 min.	7.5	4
	IM	15 min.	30-90 min.	2-4	4
	SC	10-15 min.	15-30 min.	2-4	2-3
	IV	3-5 min.	10-15 min.	2-4	4
	Rectal	15 min.	30-90 min.	3	
Levorphanol	PO	1 hr.	1½-2	4	4-8
Tartrate	IM	30-60 min.	1	2	
Levo-Dramoran®	SC	30-60	1-1½	2	
	IV	10 min.	20 min.	2	
Meperidine HCL	PO	15 min.	1-1½	300	2-3
Demerol®	IM	10-15 min.	30-50 min.	50-150	
	SC	10-15 min.	5-7 min.	50-150	
	IV	1 min.			
Methadone HCL	PO	30-60 min.	1½-2	20	4-8*
Dolophine®	IM	10-20 min.	1-2	10	4-8*
Westadone®	SC	10-20 min.	1-2	10	4-8*
	IV	10 min.	15-30 min.	10	3-4
Morphine Sulfate	PO	1-1½ hrs.	1-2	60	4-5
Immediate Release	IM	10-30 min.	30-60 min.	10	
	SC	10-30 min.	50-90 min.	10	
	IV	10 min.	20 min.	5	
	Rectal	1-1½ hrs.	1½-2	10	
Sustained Release					
Roxonol®	PO	1-1½ hrs.	60 min.	60	8-12
MS Contin®	PO	1-1½ hrs.	60 min.	15-30	12
Nalbuphine HCL					
Nubain®	IM	15 min.	1	10mg/kg	3-6
	SC	15 min.	1	10mg/kg	3-6
	IV	2-3 min.	30 min.	10mg/kg	3-4
Oxycodone					
Roxicodone®	PO	30 min.	1 hr.	5	3-4
Percodan®	PO	30 min.	1 hr.	4.88	3-4
Percocet®	PO	30 min.	1 hr.	4.88	3-4
Tylox®	PO	30 min.	1 hr.	5	3-4
Oxymorphone HCL					
Numorphan®	IM	10-15 min.	30-90 min.	1-1.5	3-6
	SC	10-20 min.	30-90 min.	1-1.5	3-6
	IV	5-10 min.	15-30 min.	.5-1	3-4
	Rectal	15-30 min.	1½-2	5-10	3-6
Pentazocine	PO	15-30 min.	1-1½	50-180	3
Talwin®	IM	15-20 min.	30-60 min.	30-60	2-3
	SC	15-20 min.	30-60 min.	30-60	2-3
	IV	2-3 min.	15-30 min.	30-60	2-3
Propoxphene HCL					
Darvon®	PO	15-60 min.	2	65	4
Dolene®	PO	15-60 min.	2	65	4
Paragesic®	PO	15-60 min.	2	65	4
Progesic®	PO	15-60 min.	2	65	4
Proxagesic®	PO	15-60 min.	2	65	4
Propoxphene Napsylate					
Darvon N®	PO	15-60 min.	2	100	4

*4 hrs. initially, then 6-8 hrs.

Nonpharmacologic Management

Nonpharmacologic pain management approaches include surgery, radiation, neurological and neurosurgical interventions, behavioral techniques, and nursing interventions.

Both radiation therapy and surgery may be used for cancer patients with enlarging tumors or advanced disease to decrease the tumor mass and reduce painful compression of adjacent structures. These procedures are conducted for palliative purposes only.

Neurosurgical interventions are generally reserved for patients who cannot obtain adequate relief with analgesics, palliative radiotherapy, or surgery. Most neurosurgical procedures involve interruption or destruction of the pain pathway at some point along the route to the brain or in the brain itself. The risks and benefits of these techniques must be thoroughly discussed with patients because, in many cases, the patient will have residual motor or sensory deficits.

Neurostimulation techniques are based on the "gate-control" theory of pain. Some research indicates that the pathways in the spinal cord can accommodate only a certain amount of stimulation before sensory overload occurs. With neurostimulation, competitive nonpainful (e.g., vibratory) impulses are used to block the transmission of painful impulses along nerve pathways. Neurostimulation can be applied transcutaneously (as occurs with transcutaneous electrical nerve stimulation, or TENS) or via surgically implanted electrodes in the spinal cord.

Behavioral techniques such as relaxation, distraction, biofeedback, imagery, and hypnosis are now widely used by nurses to manage cancer-related pain. In general, behavioral techniques are designed to alter the patient's response to pain by fostering deep relaxation and a shifting of attention to something other than the pain. These approaches should be used in combination with, and not as a substitute for, appropriate medications. Nurses should not misinterpret the efficacy of these techniques as an indication that the patient was not really experiencing pain.

Bibliography

Bonica, J. (1988). *Effective pain management for cancer patients.* St. Paul: Pharmacia Deltec Inc.

Carson, B. S. (1987). Neurologic and neurosurgical approaches to cancer pain. In D. McGuire & C. Yarbro (Eds.), *Cancer pain management* (pp. 223–243). Orlando: Grune & Stratton, Inc.

Catalano, R. B. (1987). Pharmacologic management in the treatment of pain. In D. McGuire & C. Yarbro (Eds.), *Cancer pain management* (pp. 151–201). Orlando: Grune & Stratton, Inc.

Cleeland, C. S. (1987). Nonpharmacological management of cancer pain. *Journal of Pain and Symptom Management, 2*, 523-528.

Daut, R. L. & Cleeland, C. S. (1982). The prevalence and severity of pain in cancer. *Cancer, 50*, 1913-1918.

Enck, R. (1988). Pain management: An overview. *The American Journal of Hospice Care, 5*, 17-19.

Foley, K. (1986). The treatment of pain in the patient with cancer. *CA—A Cancer Journal for Clinicians, 36*, 194-215.

McCaffery, M., & Beebe A. (1989). *Pain: Clinical manual for nursing practice.* St. Louis, MO: The C. V. Mosby Co.

McCaffery, J. (1985). *Nursing management of the patient with pain.* Philadelphia: J.B. Lippincott Co.

Spross, J. A., McGuire, D. B., & Schmitt, R. M. (1990). Oncology Nursing Society position paper on cancer pain. *Oncology Nursing Forum*, (Published in three parts) *17*(4), 595-614; 17(5), 751-760; 17(6), 943-955.

Twycross, R. G. (1984). Incidence of pain. In R. G. Twycross (Ed.), *Clinics in oncology; Pain relief in cancer* (pp. 5-16). London: W. B. Saunders.

World Health Organization. (1987). *Cancer Pain Relief.* Geneva, Switzerland: Author.

3 NUTRITIONAL SUPPORT

Karen V. Barale

Malnutrition is a major cause of morbidity and mortality in patients with cancer. It can result from nutritional effects of the cancer itself or from the toxicities of antitumor therapies (surgery, chemotherapy, radiation therapy, and biological therapy). Treatment can cause mild, transient nutritional changes in the patient, such as mucositis from chemotherapy, or may lead to severe, permanent nutritional problems, as is the case with abdominal resection. These problems require ongoing assessment, counseling, and intervention.

NUTRITIONAL EFFECTS OF CANCER

Anorexia, the loss of appetite, is a frequent problem for patients with cancer. Changes in hypothalamic function or in taste, the development of food aversions, early satiety, and the psychological stress of the cancer diagnosis have been suggested as causes of anorexia. Ultimately, they affect the patient's ability to consume enough nutrients to maintain a normal weight.

Cancer *cachexia*, a complex metabolic problem, is seen in the majority of patients with advanced cancer. Cachexia is characterized clinically by anorexia, early satiety, weight loss, electrolyte and water abnormalities, and a progressive weakening of vital functions. The various factors contributing to this problem are shown in Figure 1. The tumor itself is responsible for initiating cachexia; only by controlling the disease can the syndrome be reversed.

The weight loss seen in cachexia is the result of a negative balance between caloric intake and expenditure. However, decreased intake cannot entirely explain the progressive weight loss manifested in patients with cancer. The body's normal response to decreased food intake is the lowering of the basal metabolic rate (BMR). Although rarely seen, some patients with cancer exhibit a significant increase in BMR and total energy expenditure, possibly as a result of tumor growth and host metabolic alterations. However, not all patients with cancer manifest increased energy needs.

Poor utilization of nutrients, another major cause of cancer cachexia, involves altered metabolism of glucose, protein, and fat. Cachectic patients' inability to gain and increase their lean body

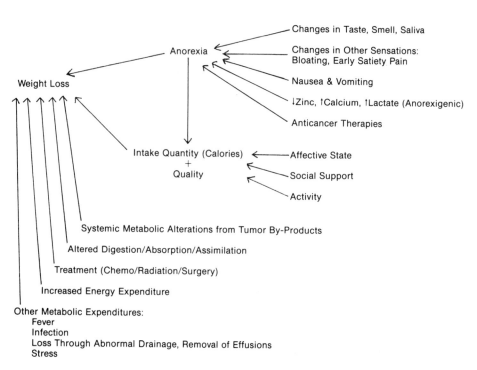

Figure 1. Factors influencing weight loss in cachexia.
Source: From "Cancer cachexia: Effects of the disease and its treatment" by A. M. Lindsey, 1986, *Seminars in Oncology Nursing, 2,* pp. 1929. Reprinted with permission of Grune & Stratton, Inc.

mass despite adequate nutritional support is due partly to these metabolic changes.

The etiology of electrolyte disturbances is usually complex and tumor-specific. Weight loss and increased catabolism cause additional sodium and potassium losses. Gastrointestinal (GI) tract obstruction or increased intracranial pressure from tumor growth can cause vomiting, resulting in fluid and electrolyte losses. Small-bowel fistulas can result in major losses of sodium, bicarbonate, potassium, magnesium, and zinc.

Patients with hepatic or cardiac metastases or obstruction of the urinary, lymphatic, or venous tracts will also have fluid and electrolyte imbalances. Hormone-secreting tumors that impair renal function cause similar changes. For example, small-cell carcinomas of the lung and hypothalamic tumors both result in inappropriate secretion of antidiuretic hormone, water retention, and hyponatremia. The adrenocorticotropic hormone produced by some tumors also causes fluid and electrolyte abnormalities.

Bone destruction or hormonal changes can cause calcium metabolism alterations. Hypocalcemia also occurs as a result of malnutrition; however, when coupled with hypoalbuminemia, the ionized part of the total calcium remains normal. Hypercalcemia is associated with parathyroid tumors, primary tumors of the breast or thyroid that metastasize to the bone, and multiple endocrine adenomatosis (See Unit IV, Chapter 4).

A patient's fluid needs will increase with fever or with any GI disturbance, such as vomiting or diarrhea. Patients with advanced cancer exhibit increased intracellular and extracellular water content. This water retention may partially obscure an actual loss of lean body mass and mislead the observer who uses the patient's weight as an index of nutritional status.

NUTRITIONAL EFFECTS OF TREATMENT

Treatment modalities used to control cancer can have an adverse effect on the already impaired nutritional status of the patient.

Surgery

Radical surgery of the head and neck regions frequently results in impaired mastication and swallowing. Fat malabsorption, gastric stasis secondary to vagotomy, and diarrhea may occur after esophagectomy. In addition to hypoglycemia and malabsorption, dumping syndrome is common following partial gastrectomy and gastrojejunostomy. *Dumping syndrome* is a complex reaction, probably due to an excessive, rapid emptying of the contents of the GI tract. Symptoms include nausea, weakness, sweating, palpitation, varying degrees of syncope, often a sensation of warmth, and sometimes diarrhea, occurring after the ingestion of food. Patients with this syndrome require careful nutritional management to prevent chronic deficiencies of iron, calcium, and the fat-soluble vitamins.

Patients generally experience substantial sodium and water losses immediately after ileostomy. The losses usually decrease within 7 to 20 days, approaching the range seen in otherwise healthy individuals on stable diets. Patients who have had massive small bowel resection (leaving a functional small bowel of 3 feet or less) have serious long-term problems with maintenance of adequate nutrition.

Total pancreatectomy and the resulting absence of pancreatic digestive enzymes lead to diabetes mellitus, as well as malabsorption of fats, proteins, fat-soluble vitamins, and minerals. Nutritional problems resulting from radical surgeries are shown in Table 1.

Radiation

One type of radiation treatment that often compromises nutrition is radiation to the head and neck. Radiation injury to the salivary glands, oral mucosa, oral musculature, and alveolar bone manifests as *xerostomia* (mouth dryness), loss of taste ("mouth blindness"), dental caries, mucositis, osteoradionecrosis, oral infection, and production of thick, viscous saliva. The consistency of food should be adjusted for patients with viscous mucus to facilitate swallowing. When swallowing is impossible, total parenteral nutrition or tube feeding may be necessary. Residual mucous often settles into the throat and sinuses, causing nausea. Additional effects, including mouth sores, dysphagia, or nausea and vomiting may make eating painful or unpleasant, exacerbating anorexia. Radiation damage to the esophagopharyngeal area may also lead to reduced oral intake, dysphagia, and *odynophagia*, or painful swallowing.

The small-bowel epithelium is very sensitive to radiation. Changes in intestinal function as a result of pelvic or abdominal radiotherapy include radiation induced enterocolitis, diarrhea, stricture formation, and fistulas. Symptoms of this damage, such as abdominal pain, nausea, vomiting, and malabsorption, threaten adequate oral intake and nutritional status.

Chemotherapy

Most of chemotherapy's effects upon nutrition are the result of interference in normal cellular activities. The effects produced depend on the type of drug, dosage, duration of treatment, rates of excretion, and individual susceptibility. Among the most common effects of chemotherapy are diarrhea, nausea, and vomiting. Diarrhea and vomiting can lead to fluid and electrolyte imbalances and, if prolonged, dehydration and metabolic alkalosis. Persistent vomiting or diarrhea mandate nutritional intervention. Other common alimentary tract problems caused by chemotherapeutic agents include altered taste and smell, mucositis, stomatitis, and constipation.

Table 1. Nutritional Consequences of "Radical" Resection

Organs Resected	Nutritional Sequelae
Oral cavity and pharynx	Dependency on tube feedings
Thoracic esophagus	Gastric stasis (secondary to vagotomy)
	Fat malabsorption
	Gastrostomy feedings in patients without reconstruction
Stomach	Dumping syndrome
	Fat absorption
	Anemia
Small intestine	
Duodenum	Pancreatobiliary deficiency with fat malabsorption
Jejunum	Decrease in efficiency of absorption (general)
Ileum	Vitamin B_{12} malabsorption and bile salt absorption
Massive (>75%)	Fat malabsorption and diarrhea; vitamin B_{12} malabsorption; gastric hypersecretion
Colon (total or subtotal)	Water and electrolyte loss

Source: From "Nutritional consequences of surgical resection of the gastrointestinal tract for cancer" by W. Lawrence, Jr., 1977, Cancer Research, 37, pp. 2379–2386. Reprinted with permission of Cancer Research, Inc.

DEVELOPMENT OF THE CARE PLAN

Protein malnutrition is frequently seen in hospitalized patients with cancer. This can interfere with the response to treatment and affect the patient's overall quality of life. The goals of nutritional care of these patients are to prevent or correct nutritional deficiencies and minimize weight loss.

The first step in planning nutritional care of the patient is an assessment of nutritional status. Although the assessment may consider several factors, it is performed primarily to determine the degree to which the patient's need for nutrients is being met by his or her food intake. Table 2 outlines the components of the nutritional assessment. This assessment serves as the basis for a care plan that includes monitoring, evaluation, and education.

Optimally, the dietitian reviews information from the patient's chart and conducts the full assessment. However when available dietitian services are limited, nurses should draw upon their own knowledge of nutrition to collect and review patient data and identify those patients at a high risk for nutritional problems. Nurses can then arrange consultations between the dietitian and these high-risk patients.

Table 2. Components of The Nutritional Assessment.

Medical History	Physical Examination
Duration and type of malignancy Frequency, type, and severity of complications (infections, draining lesions, etc.) Type and duration of therapy Specific chemotherapeutic agents used Radiation sites Antibiotics used Other drugs used Surgical procedures performed (site, type, date) Side effects of therapy (diarrhea, anorexia, nausea and vomiting) Concomitant medical conditions (diabetes, heart disease, liver failure, kidney failure, infection)	General appearance Condition of hair Condition of skin Condition of teeth Condition of mouth, gums, and throat Edema Performance status Identification of nutritionally related problems (fistula, pain, stomatitis, xerostomia, infection, constipation, diarrhea, nausea and vomiting, obstruction)

Dietary History	Socioeconomic History
24-hour recall of foods eaten, including snacks Composition of food taken in 24 hours (calories and protein, caffeine, liquor) Time of day meals and snacks eaten Past or current diet modifications Self-feeding ability Special cancer diet Vitamins, minerals, or other supplements Modifications of diet or eating habits as a result of treatment or illness Foods withheld or given on the basis of personal or religious grounds (kosher, vegetarian, etc.) Food preferences Food allergies or intolerances	Number of persons living in the home (ages and relationships) Kitchen facilities Income Food purchased by Food prepared by Amount spent on food per month Outside provision of meals

Anthropometric Data	Biochemical Data
Height Weight Actual weight as percentage of ideal Weight change as percentage of usual Triceps skinfold measurement Actual triceps skinfold as percentage of standard Midarm circumference Midarm muscle circumference Actual midarm muscle circumference as percentage of standard	Hematocrit Hemoglobin Serum albumin Total iron-binding capacity or serum transferrin Creatinine Creatinine height index Total lymphocytes Delayed hypersensitivity response—skin testing Nitrogen balance Blood urea nitrogen Sodium, potassium, carbon dioxide, chloride Glucose

Source: From *Cancer nursing: Principles and practice.* (p. 157) by S. L. Groenwald (Ed.), 1987. Boston: Jones & Bartlett Publishing Co. Reprinted with permission of publisher.

NUTRITIONAL INTERVENTION AND COUNSELING

Whenever possible, the GI tract should be used for feeding the patient. Table 3 lists several suggestions for increasing oral intake of regular foods; there are also many medical nutritional products that can be used to augment reduced food intake. These products are usually high-calorie and/or high-protein liquid preparations that can supplement regular meals, be taken between meals, or serve as meal replacements. In addition, protein-fortified drinks or double-strength milk (one-quarter to one-third cup non-fat dry milk mixed with one cup fluid milk, served cold) can add protein and calories to the diet.

It is not unusual for patients to develop *lactase deficiency* following chemotherapy or abdominal radiation. Symptoms may include bloating, cramping, or gas 1 to 3 hours after eating milk products. Restricting milk products eliminates an excellent source of calories and protein. These patients may benefit from the use of Lactaid® (Lactaid, Inc., Pleasantville, NJ), an enzyme added to milk to break down the lactose or lactose-reduced dairy products.

Printed resources, such as cookbooks and guides to increasing intake, are available through the American Cancer Society or the National Cancer Institute. They can be helpful for patients attempting to increase their oral intake. These guides provide variety and ideas for patients or family members preparing foods.

ENTERAL AND PARENTERAL FEEDING

Patients unable to eat adequately for extended periods may benefit from enteral or parenteral feedings. The general rule of thumb is if the gut works, use it.

Enteral Feeding

Formula characteristics and the patient's medical status must be reviewed before choosing an enteral formula. Formula characteristics to be considered include digestibility of nutrients, osmolality, viscosity, nutritional completeness, ease of use, and cost. Formula osmolality and rate of delivery are major factors in the patient's tolerance of the tube-feeding. A decision tree for determining the type of feeding is shown in Figure 2.

Formula types fall into four major categories. Complete products are essentially meal replacements that require digestion and a relatively intact capacity for intestinal nutrient absorption. Chemically defined products require minimal or no enzymatic activity prior to absorption and are designed specifically for patients with digestion problems or severe malabsorption. These products are indicated

Table 3. Symptom-Specific Nutrition Plans for Patients With Cancer

Symptom	Etiologies	Nutrition Plan
Anorexia	Radiation; chemotherapy; metabolic or psychologic problems associated with chronic disease	• Offer small, frequent, high caloric-density feedings. • Adjust meal size to appetite. • Enhance or minimize food odors. • Create a relaxed, pleasant eating atmosphere. • Suggest small amounts of alcohol before meals.
Alterations in taste/ smell	Radiation; chemotherapy; metabolic problems; medications	• Avoid offensive foods. • Experiment with seasonings and food combinations. • Enhance or minimize food odors. • Serve foods at room temperature.
Mouth dryness	Radiation; chemotherapy; medications	• Puree or liquefy foods. • Use artificial salivas. • Add sauces, gravies, and juices. • Serve liquids with meals. • Experiment with food temperature.
Dysphagia/odynophagia (painful swallowing)	Radiation; chemotherapy	• Modify foods to a soft consistency. • Avoid highly seasoned, spiced, or acidic foods. • Adjust food temperature to tolerance.
Early satiety	Surgery; anorexia; tumor involvement	• Offer small, frequent, high caloric-density feedings. • Limit liquids with meals. • Minimize intake of low caloric-density foods and liquids. • Exercise between meals.
Nausea/vomiting	Multifactorial	• Eat dry, bland foods (e.g. crackers, toast) before meals. • Avoid offensive foods. • Minimize food odors. • Shorten food preparation time. • Consume larger portions when nausea subsides. • Eat bland, easy-to digest meals several hours before treatment. • Eat and drink slowly. • Identify best-tolerated foods; avoid poorly tolerated foods, such as fatty, spicy, overly sweet, or strongly flavored foods.
Stomatitis/mucositis (mouth sores)	Radiation; chemotherapy	• Avoid acidic, salty, or spicy foods.
Diarrhea	Surgery; chemotherapy; radiation; tumor involvement; medications; bacterial infection; malabsorption	• Use low-residue diet during acute phase. • Increase fluid consumption. • Increase potassium intake. • Avoid gas-producing foods and beverages. • Adjust lactose intake to level of tolerance; eliminate it if necessary.
Constipation	Chemotherapy; medications; low-residue diet; inadequate intake	• Increase residue as tolerated. • Increase fluid consumption.

Source: From *Dietary Modifications in Disease* (p. 15), 1983, Columbus, OH: Ross Laboratories, Reprinted with permission of Ross Laboratories.

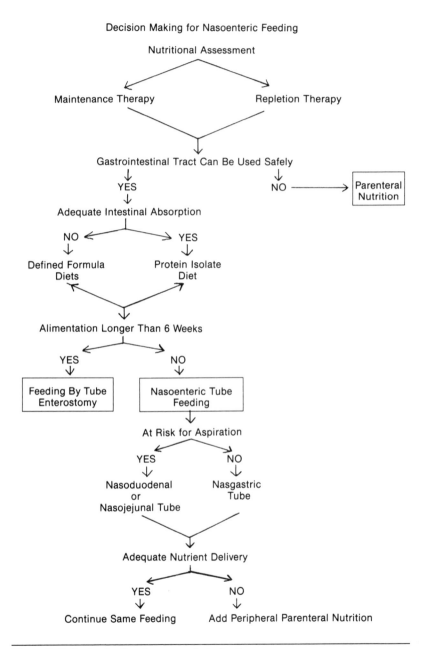

Figure 2. Patient selection for nasoenteric feeding.
Source: From *Enteral and Tube Feeding.* (p. 263) by J. Rombeau and M. Caldwell (eds.), 1983. Philadelphia: W. B. Saunders Company. Reprinted with permission of publisher.

```
┌─────────────────────────────────────────────┐
│  Non-functional GI tract                     │
│    obstruction                               │
│    ileus                                     │
│    bowel resection                           │
│    stomatitis                                │
│    dysphagia treatment                       │
│                                              │
│  Therapeutic Bowel Rest                      │
│    fistulas                                  │
│    radiation, chemotherapy enteritis         │
│                                              │
│  Head and neck surgery                       │
│                                              │
│  Prolonged unconsciousness                   │
│                                              │
│  Hypermetabolism                             │
│    fever, infection                          │
│    major surgery                             │
│                                              │
│  Malnutrition                                │
│    malabsorption                             │
│    need for rapid repletion                  │
└─────────────────────────────────────────────┘
```

Figure 3. Indications for total parenteral nutrition.

for patients with pancreatic cancer who have pancreatic exocrine insufficiency. These products may also reduce intestinal damage caused by some chemotherapeutic agents or abdominal radiation. Modular products may be combined to form an individualized feeding solution or used in conjunction with other tube feeding products to boost calorie or protein intake. Specialty products are designed for patients with hepatic or renal failure or trauma. These products vary considerably in terms of the specific amino acid, carbohydrate, and fat content and are used to tailor nutrient intake to the metabolic abnormalities that accompany major stress or organ failures.

Parenteral Nutrition

Parenteral nutrition is defined as the intravascular administration of macronutrients, vitamins, minerals, and trace elements, either peripherally or through a central line. The patient who cannot be sustained by the oral route and is not a candidate for tube feeding may benefit from this alternate support. This technique is referred to as *total parenteral nutrition* (TPN), *hyperalimentation,* or *intravenous hyperalimentation.* Either partial or total nutritional support may be provided. Indications for TPN are listed in Figure 3.

Dextrose and amino acid solutions should be infused daily. Fat emulsions should be used at least twice a week to provide essential fatty acids. Most patient care settings have developed policies and procedures for parenteral nutrition.

Bibliography

Coulston, A. M., & Darbinian, J. A. (1986). Nutrition management of patients with cancer. *Topics in Clinical Nutrition, 1,* 26-36.

Curtas, S., Chapman, G., & Meguid, M. M. (1989). Evaluation of nutritional status. *Nursing Clinics of North America, 24*(2), 301-313.

Grant, M. M. (1986). Nutritional interventions: Increasing oral intake. *Seminars in Oncology Nursing, 2*(1), 36-43.

Groenwald, S. L. (1987). Nutritional disorders. In S. L. Groenwald (Ed.), *Cancer nursing: Principles and practice* (pp. 141-170) Boston: Jones and Bartlett Publishers, Inc.

Irwin, M. M. (1986). Enteral and parenteral nutrition support. *Seminars in Oncology Nursing, 2*(1), 44-54.

Kern, K. A. & Norton, J. A. (1988). Cancer cachexia. *Journal of Parenteral and Enteral Nutrition, 12,* 286-298.

Kokal, W. A. (1985). The impact of antitumor therapy on nutrition. *Cancer* (Supplement), *55,* 273-278.

4 ONCOLOGIC EMERGENCIES

Brenda Nevidjon

People with cancer can be subject to life-threatening medical emergencies caused by complications of the disease itself or its treatments. These emergencies can be the initial manifestation of a malignancy or occur late in the course of disease. Nurses who know which patients are at risk for oncologic emergencies can promote early detection and treatment of these complications. Early intervention decreases associated morbidity and may help the patient regain functional status. In all oncologic complications, treatment of the underlying cause is crucial in preventing recurrence of the syndrome.

GENERAL NURSING CONSIDERATIONS

Nursing intervention for patients with oncologic emergencies should include careful periodic assessment of changes in the patient's status, administration of treatments, education, and emotional support. The assessments made and physical care delivered will vary with the type of emergency. If the oncologic complication is the first manifestation of disease, the patient's anxiety about symptoms of the emergency condition may be compounded by the shock of the new diagnosis of cancer. The nurse needs to provide information as well as emotional support during this period, because the patient and family will want to know about the disease and treatments once the emergency is resolved. Nurses caring for people with cancer can identify populations at risk for developing these complications, participate in early detection, and collaborate in the management once the emergency has been diagnosed.

SUPERIOR VENA CAVA SYNDROME

Superior vena cava syndrome (SVCS) is caused by the obstruction of venous drainage in the upper thorax. The superior vena cava is particularly vulnerable to obstruction because of its thin walls, low venous pressure, and anatomic location. It is surrounded by lymph nodes and enclosed in a rigid compartment formed by the mediastinum, sternum, and right mainstem bronchus. Enlarged lymph nodes or local tumor extension can compress and obstruct the vena cava extrinsically. Blood flow can also be blocked by direct invasion of the tumor into the lumen of the vessel.

Patients commonly present with shortness of breath, facial edema, swelling of the trunk and upper extremities, and less frequently with chest pain, cough, and dysphagia. Physical examination may reveal thoracic and neck vein distention, tachypnea, conjunctival edema, and central nervous system (CNS) manifestations such as headache, visual disturbances, and altered levels of consciousness.

Radiation and/or chemotherapy are the most common treatments for SVCS. Treatment selection is based on the history and size of the tumor, its responsiveness to treatment, and any prior treatment the patient may have received. Radiation therapy is usually the best method of reducing the size of a tumor. Lymphomas are more radiosensitive than carcinomas; in these cases symptomatic relief can usually be attained 3 to 4 days after the start of radiation therapy, with objective improvement occurring in 7 to 14 days.

Chemotherapy is generally used with radiation to treat tumors sensitive to antineoplastic agents. Chemotherapy is administered first to reduce the tumor and limit the normal lung tissue exposed to radiation. Occasionally chemotherapy may be used alone against tumors that are extremely sensitive to the effects of cytotoxic drugs or when the mediastinal tissues have already been irradiated the highest level the tissue can tolerate. SVCS secondary to small cell lung cancers, for example, is frequently managed in this way.

Steroids, diuretics, and anticoagulants may be used adjunctively to decrease local inflammation and edema and prevent formation of intraluminal thrombosis.

Nursing management of acute SVCS includes: maintaining airway patency, monitoring fluid and electrolyte balance, and monitoring vital signs and level of consciousness. Patients should be observed for respiratory stridor. Changes in mental status should be noted immediately, as they may indicate progressive CNS involvement. Nurses should avoid accessing veins of the involved extremity(ies) because of the potential for venous stasis, phlebitis, and thrombosis.

SPINAL CORD COMPRESSION

Spinal cord compression (SCC) can be caused by direct pressure on the spinal cord, compromise of the vascular supply to the area resulting in spinal cord infarct, or vertebral collapse. Approximately 5-10% of people with metastatic disease develop spinal cord compression.

Successful treatment of SCC depends on early diagnosis and treatment. The nervous system can be permanently damaged unless therapy is begun immediately.

Signs of SCC include progressive back pain, weakness, motor deficits, autonomic dysfunction, and sensory impairment. More than 90% of patients with SCC experience back pain, which may be localized or radicular and precede other symptoms by several months. Because of the nonspecific nature of this complaint, health care personnel should have a high index of suspicion for SCC in patients with a history of malignancy.

The majority of patients experience weakness in the lower extremities by the time SCC is diagnosed. Approximately one-half of patients will also exhibit sensory and autonomic dysfunction at diagnosis. Sensory deficits include numbness and paresthesias; autonomic dysfunction is generally associated with a poorer prognosis. Bladder dysfunction begins with hesitancy and incomplete voiding and progresses to urinary retention. Constipation is an early indication of bowel problems, and sphincter control may be lost as the cord compression worsens. SCC can also affect sexual function.

Patients with SCC symptoms require further evaluation. A myelogram can confirm the diagnosis of SCC and determine its precise location. Computerized tomography (CT) scanning can provide useful information if myelography cannot be performed or is contraindicated.

The choice of treatment is dictated by the type and location of the tumor, rapidity of symptom onset, and the patient's overall prognosis. Recent research has provided evidence that radiation therapy is the best treatment for SCC because response rates are equivalent to those with surgery, but with less morbidity. Radiation treatments are begun as soon as the diagnosis is confirmed, because delaying treatment can result in irreversible neurological deficits. Steroids are administered concomitantly to reduce local edema and improve neurological function.

Surgical decompression, which includes partial resection of the tumor and laminectomy, is performed less frequently. It is used primarily for patients with rapidly progressing dysfunction, radio-resistant tumors, or for those who have had previous maximal radiation to the involved area. Laminectomy is associated with significant morbidity and may actually aggravate the neurological deficit. Some residual tumor may remain after surgery, so radiation is generally administered to prevent tumor regrowth and optimize the restoration of neurological function.

After surgery, nurses should monitor the restoration of neurological function, provide comfort measures, and ensure hygiene. Because the spine is unstable, a log-rolling method is used to move the patient and a back brace may be ordered. If radiation is given postoperatively, the incision line should be carefully assessed before any postoperative radiation is administered because radiation impairs healing. Patients receiving treatment to the thoracic spine may experience dysphagia; topical anesthetics and dietary modifications may be helpful in this situation.

HYPERCALCEMIA

Patients with bone metastases from solid tumors are those most likely to have *hypercalcemia*. Infiltrating tumors destroy bone tissue, accelerating bone resorption and the release of large amounts of calcium. Certain hematologic malignancies involve the bone as well. Widespread osteolytic lesions occur with multiple myeloma and other plasma cell malignancies, causing hypercalcemia.

Since malignant cells are often undifferentiated and lack regulatory controls, they sometimes produce hormone-like substances. Ectopic production of parathyroid hormone (PTH) or PTH-like substances, vitamin D-like substances, or osteoclastic activation factor leads to increased serum calcium. Other factors that may contribute to hypercalcemia in this population are dehydration and immobilization.

Hypercalcemia can cause gastrointestinal, cardiac, and renal dysfunction. The clinical manifestations will vary and are usually proportional to the degree of hypercalcemia and the rate of its development (Table 1).

The goal of medical management is to reduce calcium resorption from bone and increase renal excretion of calcium. Primary treatment usually includes vigorous hydration using normal saline to restore fluid volume and increase glomerular filtration. Diuretics such as furosemide are given during hydration to promote renal excretion of calcium; however, thiazide diuretics are not recommended because they depress calcium excretion. Mithramycin, an antineoplastic agent that lowers calcium by inhibiting PTH, may be administered for severe hypercalcemia. It must be used with caution because of its effects on platelets, and renal and liver function. Other agents that caregivers may use to control hypercalcemia are glucocorticoids, oral phosphates, and calcitonin.

Nursing interventions include identification of patients at risk for developing hypercalcemia, evaluation of changes in hypercalcemia-related symptoms, administration of medical therapy, and monitoring treatment side effects. Although encouraging mobilization to promote weight-bearing can help prevent further long bone demineralization, patients with bone involvement of any weight bearing area are at risk for developing pathological fractures and may need to modify physical activity. Because hypercalcemia can occur, the nurse should instruct the patient and family about its signs and symptoms (Table 1).

Table 1. Symptoms of Hypercalcemia

System	Mechanism	Signs and Symptoms
Gastroin-testinal	Depressed smooth muscle contractility causes delayed gastric emptying and decreased intestinal motility	Early: nausea, vomiting, anorexia, constipation Late: obstipation and ileus; weight loss
Neuro-muscular	Depressed excitability of neurons	Early: lethargy, drowsiness; restlessness, mood changes Mild: mental status changes, poor calculation, decreased attention span, somnolence Late: psychotic behavior, marked confusion, slurred speech, stupor, coma
	Impaired electrical conduction and cell membrane permeability in skeletal muscles	Early: muscle weakness, fatigue Late: profound muscle weakness, hypotonia
	? PGE-mediated bone resorption	Bone pain
Renal	Interference with action of ADH on renal collecting tubules → inability to concentrate urine and then volume contraction followed by ↓ GFR	Early: polyuria Mild: polydipsia Late: prerenal azotemia
Cardio-vascular	Impaired electrical conduction and cell membrane permeability, altered intracellular metabolism; arterial vasoconstriction	Early: hypertension Mild: sinus bradycardia, prolonged PR interval, shortened QT interval, dysrhythmias especially in digitalized patients Late: Prolonged QT interval due to widened T wave, coving of ST segment, AV block, asystole.

Source: From "Hypercalcemia" by J. M. Lang-Kummer, 1990, p. 528. S. L. Groenwald, M. H. Frogge, M. Goodman, and C. H. Yarbro (Eds.), *Cancer Nursing: Principles and Practice* (2nd Edition), Boston, MA: Jones and Bartlett. Reprinted with permission of the publisher.

PERICARDIAL EFFUSION/CARDIAC TAMPONADE

Infiltration of the pericardium causes inflammation, resulting in increased production of pericardial fluid. Accumulation of fluid in the pericardial sac interferes with diastolic filling and reduces stroke volume.

Tamponade occurs when the amount and pressure of the pericardial fluid obstruct the flow of blood into the ventricle. When this condition develops gradually, the pericardium can compensate by stretching to maintain cardiac output; in this situation, large (> 1 liter) effusions can accumulate before patients become severely symptomatic. With rapidly developing effusions, however, the pericardium cannot compensate, and much smaller volumes of fluid can impair normal cardiac output. Tumor involvement and radiation side effects can also cause the pericardium to become fibrotic, leading to constrictive pericarditis. If constriction is severe, tamponade can occur without fluid accumulation.

Early symptoms are nonspecific and include dyspnea, cough, hepatomegaly, pain, orthopnea, cyanosis, venous distention, and leg edema. As cardiac function is further compromised, signs of ventricular failure are apparent: hypotension with cold, clammy skin; decrease in pulse pressure; thready pulse; and distended neck veins. As the pericardium becomes less able to compensate, blood pressure measurements will reveal increasing pulsus paradoxus, a pulse that decreases markedly in volume with inspiration.

Pericardial effusion can be confirmed by an echocardiogram; pericardiocentesis should be performed in critical cases of cardiac compromise. Unless the original cause of the effusion is treated, the fluid will reaccumulate. In many cases, sclerosing agents may be instilled to eliminate the pericardial space and prevent reaccumulation of fluid. Other surgical interventions to manage recurrent pericardial effusions include placement of an indwelling catheter, placement of pericardial windows, or pericardiectomy.

DISSEMINATED INTRAVASCULAR COAGULATION

Disseminated intravascular coagulation (DIC) is a hematologic disorder characterized by rapid formation of fibrin clots in the microcirculation, consumption of clotting factors, and stimulation of fibrinolysis, or clot degradation. The diffuse nature of this process renders the body unable to respond to tissue or vascular injury with stable clot formation, resulting in hemorrhages in the skin, mucosa, and internal organs.

Although DIC is frequently diagnosed based on laboratory findings alone, many patients will have evidence of hemorrhage. This can manifest itself as frank bleeding from any body orifice. Patients may also exhibit petechiae, ecchymosis, oozing from injection and surgical sites, hypotension, tachycardia, and confusion.

Heparin administration is the primary treatment for DIC because it inhibits thrombin activity. It is generally given by continuous infusion until DIC is controlled, but identification and treatment of the underlying cause are crucial to preventing recurrence. Concurrent administration of platelets, packed red blood cells, fresh frozen plasma, and cryoprecipitate helps to achieve hemostasis until the underlying coagulopathy is corrected.

SYNDROME OF INAPPROPRIATE ANTIDIURETIC HORMONE

The *syndrome of inappropriate antidiuretic hormone* (SIADH) is caused by release of excessive antidiuretic hormone (ADH) from the posterior pituitary gland. ADH modifies the permeability of the distal collecting tubules in the kidney, causing water retention and greater urinary sodium excretion. Normally, it is released in response to plasma volume and extracellular osmolarity. The most common disease-related cause of SIADH is the ectopic production of ADH by tumor cells. Infections, tumors, and other disorders of the central nervous system can also cause SIADH by directly stimulating the hypothalmus and posterior pituitary. Both cyclophosphamide and vincristine have also been associated with the SIADH development.

Patients present with weight gain without edema; anorexia; nausea; vomiting; and CNS manifestations of hyponatremia such as weakness, lethargy, irritability, and confusion. In severe hyponatremia, seizures and coma can occur.

Restricting fluids to 500-1000 cc a day corrects the hyponatremia in mild to moderate cases. For patients with more severe symptoms of water intoxication, administration of hypertonic saline and furosemide will rapidly correct the fluid and electrolyte imbalance. Demeclocycline, which blocks the renal tubule response to ADH, may be used to manage chronic SIADH.

SEPTIC SHOCK

Oncology patients whose immune systems are suppressed by the disease itself or by treatment toxic to the bone marrow are at a greater risk for life-threatening infections. Although gram negative bacteria are the most common causative organisms, gram positive, fungal, parasitic, and viral infections are not unusual. Pathogenic endotoxin produced by gram negative bacteria causes local damage to the endothelial lining of capillaries and activates clotting factors and the complement system. These mechanisms, in turn, trigger vasodilation and blood pooling in peripheral vascular beds. Subsequent reduction of the circulating blood volume leads to inadequate tissue perfusion and shock.

Fever is an early sign of infection and, because there are insufficient white blood cells for an adequate immune response, it may be the only indication of infection. Early symptoms of impending shock are irritability, confusion, chills, tachycardia, tachypnea, weak peripheral pulses, glycosuria, excessive thirst, nausea, warm dry skin, and hypotension. As shock progresses other symptoms can appear, including cool, dry skin which becomes cold and clammy; peripheral edema; oliguria; and further deterioration of neurological, respiratory, and cardiac function.

Early detection and management of septic shock afford the patient the best chance of reversing this disorder. Most febrile, neutropenic patients will already be receiving prophylactic antibiotic therapy; untreated patients should be started on this therapy immediately if any signs of impending shock are present. Medical management of septic shock generally includes use of vasoactive drugs to maintain cardiac output, administration of plasma expanders, respiratory support, management of metabolic acidosis associated with sepsis, and administration of high-dose steroids and antipyretics.

TUMOR LYSIS SYNDROME

When patients with rapidly dividing tumors receive cytotoxic chemotherapy, large numbers of tumor cell membranes rupture, releasing the intracellular contents into the bloodstream. This causes *tumor lysis syndrome* (TLS) characterized by elevated levels of uric acid, potassium, and phosphate, decreased levels of calcium, and other severe metabolic abnormalities.

The combination of hyperuricemia and severe electrolyte disturbances can ultimately cause renal failure and cardiac arrest. Urate crystals precipitate in and eventually obstruct the renal tubules. This is called uric acid nephropathy.

Patients at increased risk for developing TLS should be identified before the initiation of therapy. This group includes patients with high-grade lymphomas and large tumor burdens, and patients with high white blood cell counts, lymphadenopathy, and splenomegaly. Electrolytes, uric acid, and renal function should be measured before treatment is started, and should be closely monitored during therapy.

High-risk patients will generally be vigorously hydrated to decrease the concentration of uric acid in the urine. Because uric acid is more soluble and less likely to precipitate in alkaline urine, sodium bicarbonate is added to IV fluids. Diuretics are administered along with hydration measures to promote excretion of potassium and phosphate. Allopurinol, a drug that decreases uric acid levels by interfering with purine metabolism, is routinely used prophylactically in high-risk patients.

Acute tumor lysis generally resolves within 4 to 7 days after treatment is initiated, as long as renal function has been preserved and electrolyte abnormalities have been corrected.

Bibliography

Barry, S. (1989). Septic shock: Special needs of patients with cancer. *Oncology Nursing Forum, 16*(1), 23–27.

Harnett, S. (1989). Septic shock in the oncology patient. *Cancer Nursing, 12*(4), 191–201.

Hughes, C. (1986). Hypercalcemia of malignancy: Nursing responsibilities. *NITA, 9*(4), 191–201.

Lang-Kummer, J. M. (1990). Hypercalcemia. In S. L. Groenwald, M. H. Frogge, M. Goodman, & C. H. Yarbro (Eds.), *Cancer nursing: Principles and practice* (2nd edition) (p. 528). Boston, MA: Jones and Bartlett Publishers.

Poe, C., & Radford, A. (1985). The challenge of hypercalcemia in cancer. *Oncology Nursing Forum, 12*(6), 29-34.

Poe, C., & Taylor, L. (1989). Syndrome of inappropriate antidiuretic hormone: Assessment and nursing implications. *Oncology Nursing Forum, 16*(3), 373-381.

Spiegel, R. (1983). Emergencies cancer patients are heir to. *Emergency Medicine, 15*(3), 73-93.

Valentine, A. S., & Stewart, J. (1983). Oncologic emergencies. *American Journal of Nursing, 83*(9), 1282-1285.

Wilkowski, J. (1986). Spinal cord compression: An oncologic emergency. *Journal of Emergency Nursing, 12*(11), 9-12.

Wood, H. (Guest Ed.). (1985). Acute complications of cancer. *Seminars in Oncology Nursing, 1*(4), entire issue.

5 CANCER AND SEXUALITY

Terry Chamorro

Sexuality is a complex phenomenon involving emotional and social factors as well as biologic function. It is a component of everyone's character, regardless of age, gender, or culture. Health care providers often neglect or disregard changes in sexuality resulting from cancer and its treatment because they perceive that concerns about cancer treatment or the threat of death overshadow sexuality issues. Unfortunately, without appropriate counseling, sexual dysfunction can disturb relationships between patients and their partners, thereby compounding other problems experienced by the person living with cancer.

ALTERATIONS IN SEXUALITY RELATED TO CANCER

The loss of functional sex organs is not the only cause of sexual dysfunction in the cancer patient; concerns about appearance and changes in self-concept are also powerful negative influences. In addition, cancer treatment may cause a variety of complications that can interfere with any phase in the sexual response cycle: desire, excitement, orgasm, and resolution or return to the unexcited state (Tables 1 and 2). Relations that are compromised before diagnosis will be further stressed by the physical and emotional impact of planned treatment.

Changes in sexual function may occur before the underlying malignancy is discovered. Many patients complain of profound fatigue, dull or continuous pain, and general malaise. Such symptoms are seldom compatible with sexual desire or expression in either men or women who are otherwise psychologically healthy. Pain can override feelings of desire and prevent the initiation of love making. Discharge or postcoital bleeding experienced by a gynecologic cancer patient may have an offensive odor or appearance and will affect both patient and partner.

Growing tumors can affect sexual function by interfering with central or peripheral nerve supplies. Intracranial tumors involving the frontal or temporal lobe portion of the limbic system may alter sexual desire, causing a dramatic increase in or a complete loss of desire. Enlarging genitourinary cancers can compress peripheral nerves, interfering with reflex mechanisms controlling male erection

Table 1. Male Sexual Problems Caused by Cancer Treatment

Treatment	Low Sexual Desire	Erection Problems	Lack of Orgasm	Dry Orgasm	Weaker Orgasm	Infertility
Chemotherapy	Sometimes	Rarely	Rarely	Rarely	Rarely	Often
Pelvic radiation therapy	Rarely	Sometimes	Rarely	Rarely	Sometimes	Often
Retroperitoneal lymph node dissection	Rarely	Rarely	Rarely	Often	Sometimes	Often
Abdominoperineal (A-P) resection	Rarely	Often	Rarely	Often	Sometimes	Sometimes*
Radical prostatectomy	Rarely	Often	Rarely	Always	Sometimes	Always
Radical cystectomy	Rarely	Often	Rarely	Always	Sometimes	Always
Total pelvic exenteration	Rarely	Often	Rarely	Always	Sometimes	Always
Partial penectomy	Rarely	Rarely	Rarely	Never	Rarely	Never
Total penectomy	Rarely	Always	Sometimes	Never	Sometimes	Usually*
Orchiectomy (removal of one testicle)	Rarely	Rarely	Never	Never	Never	Rarely**
Orchiectomy (removal of both testicles)	Often	Often	Sometimes	Sometimes	Sometimes	Always
Hormone therapy for prostate cancer	Often	Often	Sometimes	Sometimes	Sometimes	Always

*Artificial insemination of a spouse with the man's own semen may be possible.
**Infertile only if remaining testicle is not normal.
Source: From *Sexuality and Cancer: For the Man who has Cancer and his Partner* 13, 1988, Atlanta: American Cancer Society.
Reprinted with permission of the publisher.

Table 2. Female Sexual Problems Caused by Cancer Treatment

Treatment	Low Sexual Desire	Less Vaginal Moisture	Reduced Vaginal Size	Painful Inter-course	Trouble Reaching Orgasm	Infertility
Chemotherapy	Sometimes	Often	Rarely	Often	Rarely	Often
Pelvic radiation therapy	Rarely	Often	Often	Often	Rarely	Often
Radical hysterectomy	Rarely	Often*	Often	Rarely	Rarely	Always
Radical cystectomy	Rarely	Often*	Always	Sometimes	Rarely	Always
Abdominoperineal (A-P) resection	Rarely	Often	Sometimes	Sometimes	Rarely	Sometimes
Total pelvic exenteration with vaginal reconstruction	Sometimes	Always	Sometimes	Sometimes	Sometimes	Always
Radical vulvectomy	Rarely	Never	Sometimes	Often	Sometimes	Never
Conization of the cervix	Never	Never	Never	Rarely	Never	Rarely
Oophorectomy (removal of one tube and ovary)	Rarely	Never*	Never*	Rarely	Never	Rarely
Oophorectomy (removal of both tubes and ovaries)	Rarely	Often*	Sometimes*	Sometimes*	Rarely	Always
Mastectomy or radiation to the breast	Rarely	Never	Never	Never	Rarely	Never
Anti-estrogen therapy for breast or uterine cancer	Sometimes	Often	Sometimes	Sometimes	Rarely	Often
Androgen therapy	Never	Never	Never	Never	Never	Uncertain

*Vaginal dryness and size changes should not occur if one ovary remains or if hormone replacement therapy is given.
Source: From *Sexuality and Cancer: For the Woman who has Cancer and Her Partner*. (15), 1988, Atlanta, American Cancer Society. Reprinted by permission of the publisher.

and ejaculation. Sensation in the genital area may be impaired when a growing mass compresses the spinal cord.

EFFECTS OF SURGERY

Sexual function is most often affected in cancer patients when genitalia are structurally modified. For example, surgical resection for penile or vulvar cancer can be severely disfiguring.

The treatment for advanced penile carcinoma is a partial or total penectomy with a diverted urinary outlet. The patient retains full capacity for sexual arousal, orgasm, and ejaculation, even though the penis is removed or significantly altered. Although erection and vaginal penetration are no longer possible, orgasm can be reached by stimulation of the perineal and scrotal area. Ejaculation occurs through the diverted urethrostomy. Body image may be severely affected but successful adjustment can be achieved if a healthy sexual relationship exists at the time of diagnosis.

Serious sexual problems have been reported in women who have a vulvectomy for cancer of the external genital area. Minimal surgery is required in early disease, but a radical vulvectomy is indicated when the disease is advanced. Extensive vulvar tissue—including the clitoris—is removed, significantly altering the contours of the external genitalia. Although the desire for sex is not compromised by interruption of pelvic innervation, clitorectomy may limit the capacity for sexual arousal. As many as half of these patients will cease all sexual activity because of the changed appearance of their external genitalia and because of *dyspareunia* (painful intercourse) resulting from a surgically narrowed vaginal opening. Edema and restricted mobility may result from surgical resection in the groin area and also limit sexual activity.

Female sexuality is significantly disturbed as a result of vaginal cancer. Although radiation may be the primary treatment for many patients, some are treated by surgical removal of the vagina. The vagina is reconstructed by lining the original area or vault with a very thin layer of skin grafted from the buttocks or another inconspicuous area. This reconstruction generally retains the characteristics of a normal vagina, including elasticity, if vaginal dilation is maintained. Patients will need to use lubricants before intercourse, since no secretory glands remain after vaginectomy. A less successful method of vaginal reconstruction uses muscle flaps from the inner aspects of the thighs. Vaginal intercourse can continue to be a part of sexual activity with this method of reconstruction, but problems such as overly large or small vaginas and persistent odorous discharge have been noted.

Cervical cancer may be treated with surgery, radiation, or a combination of both, depending upon the extent of disease. Fifty to seventy-five percent of patients report diminished sexual responses after these treatments. For early-stage carcinoma, a radical hysterectomy is performed in which the uterus and adjacent tissue are removed along with the fallopian tubes, ovaries, and pelvic lymph nodes. Vaginal shortening occurs with this procedure and although the vagina is a distensible structure, some women experience discomfort during sexual intercourse. When pelvic nodes are stripped during surgery, autonomic innervation can be altered, resulting in changes in vaginal engorgement and lubrication. This may affect sexual excitability and the ability to have an orgasm.

Pelvic exenteration, an extensive surgery for advanced or recurrent cervical carcinoma, involves removal of the reproductive organs, vagina, and pelvic lymph nodes. The bladder and/or rectum may also need to be removed, leaving the patient with a urinary conduit or colostomy. The patient may require intensive counseling in order to adjust to postoperative disturbances in body image, self-esteem, and sexuality.

Patients with certain types of testicular cancer may have a radical orchiectomy, a procedure involving the removal of the testicle and resection of the pelvic lymph nodes. Patients will retain erectile function and the ability to have an orgasm, but ejaculation is disturbed. Some men will recover ejaculatory function as nerve tissue recovers from the surgical trauma.

Although fertility is retained when only one testicle is removed, the surgery still has an impact on a young man's sexuality. Severe long-term sexual dysfunction has been noted in a large percentage of patients. Many complain of a decrease in the pleasure of orgasm, despite the fact that testosterone levels generally remain normal and the hormonal basis for libido is physiologically intact.

Infertility results when both testes are removed. Because testicular cancer strikes relatively young men in the prime of reproductive life, patients wishing to preserve fertility may want to consider sperm banking before starting treatment. Since the underlying disease process may decrease the sperm count, patients should be counseled that sperm banking does not assure that future artificial insemination will be successful.

The treatment of both bladder cancer and prostate cancer can result in a high incidence of impotence or erectile dysfunction related to interruption of innervation and local blood supply. Most males will be impotent following radical *cystectomy*, but the incidence of impotence following radical prostatectomy for prostate cancer has been reduced using innovative surgical techniques that spare pelvic nerves. Penile implants may be recommended in physiologically based impotence resulting from surgery. Ejaculation may also be compromised in radical prostatectomy and radical cystectomy. The surgical removal of the vas deferens causes loss of seminal fluid or ejaculate. The sensation of ejaculation and orgasm may also be altered by interruption of the lower thoracic and lumbar nerve pathways.

Abdominal-perineal (AP) resection for colorectal cancer in males can also cause "dry" orgasm by damaging the nerves that control emission. Loss of erectile function also occurs in 30-50% of men who have this surgery. Because other factors in the immediate postoperative period—fatigue, chemotherapy, and radiation therapy—may affect erection, the patient may regain normal erectile function within several months of surgery.

EFFECTS OF RADIATION THERAPY

Radiation therapy for gynecologic malignancies commonly results in direct trauma to the vaginal epithelium, causing thinning of the vaginal lining and loss of elasticity. Decreased vascular engorgement and reduced lubrication of the vaginal wall also contribute significantly to dyspareunia. In these patients, vaginal stenosis can quickly occur following localized radiation; it can be prevented by maintaining or resuming frequent sexual intercourse using water-soluble or hormonal creams as lubricants. Women without sexual partners can maintain patency by using vaginal dilators, although some patients may find this practice unacceptable. Once narrowed or closed, a patent, functional vagina can be re-established through surgery.

A high percentage of males receiving radiation for pelvic malignancies becomes impotent. Loss of erectile function results from fibrosis of the pelvic vascular system or direct radiation damage to nerve pathways. The permanency of the loss is related to the radiation dose as well as the individual's pretreatment functional ability. A patient with diminished erectile function before treatment has a reduced chance of regaining optimal function.

EFFECTS OF CHEMOTHERAPY

The ability to produce children is an integral component of a person's sexuality. Chemotherapy can be directly toxic to the gonads, producing temporary or permanent sterility. Before starting chemotherapy, male patients may wish to consider semen preservation for future artificial insemination or in vitro fertilization.

Health care staff should also keep in mind the teratogenic and mutagenic effects of certain chemotherapy agents. Children conceived during treatment can have severe genetic abnormalities. For this reason, patients should be advised to use birth control during treatment and for 2 years after treatment.

Some chemotherapy drugs also affect sensation in peripheral nerves; this may impair the ability to have or maintain an erection.

EFFECTS OF HORMONAL ALTERATIONS

Irradiation, chemotherapy, and surgical resection can impair hormone production in the ovaries or testicles. Bilateral oophorectomy results in immediate cessation of estrogen and progestin production in premenopausal women. Women receiving pelvic or abdominal irradiation may also exhibit ovarian failure shortly after treatment unless the ovaries are surgically repositioned before the irradiation. Symptoms of estrogen loss include depression, irritability, hot flashes, insomnia, and diminished lubrication of the vagina that may result in dyspareunia. Estrogen replacement, frequently prescribed after normal menopause, is not indicated for patients with breast and certain gynecologic malignancies because of its potential to trigger tumor growth.

Administration of estrogen therapy to men with prostate cancer can cause decreased libido and erectile function and penile atrophy. *Gynecomastia*, or breast growth, will also occur and can significantly affect self-image. This can be prevented by pretreatment irradiation of the breast tissue.

The loss of testosterone, a hormone produced in the male by the testes and in the female by the adrenal glands and ovaries, can affect sexual desire and libido. In addition to loss of libido, men sometimes encounter difficulty with erection when testosterone is diminished.

ALTERATIONS IN BODY IMAGE AND SELF-ESTEEM

Although negative body image is prevalent among people suffering from sexual dysfunction who have no organic illness, body image alterations are often overlooked as a prime cause of sexual dysfunction in patients living with cancer. Nurses should be aware that the patient who feels physically unattractive or repulsive may have little chance of functioning in sexual relations without disturbances.

A variety of factors can lead to body image and self-esteem disturbances in the patient with cancer. Alopecia, although usually temporary, can often affect self-image. Infertility secondary to treatment may cause an identity crisis that indirectly affects sexual response. Patients with ostomies might feel self-conscious about their body excretions. Patients who had disfiguring surgery or a body part removed (i.e. head and neck, mastectomy, limb loss from bone cancer) may feel less desire to engage in sexual relations because of the fear of rejection. When damage to sexual identity leaves an individual feeling unable to respond sexually, behavioral changes are often seen.

Loss of libido may accompany the continual state of high anxiety most patients feel about the ultimate treatment outcome. The threat of impaired function or even death will negatively affect sexual desire and performance. In addition, patients' sexual partners may react to the strain of living with the disease by withdrawing emotionally or actually abandoning the patient. Patients fear this occurrence, especially when the malignancy or its treatment impairs sexual function. Spouses or significant others may be very supportive of the patient through cancer diagnosis and treatment, but in a conscious effort to avoid inflicting further stress eliminate sexual relations altogether. A major source of personal value to many individuals revolves around sharing intimacy and giving pleasure to a partner.

COUNSELING

Nurses have generally been reluctant to provide guidance and advice about sexuality issues because of a lack of knowledge about this critical area. Attitudes about sexuality, combined with a natural reluctance to intrude into matters of personal privacy, create additional barriers to the discussion of sexual matters. To improve communication with patients about sexual issues, nurses can increase their understanding of the physical and psychological changes that can directly or indirectly affect sexual behavior. Providing information and guidance may be one of the most important nursing interventions for oncology patients with sexual dysfunction. When the nurse provides general information during the initial discussion, patients may be motivated to return with more definitive and intimate questions as they become more comfortable and trusting.

Nurses can reassure patients that when sexual desire decreases, the need for non-sexual intimacy increases. Encouraging comunication between patients and their sexual partners is vital, since many problems will be solved merely by the chance to discuss them. When individual problems extend beyond these simple strategies, nurses should refer these patients to competent specialists who treat sexual dysfunction.

Bibliography

Anderson, B. & Hackes, N. (1983). Psychosexual adjustment after vulvar surgery. *Obstetrics and Gynecology, 62,* 457-462.

Edlund, B. (1982). The needs of women with gynecological malignancies. *Nursing Clinics of North America, 17,* 165-177.

Fisher, S. G. (1985). Sexuality. In B. L. Johnson, & J. Gross, (Eds.). *Handbook of oncology nursing* (pp. 363-379). New York: John Wiley and Sons.

Frank-Stromborg, M. (1985). Sexuality and the elderly cancer patient. *Seminars in Oncology Nursing, 1*(1), 49-55.

Heinrich-Rynning, T. (1987). Prostatic cancer treatments and their effects on sexual functioning. *Oncology Nursing Forum, 14*(6), 37-41.

MacElveen-Hoehn, P., & McCorkle, R. (1985) Understanding sexuality in progressive cancer. *Seminars in Oncology Nursing,* 1(1), 56-62.

Metcalfe, M., & Fischman, S. (1985). Factors affecting the sexuality of patients with head and neck cancer. *Oncology Nursing Forum, 12*(2), 21-25.

Schover, L. R., Schain, W. S., & Montague, D. K. (1989). Sexual problems of patients with cancer. In V. T. DeVita, S. Hellman, & S. Rosenberg (Eds.), *Cancer principles and practice of oncology,* pp. 2206-2224. Philadelphia: J. B. Lippincott Co.

Schwarz-Applebaum, J., Dedrick, J., Jusenius, K., & Kirchner, C. W. (1984). Nursing care plans: Sexuality and treatment of breast cancer. *Oncology Nursing Forum, 11*(6), 16-24.

Springer, M. (1982). Radical vulvectomy: Physical, psychological, social and sexual implications. *Oncology Nursing Forum, 9*(2), 19-21.

Wood, R. Y. (1978). Penile implants for impotence. *American Journal of Nursing, 78,* 234-239.

6 PSYCHOSOCIAL SUPPORT

Ginette Ferszt and Frances K. Barg

INCIDENCE

Despite dramatic progress in cancer treatment in recent decades, cancer continues to be one of the most feared of all diseases. Many people still associate cancer with death, suffering, or disfigurement. Some people with cancer fear being ostracized, treated differently, or misunderstood. As a result, they may experience the additional psychological burden of keeping their illness a secret from others.

Cancer affects the entire family system, and may upset its balance. The result may be increased tension and stress for the person with cancer, other members of the family, and even those not living with the patient. Family members' responses to the illness can have a significant impact on the patient's adaptation. To most effectively assist the patient, nursing interventions should address the problems and needs of the entire family.

SUPPORT AND THERAPY

Support

It is important to distinguish between support and therapy when considering psychosocial interventions. *Support* can be characterized as an informed empathic response to patients and families. Nurses have many opportunities during their contacts with patients and families to assist in dealing with the daily stresses associated with living with cancer. Nurses can also identify patients who may require more aggressive psychosocial interventions. Listening actively, providing information, and assisting in problem solving are all integral to the nurse's supportive role. The nurse can also foster hope by actively involving the patient in goal setting, incorporating therapeutic humor, fostering spirituality, and mobilizing the patient's own support systems. This support should always build on the patient's issues and values, not on those of the professional caregiver.

To be supportive, the nurse may need to adopt several roles. When patients and families hear emotionally laden information, such as news about diagnosis, treatment plans, or prognosis, they may become anxious and therefore less able to think critically and solve problems. Nurses in this situation can function as interpreters, demystifying the experience by translating and explaining the foreign language of medical care while offering support and reassurance.

Nurses also provide support by listening to what the patient says about the personal meaning of the disease, and making referrals for counseling if needed. Some patients feel that the cancer is punishment or that suffering is a spiritual obligation. Children may feel responsible for causing the illness. At these times a referral for counseling or spiritual guidance may be helpful.

One major objective of the supportive nurse is to help families, patients, and staff understand uncomfortable emotions. Families need to know that the anger their loved one expresses toward them may be displaced anger. Physicians may not realize that a patient's noncompliance is really a function of his anxiety. Patients may misinterpret a spouse's depression as apathy.

Attempts to provide support, while generally positive, can encounter pitfalls. Support is intended to help people feel better by providing help with concrete problem solving and lessening feelings of abandonment that may be prominent. A nurse's first impulse may be to make patients happy or "cheer them up," but this approach may fail to acknowledge the patient's actual feelings. Nurses may be reluctant to discuss powerful and painful emotions for fear of depressing the patient; but allowing ventilation of these feelings validates them. The nurse can often offer an objective ear that families may not be able to give.

Therapy

Unlike support, *therapy* is characterized by a deliberate attempt to facilitate intrapsychic change. Psychotherapy may be productive when multiple stresses impede adaptive coping. A psychological evaluation should be considered when the patient has a history of psychiatric problems or exhibits one or more of the following behaviors:

- persistent refusal of or noncompliance with suggested treatment,
- persistent anxiety or depression unresponsive to support and/ or reassurance,
- suicidal ideation, or
- excessive self-blame for illness.

Nurses can refer patients to a psychiatric mental health nurse, social worker, psychologist, or psychiatrist. Individual or group therapy may be helpful.

ISSUES ALONG THE DISEASE CONTINUUM

Patients with cancer will deal with different psychosocial issues and needs in each phase of the disease process.

Diagnosis

The initial or diagnostic phase includes diagnosis and early treatment. The reaction to diagnosis is complex. Shock reverberates throughout the family system as members try to absorb vast amounts of threatening information. Anxiety, preoccupation, sadness, agitation, fear, and withdrawal are common reactions. The patient and family try to regain control of an overwhelming situation, often by seeking extensive information.

Sometimes intellectual and emotional responses are incongruent with the severity of the disease and may be mistaken for denial. The patient may choose not to deal with the entire situation in order to conserve psychological energy for what lies ahead. Thus, denial may be a useful mechanism. The patient and family need time to fully comprehend what has happened in order to progress past the initial shock and mobilize the psychological resources necessary to deal with the illness.

The initial treatment phase is another frightening period. Often, the patient and family had no prior relationship with their health care providers, yet are now dependent on several of them for care and treatment. This may increase the patient's and family's anxiety.

Multiple losses and changes take place during this period, often provoking feelings of sadness and grief. Patients and families commonly face issues such as loss of control, changes in body image, and changes in roles and relationships. Frequently, their lives become focused on the illness and the initial treatment process. It is critical that nurses provide structure and systematic information about treatment and management of side effects at this time. In most cases, when patients know what to expect, their distress decreases.

Treatment

Many people are able to continue active, productive lives during and following cancer treatment. However, the patient and family are challenged to maintain a sense of normalcy in an abnormal situation.

Patients need open discussion and comprehensible, timely information in order to make decisions about initial treatment and treatment options. However, anxiety and information overload may make it difficult for the patient to concentrate and make decisions. Health care providers will be challenged to correct cancer myths and address the unknown by giving the correct balance of information. Suggesting that the patient write a list of questions, or asking, "what questions do you have?" may help the patient and family gain focus and use problem-solving skills. Many patients are afraid to ask their doctors direct questions because they fear the answers or worry about imposing on an important care provider. Nurses can help the patient communicate with the physician.

A second opinion could be valuable to the patient at this time. It is important for the nurse and other health care providers to support a patient's and family's search for such an opinion.

Patients and families may consider unproven methods of treatment before or during cancer therapy. Those who typically seek unproven methods tend to feel unsupported by the traditional medical system. They are generally, although not exclusively, well-educated adults of higher socioeconomic status. Nurses may be asked for information about various unproven methods or for assistance in decision-making. The American Cancer Society and the Cancer Information Service (see Unit VI) are both good sources of information about the purported basis for such methods, risks, advisability, and availability.

Treatment regimens can place heavy demands on the patient's and family's time and energy; frequently the treatment also leads to some discomfort. Treatment side effects and distressing symptoms such as nausea, alopecia, and fatigue often necessitate lifestyle changes, such as buying clothing to accommodate body changes or reassigning responsibilities to conserve physical energy. Innovation and creativity, and supportive resources can make dealing with these changes easier. Cosmetic and fashion specialists, nutritionists, clinical nurse specialists, social workers, clergy, and support groups can be valuable resources for solutions to difficult problems. Overall, however, a treatment regimen will not be a success unless the patient and family accept it.

Sometimes the patient's distress and need for information will not peak until 4 or 6 weeks after diagnosis. Typically, the patient will be at home at this point, without the easy access to health professionals available in the hospital. Nurses should discuss the possibility of this problem with the patients and families and provide concrete suggestions about how to gain access to resources.

Survivorship and Recurrence

Survivorship connotes the positive aspects of conquering a physical disease; however, survivors of cancer often experience their own brand of disease-related stress. Many describe feeling the "sword of Damocles" hanging over their heads, never completely erasing the fear of recurrence. Every subsequent cold or headache may be interpreted as a return of the disease.

Disease recurrence usually has a greater emotional impact on patients and families than the initial diagnosis. While the initial diagnosis and treatment carry the implication that the cancer can be conquered, recurrence may refute that hope. New goals need to be established with the patient and new avenues of hope need to be explored.

Advancing disease is usually characterized by increased symptom distress. If symptoms such as pain, nausea, dyspnea, anorexia, stomatitis, or skin excoriation cannot be controlled, patients and families may begin to feel helpless and hopeless. Because the link between physical disease and emotional status is so strong, it is difficult to separate symptom distress from depression. Adequate symptom management is crucial during this period, because it frees patients to explore their feelings about the illness. When family members can be involved in alleviating or managing distressing symptoms, they may feel less helpless.

The impaired mobility, disfigurement, and loss of energy that accompany difficult, prolonged treatment or advancing disease can lead to the patient's social isolation. The physical and emotional toll on the patient and family can manifest as psychological, marital, or family problems.

Families coping with prolonged, deteriorating illnesses must learn to redistribute their work load and change their life expectations. Today's American family is often fairly isolated, functioning without supportive networks that can absorb this work load. In this situation families are often stretched too far, and the unrelenting stress and strains can cause guilt, anger, and resentment. The patient may feel guilty for being a burden, and family members may be angry because their own needs go unmet. Financial pressures may result from lost income and the burden of health care costs. Nurses need to keep in mind the wide variety of sources of stress and help families identify their specific areas of concern and where assistance may be available.

Terminal Illness

The terminal phase of the illness brings a new set of major decisions that the patient and family must confront: active treatment or palliation; death at home or in the hospital. The patient and family are also faced with impending separation and death. Throughout the terminal phase and the dying process, they may experience a range of emotions, including mood swings, sadness, depression, anger, guilt, powerlessness, withdrawal, and relief. During this period, the patient and family often search for meaning in life arid experience suffering and loss. Some families may feel a renewed commitment or connection to their religion.

Approaching death makes some patients and families realize for the first time the significance of their relationship and how deep the loss will be. Patients and families in troubled relationships may grieve because problems in the relationship will never be resolved. And for others, death is a welcome relief.

The actual death can be a very stressful time. Physical evidence of the dying process can be difficult to witness for families who are not prepared for what they will see and hear. Families may react impulsively, demanding extraordinary measures they may have eschewed earlier. If the patient is at home, a specific, written action plan with phone numbers and names of contacts to call when death is imminent can be very useful.

In some situations the family struggles with its wish to hold on. At times, it may be more difficult for the family to let go than it is for the patient to die. Families may not understand and feel hurt by the patient's emotional withdrawal in the final days. Explaining emotional reactions to families and outlining what they can do for their loved one are often helpful.

Some families may have unfinished business. Some will be able to say their last goodbyes and plan for their funeral services. In other families, the patient will die without ever having talked about it openly. It is important for the nurse to respect families' need to grieve and express emotion in a way consistent with their own traditions.

Hospice care should be considered when cure is no longer a treatment goal. Criteria for hospice admission vary, but eligible patients generally have a prognosis of less than six months to live. These programs address the physical, social, emotional, and spiritual needs of the patient and family, with a focus on pain and symptom control, respite care, volunteer support, and extended support at home. Most hospice programs provide bereavement follow-up for a limited period of time after the patient's death.

Hospice programs are typically home care programs; a small percentage of United States hospices are inpatient facilities with home care components.

COPING AND COMMUNICATION

In the course of the disease, patients need to feel that their family and caregivers understand them and will respond to their needs. Nurses can cultivate, and encourage families to cultivate, several communication skills that support the patient.

Communication

Active listening is a skill that asks the caregiver to "be there" for the patient physically and emotionally. Nurses who listen with unconditioned positive regard and state what they think the patient is feeling allow the patient to clarify salient issues for himself or herself. The role of the nurse here is not to solve problems, but to assist the patient's inward search for solutions to major issues.

The nurse can control the direction of communication to a certain extent by focusing on the content of the message. If the patient says, "I don't feel like eating today," the nurse can respond to the *fact* in the statement by asking questions about diet and frequency of meals. Or, the nurse may address the *feeling* in the statement by replying, "It sounds as if you aren't interested in much of anything today. Is there something you are upset or worried about?" Responding to the facts in the statement limits the response. The nurse who attends to the emotions in the patient's statement encourages the patient to reflect on the problem and to express feelings.

Research findings indicate that the role changes typically found in families living with cancer are handled best in families that communicate openly about the disease. Adolescents with cancer report greater trust in their families when the diagnosis was explained early in the disease. Families can be encouraged to communicate rather than retreat from each other when cohesion is needed most. The nurse can be a role model for open communication between patients and families, and family meetings can be valuable forums for family needs and problems.

Coping

Patients' and families' responses to the diagnosis of cancer will usually resemble their responses to past crises. Everyone copes differently; variations in coping ability are often a function of the individual's religious and cultural background and early life experiences. Some patients and families even describe the overall cancer experience in positive terms, because the process of coping reveals inner strengths and establishes, in a dramatic way, the priorities of life.

Research has identified beneficial and poor coping mechanisms among patients. The onset of cancer makes many patients feel they have lost control of their lives. Restoration of this control or sense of mastery over one's environment can give patients coping strength and is therefore a major goal of psychosocial intervention.

People who face their cancer with an active, participatory frame of mind tend to cope well. Patients who seek information or share their feelings tend to cope well also, as long as they seek information from legitimate sources and share their concerns with empathic individuals who provide support without escalating negative emotions such as fear or anger.

Denial can be an adaptive coping style at certain points along the disease continuum, but becomes a concern when it is prolonged or interferes with the patient's treatment, functioning, or problem-solving ability. Withdrawal occurs when a person retreats from personal and professional caregivers, leading to further isolation and distress. Displacement, or the projection of a feeling such as anger to an inappropriate person or object, is often misunderstood and leads to interpersonal conflict. Passivity and impulsivity are other, less adaptive coping styles that may lead to a sense of powerlessness.

Certain patients are at a higher risk for psychosocial distress than others. Younger patients, or patients in families with young children, are at a higher risk because it can be difficult to balance the needs of young children with the needs of a sick family member. For example, shifts in family duties may mean asking children to assume too much responsibility for their developmental stage. Recurrent disease, diagnosis at an advanced stage of illness, or unresolved symptom distress also increases the potential for emotional distress. Families with concurrent losses, substance abuse, or a multitude of problems are also predisposed to distress. When the nurse identifies a patient who may be having trouble coping, or identifies a patient and family at high risk for distress, a referral should be made to an appropriate counselor or therapist for assessment and treatment.

HEALTH PROFESSIONALS AS A SUPPORT NETWORK

Cancer care can be both rewarding and stressful for the health professional. A nurse's professional life can be enriched by opportunities to use knowledge and skills and to maintain significant relationships with patients and families. However, caring for patients and families who are suffering physically, emotionally, and spiritually is emotionally draining. Nurses may identify with patients or feel sad or inadequate. As nurses provide care for people with multiple losses, personal loss issues can be brought to the surface.

Maintaining a balanced life and developing supportive networks in and out of the workplace are important strategies for all health care professionals. It is also helpful to realize that nurses work in groups with norms and sanctions just like any other group. If the values and rules of the group are incongruent with a nurse's personal values and rules, the nurse will experience dissonance. Nurses may find it helpful to examine the groups in which they work to determine the degree to which their personal needs are supported by that group. Similarly, it is important to recognize that the roles performed in a given situation may vary from patient to patient. Just as families often need to renegotiate roles when cancer occurs, members of the health care team frequently renegotiate roles too. Developing collaborative relationships takes time and commitment. By participating in interdisciplinary rounds and conferences, and taking time to celebrate informally together in the work place, nurses can foster mutual respect and recognition for the contributions that each discipline offers.

Bibliography
American Cancer Society (1988). Psychosocial issues and cancer. *CA: A Cancer Journal for Clinicians, 38*(3), 130-186.
Blank, J., Clark, L., Longman, A. J., & Atwood, J. R. (1989). Perceived home care needs of cancer patients and their caregivers. *Cancer Nursing, 12*(2), 78-84.
De Pastino, E. (1984). The nurse as counselor. *Oncology Nursing Forum, 11*(4), 93-96.
Frank-Stromborg, M., Wright, P. S., Segalla, M., & Diekmann, J. (1984). Psychological impact of the cancer diagnosis. *Oncology Nursing Forum, 11*(3), 16-22.
Fredette, S. L., & Beattie, H. M. (1986). Living with cancer. A patient education program. *Cancer Nursing, 9*(6), 308-316.
Heiney, S. P., & Wells, L. M. (1989). Strategies for organizing and maintaining successful support groups. *Oncology Nursing Forum, 16*(6), 803-809.
Hickey, S. (1986). Enabling hope. *Cancer Nursing, 9*(3), 133-137.
Lewandowski, W., & Jones, S. (1988). The family with cancer. Nursing interventions throughout the course of living with cancer. *Cancer Nursing, 11*(6), 313-321.
Miaskowski, C. A., & Nielsen, B. (1985). A cancer nursing assesment tool. *Oncology Nursing Forum, 12*(6), 36-42.
Tringali, C. A. (1986). The needs of family members of cancer patients. *Oncology Nursing Forum, 13*(6), 65-70.

7 REHABILITATION

Frances Barg and Laura Heard

Improved cancer treatment has resulted in more patients living longer than ever before. As a result, cancer is now frequently considered a chronic illness with episodic physical and emotional effects.

Rehabilitation is a dynamic, ongoing process, intended to maximize individuals' functional capabilities within the limitations of their disease or disability. Cancer has the potential to affect the physical, emotional, and social aspects of a patient's life. The patient's relationships with other family members, coworkers, and employers may be affected by the consequences of the disease and its treatment. However, the nurse, in collaboration with the patient, family, and health care team, can help patients become independent and enable them to live productive, satisfying lives whether their cancer is cured, controlled, or palliated.

THE FAMILY AS THE UNIT OF CARE

A basic tenet of cancer rehabilitation is that the patient and family are treated as a single unit. Most patients do not experience cancer by themselves, but as part of a family, neighborhood, school, work setting, or religious group. The patient's health may vary with the effects of disease or treatment, and the family and others will need to understand the reasons for these changes and realistically adjust their expectations of the patient. Nurses can assist the patient and family in clarifying goals, values, and needs when planning rehabilitation activities.

Goal Setting

Setting realistic goals is one of the most important factors in cancer rehabilitation. Although cancer can be characterized by significant loss, rehabilitation shifts the focus from what has been lost to what can be done with the remaining strengths and abilities. Goal development can start with an interdisciplinary assessment of deficits, strengths, and potential gains. Rehabilitation goals should be consistent with the specific type and stage of cancer and with goals for cancer treatment. Goals should also address aspects of prevention, restoration, maintenance, and palliation as appropriate.

BARRIERS TO REHABILITATION

Despite substantial progress, significant barriers to successful rehabilitation exist. Cancer is one of the most feared diseases. Fears of contagion, worker unproductivity, acceptance of the employee by coworkers, and inevitable death prevent many from considering cancer rehabilitation possible.

Few cancer treatment centers offer comprehensive rehabilitation services. Rehabilitation care is often fragmented. Houts and his colleagues in Pennsylvania recently studied unmet rehabilitation needs of cancer patients and found that 57% of the 629 patients studied had at least one unmet rehabilitation need. Most frequently lacking were emotional support services. Social support has been identified as an important variable influencing coping and rehabilitation.

Cancer pain can also limit successful rehabilitation. Despite efforts to disseminate accurate information, cancer pain is frequently undertreated because patients and health professionals lack expertise in managing pain and persist in their fears about addiction and the use of narcotics.

Patients with cancer frequently experience fatigue and fluctuating endurance. These factors must be considered when planning rehabilitation activities, especially activities of daily living and mobility.

The fear of disease recurrence can also pose a barrier to rehabilitation. Some patients have difficulty believing they are cured. These patients may be less willing to plan long-term intervention based on their current status. Because the disease can recur, many patients may resist rehabilitation activities, thinking, "What's the use?" The nurse can help patients explore their fears about recurrence and set realistic rehabilitation goals. Consistent advocacy of self-care, independence, and self-determination is important regardless of the stage of disease.

REHABILITATION AS AN INTERDISCIPLINARY PROCESS

Considering the complex and chronic nature of cancer patient care, the range of potential areas of rehabilitation is vast. Some aspects of care and rehabilitation are short-term activities, such as the management of temporary alopecia from chemotherapy. Other rehabilitative activities will need to address permanent changes, such as those resulting from a laryngectomy or colostomy. An interdisciplinary approach is best for addressing the range of possible patient and family needs. Depending on the needs to be addressed, the team may include nurses, physicians, psychologists, social workers, physical therapists, occupational therapists, speech

Table 1. Topics for Consideration by the Rehabilitation Team

Areas of Activity	Specific Tasks and Needs
Discharge planning	Follow-up care, community resources, contingency plans
Activities of daily living	Bathing, dressing, feeding, grooming, medication administration, adaptive equipment
	Bed mobility, transfers, ambulation, range of motion, strength, endurance, community access, transportation
Nutrition/swallowing	Enteral and parenteral nutrition, supplements, barriers to swallowing, anorexia
Symptom management	Pain, fatigue, weakness, nausea, sensory alterations, constipation, diarrhea, lymphedema, mucositis, dyspnea
Living environment/home maintenance	Distance from resources, presence of stairs or other architectural barriers, need for help at home, need for special equipment at home
Body functions	Bowel and bladder management, care of skin and mucous membranes
Communication	Speech and language functions
Psychosocial relations	Relations with family members, support systems for patient and family, sexuality, body image, coping skills, role reversal
Financial considerations	Insurance coverage, job security
Vocational/avocational	Concerns about the return to work, discrimination, adaptation necessary for current job, need for re-education to obtain a new job, identity issues
Spirituality	Existential issues

pathologists, vocational counselors, prosthetists/orthotists, pharmacists, chaplains, enterostomal therapists, dietitians, and of course the patient and family. By functioning as a team all members can coordinate goals, support and teach each other, enhance communication among the disciplines, and provide a vehicle for accountability. The patient care conference or rehabilitation team conference provides a forum for discussions of a variety of problem areas. Table 1 lists common topics.

WORK AND IDENTITY

Americans are bound to the work ethic, so work/productivity issues can pose additional barriers to rehabilitation. Personal identity is intimately linked with occupation. When a person's role changes because of limitations imposed by the disease or its treatment, self-esteem and mood will be affected. Rehabilitation embraces the concept that a return to productive function, paid or unpaid, will enhance patients' feelings of mastery, control, and self-esteem.

Workplace discrimination against people with cancer may be overt or covert. Discriminatory employers may be motivated by fears that recovering or recovered cancer patients will be unable to do their jobs, that their turnover and absentee rates will be high, or that their disease will be fatal. Yet anecdotal evidence suggests that turnover and absenteeism are frequently no higher for the employee with cancer than for other employees. The funds employers pay to worker compensation are unaffected, because this program provides insurance for industrial accidents.

The Rehabilitation Act of 1973 prohibits discrimination against people with cancer by classifying cancer as a handicap under the law. Section 503 of this act prohibits federally funded employers from discriminating against people with cancer in hiring, promotions, transfers, recruitment, layoffs, termination, pay scales, and selection for training. Section 504 prohibits federally funded schools, colleges, and hospitals from discriminating against people with cancer in hiring practices or the provision of health, welfare, and social service benefits.

State Offices of Vocational Rehabilitation (OVR) may be valuable resources in helping people with cancer return to work when skill modification or retraining is needed. OVR can also help employers modify the workplace to accommodate worker disability and to educate other employees about cancer. The services available through state vocational rehabilitation and knowledge and services specific to cancer vary from state to state.

SITE-SPECIFIC REHABILITATION MEASURES

The type of cancer will partly determine the kinds of rehabilitation services a patient needs. For example, a person with a laryngectomy will need information on and assistance with stoma care and communication. A woman who has had a mastectomy will want information about exercises, wound care, prostheses, and possibly reconstruction. Rehabilitation issues associated with common sites of cancer are highlighted in Table 2. A common problem in cancer rehabilitation is that attention is focused on sites when specific disability is obvious, especially those requiring prostheses or appliances. However, comprehensive rehabilitation plans should include identification of more subtle needs and specific interventions to address them. Resources that may be useful are listed in Unit VI. The chapter bibliographies also provide sources of further information on rehabilitation measures that can enhance self-esteem, increase function, and add to productivity.

Table 2. Rehabilitation Issues Associated with Specific Cancer Sites

Cancer Site	Rehabilitation Issues
Head and neck cancers	Maintenance of optimal nutrition and deglutition Shoulder dysfunction rehabilitation Neck dysfunction rehabilitation Self-care considerations Speech/communication Restoring acceptable appearance and function
Breast cancer	Physical restoration of affected arm Psychosocial rehabilitation regarding loss, body image alterations, and sexuality Cosmetic rehabilitation with form, prosthesis, or reconstruction
Bone and soft tissue malignancies	Restore near-normal function through prostheses, appliances, and aids to ambulation Restore acceptable appearance Vocational rehabilitation Psychosocial restoration
Lung cancer	Preoperative rehabilitation emphasizes breathing retraining Pulmonary disability prevention after radiation or surgery
Colorectal and bladder malignancies resulting in ostomies	Self-concept adjustment Elimination control and ostomy adjustment Self-care considerations Psychosocial rehabilitation Effective skin care
Central nervous system	Preventing unnecessary loss of function and diminished quality of life Cognitive function evaluation Mobility modifications Retraining for activities of daily living Bowel and bladder management

Source: From "Rehabilitation of the Cancer Patient" by J. A. DeLisa, R. M. Miller, R. R. Melnick, L. H. Gerber, and A. B. Hillel. 1989, pp. 2341–2364. In V. T. DeVita, S. Hellman, and S. A. Rosenberg (Eds.), Cancer: Principles and Practice, Philadelphia: J. B. Lippincott Co. Adapted by permission.

NURSING'S CONTRIBUTION

Nurses can readily enhance patient and professional awareness of cancer rehabilitation needs. Dudas and Carlson described five areas in which nurses can have a positive impact: promoting a positive attitude toward cancer rehabilitation by emphasizing cancer as a chronic disease; incorporating potential rehabilitation needs into initial patient assessments; exposing nursing students to cancer "success" stories; promoting the independence of people with cancer by referring them to established education and volunteer groups such as *I Can Cope* or *Reach to Recovery* and by working with other disciplines; and maximizing functional status by helping patients anticipate potential obstacles and solutions to surmounting them. Long-term survival has become a reality for an increasing number of people with cancer. The needs of cancer survivors are being articulated by both survivor groups and organizations such as the American Cancer Society. The National Coalition for Cancer Survivors has outlined areas of need specifically concerning work and community. The coalition also identified a need for health surveillance guidelines and long-term support. Nurses have opportunities through their work or community roles to help survivors return to usual activities and to educate the public about the positive advances in cancer survival and rehabilitation.

Bibliography

Anderson, J. L. (1989). The nurse's role in cancer rehabilitation. *Cancer Nursing, 12*(2), 85–94.

DeLisa, J. A., Miller, R. M., Melnick, R. R., Gerber, L. H., & Hillel, A. B. (1989). Rehabilitation of the cancer patient. In V. T. DeVita, S. Hellman, & S. A. Rosenberg (Eds.), *Cancer: Principles and practice of oncology* (3rd ed.) (pp. 2333–2368). Philadelphia: J. B. Lippincott.

Dudas, S. & Carlson, C. E. (1988). Cancer rehabilitation. *Oncology Nursing Forum, 15*(2), 183–188.

Dudas, S. (1986). Psychosocial aspects of patient care. In D. B. Smith & D. Johnson (Eds.), *Ostomy care and the cancer patient* (pp. 93–102). Orlando: Grune & Stratton.

Harvey, R. F., Jellinek, H. M., & Habeck, R. V. (1982). Cancer rehabilitation: An analysis of 36 program approaches. *JAMA, 247,* 2127–2131.

Hoffman, B. (1989). Cancer survivors at work: Job problems and illegal job discrimination. *Oncology Nursing Forum, 16*(1), 39–43.

Houts, P., Yasko, J., Kahn, B., Schelzel, G., & Marconi, K. (1986). Unmet psychological, social, and economic needs of persons with cancer in Pennsylvania. *Cancer, 58,* 2355–2361.

Millette, S. J. (1989). Rehabilitation issues for cancer survivors. *Journal of Psychosocial Oncology, 7*(4), 93–110.

Romsaas, E. P., Juliana, L. M., Briggs, A. L., Wysocki, G., & Moorman, J. (1983). A method for assessing the rehabilitation needs of oncology outpatients. *Oncology Nursing Forum, 10*(3), 17–23.

Stanwood, J. E., Rich, S., Frymark, S., Moore, E., Cowsky, K., Kaplan, L., & Weggerman, D. (1978). *Cancer rehabilitation care plans for cancer rehabilitation program.* Portland, OR: Good Samaritan Hospital and Medical Center and Emmanuel Hospital.

Watson, P. (1990). Cancer rehabilitation: The evolution of a concept. *Cancer Nursing, 13*(1), 2–8.

Worden, J. W. (1989). The experience of recurrent cancer. *Ca—A Cancer Journal for Clinicians, 39*(5), 305–310.

UNIT 5

Treatment of Specific Neoplasms

The chapters in this unit describe specific neoplasms. Nurses should understand the incidence and risk factors of different cancers and have a sense of the types of cancer they are likely to encounter in their practices. Risk factors are fairly well delineated for most cancers, and for some, specific preventive behaviors have been outlined. Information on detection methods and staging is extremely useful to the nurse when preparing patients for diagnostic procedures and when helping patients and families to interpret results.

These chapters also describe the treatment approaches for different cancers, building on the principles of treatment contained in Unit III. Patients and families will often seek assistance in understanding the implications of treatment and in weighing choices. Nurses need to keep in mind that although the basic information about each cancer site is well established, treatment approaches are always being refined. Nurses will want to identify ways to keep their knowledge current.

1 CANCERS OF THE HEAD AND NECK

Barbara E. Albertson

INCIDENCE

Cancers of the head and neck region are those tumors arising in the oral cavity, oropharynx, nasopharynx, paranasal sinuses, hypopharynx, and larynx (See Table 1). Although these cancers constitute less than 5% of all malignancies, treatment may cause pronounced cosmetic deformities and impair such essential functions as eating and speaking. Head and neck cancer may occur at any age, but incidence is highest after age 40, among males, and in individuals with a history of tobacco use and/or heavy alcohol consumption.

RISK FACTORS

Researchers have established a strong relationship between tobacco use or alcohol intake and development of cancers of the head and neck. In fact, tobacco and alcohol are thought to have a synergistic effect in increasing the risk of developing these tumors. Pipe smoking and chronic exposure to sunlight have also been linked to an increased incidence of lip cancer. "Smokeless" or chewing tobacco use has been identified as a risk factor for oral cancer. Although chronic oral irritation has been implicated as a factor in the development of intraoral cancers, it is doubtful that trauma alone can induce the cellular changes responsible for the development of cancer.

PREVENTION AND DETECTION

The nurse's role in prevention and detection includes public education about the potential risks of tobacco and chronic, excessive alcohol use. The recent increased use of "smokeless" tobacco by adolescents is of special concern to nurses working with this age group. Nurses should also participate in screening programs for the early detection of head and neck cancers. Because stage of disease at the time of diagnosis is the most important prognostic factor, early detection can significantly affect the disease outcome. Nurses can encourage early identification and evaluation of premalignant or malignant tissue changes by educating patients about

Table 1. Possible Primary Sites of Head and Neck Tumors

Larynx Supraglottic Glottic Subglottic
Oral Cavity Lip Gums (Gingivae) Hard Palate Retromolar Trigone Anterior 2/3 of tongue Buccal Mucosa Floor of Mouth

Oropharynx
Soft Palate
Base of Tongue
Tonsil
Lateral and
    Posterior
    Pharyngeal Wall

Hypopharynx Postcricoid Pyriform Fossa
Others Nasopharynx Paranasal Sinuses   (Ethmoid, Sphenoid, Maxillary) Nasal Cavity

Source: From *Cancer of the Head and Neck* (p. 15) 1984, Atlanta: American Cancer Society. Reprinted with permission of the publishers.

the warning signs of head and neck cancers: sores that do not heal, chronic changes in the appearance of oral mucous membranes, persistent hoarseness or changes in voice quality, and lumps or swelling in the mouth or neck. Nurses should have a high index of suspicion about such signs and symptoms in all patients, but especially in those who are middle aged or older and those who use tobacco products or drink heavily.

Health professionals may discover asymptomatic lesions during a routine oral examination by an oral hygienist, dentist, physician, or nurse practitioner. Easy visualization of structures within the oral cavity makes identification of many precancerous or early malignant lesions possible. Although *leukoplakia* (thickened, whitish patches on the tongue or mucous membranes), has been regarded as the most common premalignant lesion, *mucosal erythroplasia* (red, inflammatory lesions) is actually the earliest visual sign of oral and pharyngeal cancers.

Unfortunately, most lesions are detected only after they increase in size and become symptomatic, and some are only visible through instrumentation or during surgery. Patients presenting with hoarseness, painful *(odynophagia)* or difficult swallowing *(dysphagia)*, or a feeling of a foreign body in the throat require immediate further evaluation.

Diagnostic examination may include direct, indirect, and fiberoptic laryngoscopy, esophagoscopy, CT scan, and biopsy of suspicious tissue.

TREATMENT

In most early-stage head and neck cancers the prognosis is very favorable. Comparable cure rates can be achieved with either surgery or radiation; each modality has advantages that must be weighed before making treatment recommendations (Table 2). Factors influencing the selection of a treatment modality include: location and extent of disease, prior treatment, the patient's general state of health, projected functional and cosmetic impairment following treatment, and the patient's preference. The goal of treatment is to produce maximal cure rates with minimal disability and disfigurement.

Table 2.   Advantages of Treatment Modalities in the Treatment of Head/Neck Cancers

Therapy	Advantages
Surgery	Limited amount of tissue exposed to treatment
	Shorter treatment time
	Avoids risk of radiation-related side effects
	Pathologic examination of tissue borders permits identification of patients with more extensive disease who require postoperative radiation therapy
	Permits later use of radiation as salvage therapy for surgical failures
Radiation therapy	Avoids operative mortality (1–2%)
	Avoids surgical resection, which may result in cosmetic or functional deformity
	Lymph nodes can be treated along with the primary site
	Permits later use of surgery as salvage therapy for radiation failures

Table 3.   Common Surgical Procedures for Cancers of the Head and Neck

Procedure	Structures involved
Neck dissection (simple, radical)	Removal of cervical lymph nodes and surrounding tissue
Composite resection	May include radical neck dissection, resection of part of floor of mouth, tongue, cheek, or tonsillar area, and mandibulectomy
Glossectomy (total, hemi-)	Removal of all or part of the tongue
Laryngectomy (total, supraglottic)	Removal of all or part of the larynx
Maxillectomy, mandibulectomy	Removal of some portion of the upper or lower jaw bone

Surgery

Large tumors or those that extend into adjacent structures may necessitate surgical resection of portions of bone, muscle, and soft tissue. Common surgical procedures are outlined in Table 3. Surgery for cancers of the head and neck may result in impaired chewing, swallowing, speech articulation, or control of saliva, as well as cosmetic defects. Through advanced surgical techniques, such defects can be reconstructed using grafts and myocutaneous flaps, allowing for improved function and appearance. Reconstruction may be performed during the initial surgery or delayed. Often, maxillofacial prosthetic devices are used to correct intraoral defects, particularly those involving the hard palate and nasal fossa. Closure of a hard palate with an obturator can prevent passage of food into the nasal fossa and improve the quality of speech.

Because of refined surgical procedures, total laryngectomy may not be necessary for some patients with laryngeal cancers. Depending on the size and location of the lesion, a less radical surgical procedure that permits preservation of parts of the laryngeal tissue and partial conservation of the natural voice may be possible.

Cryosurgery and laser excision may also help to control tumor growth. Cryosurgery is often useful in treating recurrent tumors in patients who have already had radiation. Laser excision is useful in treating small lesions.

Radiation

When adjacent lymph nodes are involved, a simple or radical neck dissection is frequently performed to prevent distant metastasis. In these patients, surgery is usually followed by radiation therapy to the involved nodes. Radiation may also be used as the primary treatment for early lesions.

In radiation therapy for head and neck cancers the principle of shrinking fields is used to minimize the toxic effects of radiation to large volumes of tissue. With this approach, the maximal dose is delivered to the tumor site while smaller doses are given to the surrounding tissue and lymph nodes. *Brachytherapy* (the use of radioactive implants) is sometimes used to supplement external beam irradiation.

All patients receiving treatment to the oral cavity and salivary glands should first obtain a dental consult, because of the potential for radiation-induced dental disease and *xerostomia*, an abnormal dryness of the mouth due to insufficient secretions. *Osteoradionecrosis* of the mandible, a necrosis of the bone following irradiation, is a potential complication of high-dose irradiation of the mandible. In severe cases that are unresponsive to conservative therapy with antibiotics and oral hygiene measures, surgical resection of involved bone may be required.

Chemotherapy

Because chemotherapy is not curative in head and neck cancers, its use is generally reserved for patients with advanced disease or those who have failed other forms of treatment. Researchers are currently exploring the role of chemotherapy as an adjunct to either surgery or radiation. When combined with surgery, chemotherapy is given preoperatively to reduce tumor size, thus permitting less extensive surgical resection and minimizing subsequent functional impairment and deformity.

Investigators are also examining the role of intra-arterial infusion of chemotherapy agents in the management of head and neck cancers. Although this approach brings higher concentrations of chemotherapeutic agents directly to the tumor site, there is a risk of catheter-related complications such as stroke, bleeding, and infection.

NURSING CONSIDERATIONS

Potential problems related to uncontrolled tumor growth include airway obstruction, difficulty with chewing and swallowing, impaired speaking ability, pain, odor, and cosmetic changes. Untreated tumors cause death through starvation, airway obstruction, or massive hemorrhage following carotid artery rupture.

Treatment itself can also result in problems that ultimately affect the patient's ability to eat or communicate, and pose a major threat to an individual's body image and sexuality. Additional problems related to surgical intervention include an increased risk of aspiration with surgery involving the hypopharynx, and possible impairment of shoulder function because of trauma to the accessory nerve during radical neck surgery.

With the current trend toward shortened hospital stays, patients with head and neck cancer are being discharged sooner to their homes or continuing care facilities. Many leave the hospital with artificial airways or feeding tubes in place, or after having only a short time to learn the new skills required to handle changes caused by treatment. Follow-up nursing care by community-based nursing agencies is extremely important if these patients are to manage at home. Nursing care may consist of regular visits for wound care, to monitor feedings or respiratory status, to provide equipment or supplies, or for further teaching of self-care skills.

There is a high incidence of subsequent new primary cancers in patients cured of their original head and neck cancer. Many of these new lesions occur in the head and neck area and may be related to continued alcohol and tobacco use. For this reason, patients should be strongly encouraged to discontinue smoking and alcohol ingestion. Support groups such as Alcoholics Anonymous or stop smoking programs may be helpful.

Alteration in Airway

Surgery to remove large tumors often results in edema of the upper airway with the need for a temporary tracheostomy. In cases where total laryngectomy is required, the patient must learn to care for a permanent tracheostomy. Nurses should assess respiratory status, manage the tracheostomy, and assist with use of an alternative means of communication while the tracheostomy is in place. When tracheostomy is used for long-term airway management, home care teaching and follow-up referral to community agencies is required. In addition, the patient may need specialized equipment following discharge.

These patients frequently experience strange sensations associated with the tube, fear of suffocation, and anxiety about not being able to talk. Nurses can increase these patients' confidence by involving them in self-care as early as possible and allowing sufficient time for learning new skills.

Altered Nutrition

Head and neck patients with advanced tumors and those with intraoral defects or swallowing problems following tumor resection may have difficulty maintaining adequate oral intake. Postoperatively, patients are frequently fed enterally (nutrition administered directly to the stomach or small intestine) to prevent stress on intraoral or pharyngeal suture lines, to reduce the risk of aspiration, or to bypass an interruption in the alimentary canal. While a nasogastric tube is most commonly employed, esophagostomy or gastrostomy/jejunostomy tubes are also used. Enteral nutrition is continued until the patient is able to safely resume oral feedings.

Nursing care involves providing high-protein liquid tube feedings and monitoring the patient for complications such as tube blockage or dislodgement, aspiration, intolerance of the feedings, and fluid and electrolyte disturbances. Many patients can be taught to administer their own feedings. If the individual is to be discharged with a feeding tube in place, commercially prepared liquid diets or blenderized foods may be administered at home. In addition, a speech pathologist or occupational therapist may be involved in retraining patients whose ability to swallow has been altered.

Wound Management

Head and neck surgery often results in swelling of the face and neck and extensive, highly visible suture lines. Nurses can reduce the distress that patients and families may initially feel at the postoperative appearance by providing preoperative explanations of normal healing and tissue response to trauma. To decrease swelling and promote healing, nurses can help the patient elevate the head, avoid constricting clothing or ties around the neck, and maintain adequate oxygen exchange and optimal nutritional status. Large wounds require suction drainage systems to prevent hematoma formation under skin flaps. If vascular flaps and grafts have been used in reconstruction, special care must be taken to avoid pressure on the flap beds and pedicles, and the neck should not be hyperextended or twisted.

Health care professionals should frequently check these wounds — like any other wounds — for evidence of impaired healing. If the patient received radiation prior to surgery, the risk of delayed healing is increased. Unusual drainage may indicate the development of a fistula. Once formed, fistulae are difficult to heal and may require additional surgery. Requirements for special wound care vary. Stress on suture lines within the oral cavity should be reduced by avoiding undue trauma from oral care, suctioning, or eating until healing has progressed. With the surgeon's permission all patients should begin a program of oral care. Wound management may also involve teaching a patient to use and care for an intraoral prosthesis.

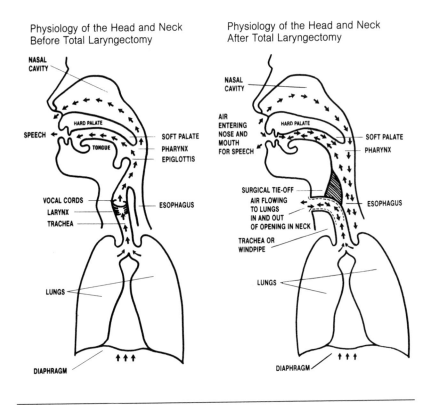

Physiology of the Head and Neck
Before Total Laryngectomy

Physiology of the Head and Neck
After Total Laryngectomy

Figure 1. Anatomical structures before and after total laryngectomy surgery.
Source: From *Rehabilitating Laryngectomies*, (pp. 5–6) 1988, Atlanta: American Cancer Society.
Reprinted with permission of the publisher.

Head and neck cancer patients with visible scars and defects and alterations in "public" functions such as eating and speaking may feel stigmatized and reluctant to resume former activities. Nurses must address concerns related to body image in order to decrease patients' isolation and promote their reintegration into the community.

Altered Communication

Loss of ability to speak, even temporarily, is one of the most frightening aspects of head and neck cancer surgery. It is vital that an alternate method of communication be devised before surgery.

Magic slates, writing tablets, picture boards, or hand signals can all be used. Since it will take longer to communicate with the patient, nurses must be sure to allocate adequate time when giving care.

The tracheostomy patient will eventually be able to speak again; the patient with glossectomy or maxillectomy frequently has problems with speech articulation and may require referral to a speech therapist. A patient undergoing total laryngectomy has lost the natural organ of speech and will have to establish another form of communication. The anatomic and functional changes that occur after total laryngectomy are illustrated in Figure 1.

Alternative forms of speech for the laryngectomy patient include esophageal speech, the use of a voice prosthesis, or the use of an external mechanical device such as the electrolarynx. A member of the Lost Chord Club can visit the patient to provide support, encouragement, and practical advice. Information about the Lost Chord Club and written materials and supplies for laryngectomy patients are available from the local American Cancer Society unit.

An additional source of information on caring for the patient with head and neck cancer is the Society of Otorhinolaryngology and Head-Neck Nurses (SOHN). Members of this national nursing organization work with head and neck cancer patients. Their address is SOHN National Headquarters, 439 N. Causeway, New Smyrna Beach, FL 32069.

Bibliography

Anderson, K. (1986). Neoplastic disorders related to respiratory function: Cancer of the larynx. In M. Patrick, W. Woods, R. Craven, J. Rokosky, & P. Bruno (Eds.), *Medical-surgical nursing: Pathophysiological concepts* (pp. 419-426). Philadelphia: J. B. Lippincott.

Baker, K. H., & Feldman, J. E. (1987). Cancers of the head and neck. *Cancer Nursing, 10*, 293-299.

Burke, J. (1989). Maintaining adequate nutrition in the head and neck patient undergoing radiation therapy. *The Journal (Official Publication of the Society of Otorhinolaryngology and Head-Neck Nurses), 7*(1), 8-11.

Droughton, M. L., & Verbic, M. (1988). Body image reintegration after head and neck surgery: Application and evaluation of three nursing interventions. *The Journal (Official Publication of the Society of Otorhinolaryngology and Head-Neck Nurses), 6*(1), 19-22.

Griffin, C. & Lockhart, S. (1987). Learning to swallow again. *American Journal of Nursing, 87*, 314-317.

Larsen, G. (1982). Rehabilitation for the patient with head and neck cancer. *American Journal of Nursing, 82*, 118-122.

Lesage, C. (1986). Carotid artery rupture: Prediction, prevention and preparation. *Cancer Nursing, 9*(1), 1-7.

Mahon, S. M. (1987). Nursing interventions for the patient with a myocutaneous flap. *Cancer Nursing, 10*, 21-31.

Metcalfe, M. C., & Fischman, S. H. (1985). Factors affecting the sexuality of patients with head and neck cancer. *Oncology Nursing Forum, 12*(2), 21-25.

Sigler, B. (1987). Nursing care for head and neck tumor patients. In S. Thawley & W. Panje (Eds.), *Comprehensive management of head and neck tumors* (pp. 79-99). Philadelphia: W. B. Saunders.

2 LUNG CANCER

Elizabeth J. White

Primary lung cancers account for 25% of all cancer deaths in the United States. Lung cancer is the leading cause of cancer deaths in both men and women. Although the incidence of lung cancer is almost two times greater for men than for women, the incidence continues to increase for women.

RISK FACTORS

The most important risk factor in the development of lung cancer is cigarette smoking, with an estimated 80-90% of cases attributable to the carcinogens in tobacco smoke. The risk of developing lung cancer is related to the age when smoking started (younger age increases the risk), the degree of inhalation, the number of packs per day, and the number of years of smoking. New research also shows a positive correlation between lung disease and exposure to secondary or passive smoke in the environment.

To help patients in their decision to quit, nurses can provide information on smoking cessation materials and resources in the community, such as American Cancer Society and American Lung Association programs. Behavioral approaches that have been helpful to those attempting to quit smoking are listed in Table 1.

Other factors associated with the development of lung cancer include exposure to industrial and environmental carcinogens: asbestos, coal tar, nickel, silver, radon, chloromethyl ethers, chromate, and vinyl chlorides. Controversy exists over the influence of genetic factors alone or in combination with pollutants in causing cancer of the lung.

PATHOLOGY

The prognosis for lung cancer is poor, with only 13% of patients surviving 5 years. This is due, in part, to the fact that approximately 80% of patients have regional or distant metastases at the time of diagnosis.

The four major types of primary lung cancers are epidermoid or squamous-cell carcinoma, adenocarcinoma, large-cell undifferentiated cancer, and small-cell or oat-cell carcinoma.

Table 1. Major Behavior Modification Strategies and Sample Activities Applied to Smoking Cessation Counseling

Strategies	Sample activities
Adversive techniques	Before quitting, associate smoking with negative consequences (e.g., use rapid smoking without inhaling, snap wrist with rubber band when desire to smoke is felt).
Self monitoring	Log cigarettes smoked using wrap-sheet around pack, recording time smoked, location and activity while smoking, and importance of cigarette. Identify smoking trigger.
Contingency management/ reinforcement	Plan daily and long-term rewards, often monetary, for taking steps towards quitting.
Stimulus control	Disrupt usual routine. Reduce or eliminate trigger situations (e.g., coffee, alcohol, smoking friends). Spend more time with non-smoking friends.
Response substitutions	Plan substitutes for smoking in trigger situations (e.g., chew gum, raw vegetables, use deep breathing. Increase positive addictions (e.g., exercise). Discard smoking paraphernalia.
Increase personal commitment to quit	Make a list of quitting benefits. Announce quit plans to family and friends. Sign a contract with self-specified quit date.
Enlist social support	Quit with a friend. Join a group program. Identify family member as helper.
Anxiety management	Learn meditation or relaxation techniques. Take 5-10 deep breaths when craving smoking. Begin regular exercise program.
Coping response training/ cognitive rehearsal	Think positively. Practice ways of turning down offered cigarettes. Have plans for common trigger situations. Rehearse non-smoking coping response for anticipated barriers. Use mental imagery, picturing self as non-smoker.

Source: From "Prevention of Lung Cancer: Stopping Smoking" by N. L. Rissner, 1987, *Seminars in Oncology Nursing, 3,* p. 231. Reprinted with permission of W. B. Saunders.

Epidermoid carcinoma accounts for approximately 40-50% of all pulmonary malignancies, and is more common in men. These tumors usually start in the periphery of the lung, and have usually invaded the large and main stem bronchi by the time they are detected. Bronchial obstruction frequently results from centrally located metastases.

Adenocarcinoma of the lung usually starts and remains in a peripheral location, making diagnosis by bronchoscope very difficult. This type of disease comprises 25% of all lung cancers, and

Table 2. Common Paraneoplastic Syndromes

Syndrome	Ectopic Substance Produced	Clinical Manifestations	Predominant Tumor Type
Inappropriate ADH Syndrome	Antidiuretic hormone (ADH)	Hyponatremia, hypo-osmolality weakness, lethargy, confusion, coma, and generalized seizures.	Small-cell
Cushing's Syndrome	Adrenocorticotropic hormone (ACTH)	Severe muscle weakness, fatigue, weight loss, metabolic alkalosis, hypokalemia, glucose intolerance, mild hypertension, hyperpigmentation.	Small-cell, Bronchial carcinoid
Hypercalcemia	Parathormone, Prostaglandins	Increased blood calcium levels, increased urinary secretion of calcium, phosphorus, and cyclic AMP, depressed blood phosphorus, increased constipation, confusion, and pain.	Squamous cell (Epidermoid)
Hypertonic osteoarthropathy, digital clubbing	Growth hormone	Digital clubbing, periostial proliferation, arthritic joint pain.	Squamous cell (Epidermoid)
Carcinoid Syndrome	Serotonin, kinins, histamine, and prostaglandins	Palpitations, facial flushing, diarrhea, abdominal cramps, wheezes, endocardial fibrosis.	Bronchial carcinoid, Small-cell

occurs more commonly in females. Frequently this type of tumor arises in areas of previous pulmonary damage or fibrosis.

Small-cell or oat-cell carcinoma accounts for 20-25% of lung tumors. It is an aggressive, centrally located tumor that usually has metastasized at the time of diagnosis. Because the cancer cells are derived from endocrine cells of the bronchial mucosa, this type of tumor can produce polypeptides that produce a variety of paraneoplastic syndromes (Table 2). These syndromes may be the first indication of the tumor's presence.

Approximately 10% of lung cancers are classified as large-cell undifferentiated cancers. These appear most frequently in the peripheral lung, with pleural and regional nodal involvement.

The most common sites of metastases for lung cancers are brain, bone, liver, cervical lymph nodes, adrenal glands, and kidneys.

Lung Cancer Manifestations

1. Cough that becomes chronic
2. Dry cough that becomes productive
3. Unilateral wheezing
4. Dyspnea
5. Pneumonia
6. Chest pain or pain in shoulder and arm (invasion of the brachial plexus by tumor)
7. Hemoptysis
8. Vocal cord paralysis
9. Atelectasis
10. Neurologic changes
11. Weight loss

Figure 1.   Clinical manifestations of lung cancer that cause people to seek medical attention.

CLINICAL MANIFESTATIONS

Lung cancers do not usually produce symptoms at the outset; early detection, therefore, is uncommon. In many cases, patients will seek medical attention only if they are experiencing one of more of the problems identified in Figure 1. Presenting symptoms are generally related to the location of the primary tumor within the lung or to metabolic abnormalities secondary to ectopic hormone production by cancer cells.

Screening programs of the general population have not been effective in detecting early lung cancers.

DIAGNOSIS

The procedures involved in the diagnostic workup for lung cancer are found in Table 3. It is particularly important to distinguish between *small-cell carcinoma of the lung* and *non-small cell carcinomas* during diagnosis because treatment approaches are different.

TREATMENT

Surgery

Surgical resection is the most effective treatment for early, local, non-small cell carcinomas of the lung. Lobectomy is the most commonly used procedure, although pneumonectomy or segmental or wedge resections may be performed. Non-small cell carcinoma is considered unresectable if esophageal obstruction, me-

Table 3.   Tests Used in the Diagnostic Work-up of Lung Cancer

Test name	Procedure
Chest radiograph (x-ray)	Posteroanterior and lateral views taken. The primary tool in diagnosing lung cancer.
Exfoliative cytologic sputum study	Microscopic examination of sloughed-off cells found in the sputum or in brush specimens or bronchial washings. Special fixative is added before the sample is centrifuged, processed, and examined.
Chest tomography & computed tomographic scanning (CT Scan)	Three-dimensional x-ray used to outline the size, shape, and location of the tumor and to evaluate enlargement of hilar and mediastinal lymph nodes. Brain and bone scans may be done if symptoms are present or if the cell type is small-cell carcinoma.
Bronchoscopy	A flexible fiberoptic instrument is passed through the throat into the bronchials, thus permitting direct visualization of centrally located tumors. Biopsies or brushings and washing for cytology can be obtained.
Lymph node biopsy	Sampling of supraclavicular fossa nodes, scalene nodes, or mediastinal nodes for histological examination. Primarily used for the staging of the tumor. Procedures can include mediastinoscopy and thoracoscopy.
Liver function test	Routine lab work. Radionuclide liver scan is done if results are abnormal or the liver is enlarged.
Bone marrow biopsy	A bone marrow sample is taken to determine whether or not small-cell carcinoma has spread.

diastinal or chest wall involvement, or distant metastases are present. In these patients, radiation or chemotherapy is used.

Surgery is not indicated for most patients with small cell carcinoma of the lung; however, the role of surgery either before or after chemotherapy to manage limited disease in selected patients is being explored.

Preoperative teaching begins as soon as the choice of surgical treatment has been determined. Nurses should provide instruction to patients on pulmonary exercises, upper and lower extremity exercises, modified postural drainage, coughing, and the use of equipment such as nebulizers. The effects of anesthesia and the loss of lung tissue when resection is performed place patients at an increased risk for postoperative respiratory complications.

Pain limits mobility as well as a patient's ability to perform coughing and deep breathing exercises, so pain management techniques must be employed after surgery. If pain should increase or change locations, the possibility of other complications such as infection, pulmonary emobolism, and thrombophlebitis should be considered.

Radiation Therapy

Although radiotherapy is sometimes used pre- or postoperatively for patients with non-small cell carcinoma of the lung, no survival advantage has been confirmed with either of these approaches. For patients with unresectable, localized non-small cell carcinomas, radiation in curative doses is given as a single treatment modality. The dose of radiation that can be administered is limited by the tolerance of the lung parenchyma and heart tissue. Divided or split-course treatment is frequently used to minimize effects of radiation and allow for a higher overall treatment dose (See Unit III, Chapter 2).

In patients with limited small-cell carcinoma of the lung, radiation may be given following chemotherapy to decrease local recurrences in the chest. This approach remains controversial because of its associated toxicity. Because of the risk of disease recurrence in the brain, prophylactic cranial radiation may be given to small-cell carcinoma patients who have responded completely to their initial treatment and are likely candidates for prolonged, disease-free survival.

Radiotherapy is used for palliation of local symptoms (e.g., bronchial obstruction, bone pain) in patients with extensive disease, regardless of tumor type.

Side effects of radiation therapy for lung cancer include esophagitis, radiation pneumonitis, skin changes, anorexia, and fatigue. Esophagitis resulting in *dysphagia* and pain may occur when the esophagus is in the treatment field. Dyclone® or viscous Xylocaine® can be administered before the patient eats to provide comfort and to improve food and fluid intake. Soft foods and liquid dietary supplements help provide calories and protein needed during treatment.

Acute radiation pneumonitis is characterized by dyspnea, hacking cough, and mild chest discomfort. Symptoms usually subside after 3-4 weeks, although larger radiation doses can result in permanent fibrotic changes. If pulmonary fibrosis occurs, symptoms develop several weeks to months after treatment. Since there is no cure for this complication, patients must learn to deal with diminished pulmonary function. The nurse should work with the physician and respiratory therapist to implement an appropriate pulmonary rehabilitation program (such as pursed lip breathing) and a progressive exercise program to improve endurance and enhance quality of life.

Cardiac toxicity is related to dose and the percentage of the heart in the radiation field. Shielding helps to reduce the incidence of cardiac damage. Cardiac toxicity increases when the patient receives both heart irradiation and chemotherapy with doxorubicin.

Chemotherapy

Patients with all stages of small-cell carcinoma of the lung are treated with aggressive, combination chemotherapy regimens. Combinations of cyclophosphamide, doxorubicin, vincristine, cisplatin, and VP-16 are most frequently used. These regimens have improved 2-year survival in patients with limited disease. Even patients with extensive disease have exhibited response rates of 75-85%; however, the duration of these has been short, and overall survival has not changed.

By combining cisplatin-containing chemotherapy regimens with surgery, the survival of patients with locally advanced non-small cell carcinomas of the lung can be prolonged. This chemotherapy is most commonly given following surgical resection. Recent studies have also suggested that preoperative chemotherapy can reduce unresectable disease to such an extent that it is operable.

Toxicity increases with the number of drugs used; therefore aggressive combination chemotherapy tends to make patients more acutely ill. Additional information on chemotherapy and symptom management can be found in Unit III, Chapter 3 and Unit IV, Chapter 1.

NURSING MANAGEMENT OF ADVANCED LUNG CANCER

Nursing interventions for patients with advanced lung cancers are aimed at decreasing the respiratory problems they experience, including dyspnea, cough, and hemoptysis.

Obstruction of airways or restriction of lung expansion most frequently leads to dyspnea for lung cancer patients, although postobstructive pneumonitis, atelectasis, pleural effusions, and treatment-related problems may also contribute to this problem. Immediate coping strategies include positioning, moving slower, use of inhalers, administration of medications, and pursed lip breathing. Distraction, meditation, guided imagery, and relaxation techniques may also be helpful in combating anxiety associated with painful breathing. Long-term adaptive strategies such as changing or decreasing the activities of daily living, transferring them to others, or scheduling them at different times of day are useful methods of conserving energy.

Other general nursing measures include increasing the patient's fluid intake to thin out secretions and educating patients about the appropriate purpose, dose, and side effects of medications used to treat dyspnea. *Anxiolytics* used during acute episodes of dyspnea can decrease the anxiety that exacerbates it. *Beta antagonists* provide symptomatic relief for patients with underlying chronic obstructive pulmonary disease. Low-dose narcotics reduce the respiratory drive and provide comfort without producing significant respiratory depression. Glucocorticosteroids like prednisone reduce edema and bronchospasm. Atropine or scopolamine can be used to dry secretions distal to an obstruction or terminal airway obstruction (death rattle).

Low flow home oxygen is indicated for patients with significant hypoxia. If the patient's blood gases are normal, insufficient oxygen in the blood is not a problem and supplemental oxygen will not help. The patient and family members may need assistance in understanding why oxygen will not be useful.

Hemoptysis, blood-tinged sputum from the lungs, is not uncommon with lung cancer patients. It results from capillary trauma, tumor sloughing, or pulmonary infection. Radiation therapy may be used to stop moderate hemoptysis. Major life-threatening hemorrhage may occur in advanced lung cancer. Whether a family decides on hospitalization or chooses to care for the patient at home, it is important that nurses help families in developing an emergency plan to reduce anxiety and increase feelings of security in the event of hemorrhage. Hemorrhage is a rare occurrence but a common fear for patients and their families when hemoptysis is present.

A cough, which frequently accompanies lung cancer, can be caused by infection, inflammation, or the tumor pressing against the bronchi or trachea. Persistent coughing disrupts sleep, increases musculoskeletal chest pain and hemoptysis, and aggravates nausea, vomiting, and anxiety. A cough may lead to pathologic rib fractures, which are an additional risk for patients with metastatic lesions to the bone or those using prednisone on a long-term basis. Since a cough is one indicator of pulmonary infection, antibiotics are appropriate for acute respiratory tract infection. Antipyretics, cough suppressants, hydration, and humidification of secretions may reduce coughing.

Bibliography

Brown, M. L., Carrieri, V., Janson-Bjerklie, S., & Dodd, M. J. (1986). Lung cancer and dyspnea: The patient's perspective. *Oncology Nursing Forum, 13*(5), 19-23.

Foote, M., Sexton, D., & Pawlik, L. (1986). Dyspnea: A distressing sensation in lung cancer. *Oncology Nursing Forum, 13*(5), 25-31.

Griffiths, M. J., Murray, K. H., & Russo, P. C. (Eds.). (1984). Cancer of the lung and mediastinum. In *Oncology nursing: Pathophysiology, assessment and intervention.* (pp.184-199), New York: MacMillan Publishing Company.

Livingston, R. (1986). Current chemotherapy of small cell lung cancer. *Chest, 89*(4), 258s-263s.

Maxwell, M. (1985). Dyspnea in advanced cancer. *American Journal of Nursing, 85,* 672-677.

Norton, L. C. (1985). Oxygenation and ventilation. In B. L. Johnson & J. Gross (Eds.), *Handbook of oncology nursing* (pp. 381-389). New York: John Wiley and Sons.

Owens, A. H., & Abeloff, M. D. (1985). Neoplasms in the lung. In P. Calabresi, P. S. Schein & S. A. Rosenberg (Eds.), *Medical oncoiogy: Basic principles and clinical management of cancer* (pp. 715-757). New York: MacMillian Publishing Company.

Pearson, F. G. (1986). Lung cancer: The past twenty-five years. *Chest Supplement, 89*(April), 200s-205s.

Risser, N. L. (1987). Prevention of lung cancer: Stopping smoking. *Seminars in Oncology Nursing, 3*(3), 228-236.

White, E. (1987). Home care of the patient with advanced lung cancer. *Seminars in Oncology Nursing, 3*(3), 216-221.

3 ESOPHAGEAL AND GASTRIC CANCER

Teresa Coluccio

ESOPHAGEAL CANCER

Esophageal cancer accounts for approximately 1.5% of all malignancies in the United States. The overall prognosis for this disease is poor, with only 5% of patients surviving 5 years after diagnosis. The bleak outlook is partly because most esophageal neoplasms have spread beyond local control when they are diagnosed.

Esophageal cancer occurs most commonly in males over age 60. The mortality rate is higher in white males than white females, and highest in black males. In addition, esophageal cancer occurs more frequently in certain geographic areas of the world, including Japan, China, Russia, Scotland, the Caspian region of Iran, and parts of eastern and southern Africa.

Risk Factors

Specific causes of esophageal cancer have not been clearly documented. However, alcohol ingestion is generally accepted as a potent risk factor, and this risk is potentiated when combined with smoking. Chronic irritation caused by a hiatal hernia and reflux esophagitis has also been implicated. Ingestion of lye or other caustic agents may also be a contributing factor. Several dietary factors have been suggested as risk factors, including heavy food seasoning, hot foods and beverages, betel nut products, and deficiencies or excesses of trace metals and vitamins.

Pathology

Approximately 90% of esophageal cancers are squamous cell (or epidermoid) tumors. The remainder are adenocarcinomas; sarcomas, small-cell cancers, and lymphomas rarely occur. Approximately 15% of these malignancies occur in the upper third of the esophagus, 50% in the middle third, and 35% in the lower third. The lymph nodes and mediastinum become involved early in the disease, and frequently the tumors are locally advanced before producing symptoms. Distant metastases are probably microscopically present at diagnosis, but do not become clinically apparent until late in the disease or at autopsy. Most commonly the liver, lungs, adrenals, bone, or kidneys are involved.

Clinical Presentation

Early symptoms of esophageal cancer are usually vague and rarely reported. Initial symptoms include a sense of pressure, indigestion, and substernal distress. As the disease progresses, dysphagia and weight loss are the most common complaints. Patients may change their diet from solids to liquids to compensate for their swallowing difficulty; eventually, even liquids may become difficult. Aspiration of food or liquids leads to aspiration pneumonia. A tracheoesophageal (T-E) fistula can occur. Tumor can encroach into nerve systems, causing hoarseness, hiccups, or paralysis of the arm or diaphragm.

Diagnostic Tests

Barium esophagram and *computerized tomography* (CT) are often used to delineate the gross appearance of the tumor. Tissue for cytologic and microscopic examination is obtained by *esophagoscopy*. Laryngoscopy and bronchoscopy may also be performed to evaluate the extent of tumor spread into the tracheobronchial tree.

Treatment

Because surgery alone has proven inadequate in the management of esophageal cancer, aggressive, combined modality therapy is being used in an attempt to improve treatment results. Surgery is often combined with radiation or chemotherapy to decrease the extent of surgical resection, treat areas that are not easily resectable, or reduce the chance of distant metastases from residual microscopic disease following surgery.

Patients who are candidates for curative treatment should be free of accompanying cardiac, renal, and pulmonary diseases; nutritionally stable; and have a localized tumor that is not fixed to adjacent structures.

Surgery: The surgical approach to lesions of the cervical esophagus, or upper third, usually includes resection of the entire larynx, thyroid, and a portion of the proximal esophagus. A unilateral radical neck dissection may also be performed if cervical lymph nodes are clinically involved. Usually, the stomach is pulled up and anastomosed to the posterior pharynx. The severe cosmetic defect resulting from surgery usually necessitates reconstructive procedures. Reconstruction may include the use of full-thickness skin grafts, formation of a gastric tube from the greater curvature of the stomach, or (less commonly) interposition of a segment of the colon.

Esophagectomy is recommended for lesions of the thoracic esophagus, or middle and lower third. The lower two-thirds of the esophagus and proximal stomach are removed, because many lesions extend into the stomach. The remaining stomach is then pulled up and anastomosed to the cervical esophagus.

Causes of morbidity following esophageal resection include anastomotic leaks, fistulae, strictures, pulmonary emboli, respiratory insufficiency, congestive heart failure, and wound infections or dehiscence. Preoperative conditions, such as poor nutritional status, can also contribute to operative morbidity.

Nursing care in the postoperative period focuses on preventing respiratory complications and protecting the integrity of the anastomotic site. Nurses should assess the suture line for evidence of a fistula, including signs of inflammation, drainage, and edema. The suture line can be damaged if suction catheters are introduced into or manipulated within the oropharyngeal cavity without knowing the location of the suture line. Pulmonary complications may dictate nasotracheal suctioning and will require extreme caution.

Reflux aspiration can occur when patients begin oral food intake after surgery. Because the normal peristaltic movement is diminished in the surgically altered esophagus, the patient needs to assist gravity to propel food into the stomach. Elevating the head of the bed to 45° even at home, ingesting food slowly, and decreasing liquids at bedtime will help prevent reflux.

In patients who have had a portion of the colon used for esophageal reconstruction, the bowel is prepared with cathartics and antibiotics before surgery to minimize the chance of infection by colonic bacterial flora. But these patients may have fecal-smelling breath despite bowel decontamination procedures. Oral hygiene and a diet aimed at reducing gas may assist in the management of this problem.

Radiation therapy: Patients who are not candidates for aggressive, combined modality treatment, such as those with inadequate cardiopulmonary function, may be treated with radiation therapy. The treatment period is prolonged, lasting 6 to 8 weeks. Treatment-induced esophagitis can be severe, requiring systemic analgesics, parenteral nutrition, and antifungal medications.

More frequently, radiation therapy is used in conjunction with surgery to improve treatment results. Preoperative radiotherapy has been used successfully to reduce tumor bulk, thereby decreasing the extent of the surgical resection and lessening the accompanying surgical risk. Postoperative irradiation is used most commonly to treat residual macroscopic or microscopic disease in unresected portions of the esophagus or at the margins of the resection. It can also be used palliatively in patients found to have unresectable disease during surgery.

Chemotherapy: Combination drug regimens administered in addition to radiotherapy and surgery are currently being evaluated. Agents that have shown some activity against esophageal cancer include methotrexate, cisplatin, 5-fluorouracil (5-FU), mitomycin C, lomustine (CCNU), doxorubicin, cyclophosphamide, and bleomycin.

Palliation: Patients with advanced or unresectable esophageal cancer may be treated to palliate pain and dysphagia and to maintain esophageal patency for food passage.

Both radiation and surgery may be used to relieve impending obstruction caused by tumor growth. In addition to using these traditional therapies, some institutions are currently using *endoscopic laser therapy* as local treatment for esophageal obstruction. This therapy provides short-term local control by vaporizing tumor tissue. Complications of this technique include perforation of the esophagus, bleeding, and fistula formation. Following any procedure to establish lumen patency, the esophagus must be dilated repeatedly to maintain patency.

To provide adequate nutrition when esophageal continuity is interrupted, a feeding gastrostomy tube can be surgically inserted. This procedure may assure adequate caloric intake, but does not treat the patient's inability to handle oral secretions. Also, a number of synthetic endoesophageal tubes have been designed to maintain a patent passage for swallowing. These are used primarily in patients who are very debilitated or have T-E fistulae or invasion of surrounding structures.

GASTRIC CANCER

Gastric cancer accounts for about 3% of all cancer deaths in the United States, but its incidence has steadily declined in this country over the past four decades. Japan and Chile, however, continue to have a very high incidence of this disease. These differences in geographic distribution remain unexplained but are generally considered to be related to the environment. In the United States and western Europe, stomach cancer occurs more frequently in lower socioeconomic groups.

Risk Factors

Dietary factors may increase the risk of developing gastric cancer: a higher incidence of this disease is noted with increased consumption of smoked and salted foods, and foods contaminated with aflatoxin.

Gastric metaplasia and dysplasia have also been associated with the development of gastric carcinoma. However, a history of gastric ulcers contributes little to the risk of this type of cancer. Also, people with blood type A may have a slightly higher risk for some types of gastric carcinoma.

Pathology

Approximately 95% of stomach cancers are epithelial tumors, predominantely adenocarcinomas. Uncommon gastric tumors include carcinoid, lymphoma, leiomyosarcoma, and lymphoid types. Approximately 50% of stomach cancers are located in the antrum and pyloric region. Disease spreads by extension along the stomach wall, through the lymphatics or the blood stream, or by direct extension to adjacent structures. The most common sites of metastasis are the liver, peritoneum, pancreas, lung, and bone.

Clinical Presentation

Vague complaints of anorexia, early satiety, weight loss, bloating, nausea, and pain are the presenting features in most cases of gastric cancer. Often, patients use home remedies and self-medication to successfully treat these symptoms for a period of time. Only symptoms of advanced disease, such as progressive weight loss, weakness, and anemia, may prompt patients to seek medical intervention. A palpable abdominal mass is usually a late physical finding. Patients may also present with ulcer-like symptoms, hemorrhage, obstruction, or symptoms related to metastatic disease.

Diagnosis

Initial screening usually involves a barium upper gastrointestinal series to evaluate the stomach for evidence of a mass. Endoscopy is then routinely done to better visualize the lesion and obtain tissue for cytologic examination. Levels of tumor markers such as *carcinoembryonic antigen* (CEA) and *alpha fetoprotein* (AFP) are of limited value in the diagnosis and follow-up of gastric cancer, because these values may be elevated in other benign and malignant diseases.

Treatment

The treatment for gastric cancer depends on the stage of disease and may incorporate a combined modality approach. Localized gastric cancers are usually treated with surgical resection, sometimes in combination with chemotherapy and/or radiotherapy.

Surgery: The extent of surgery depends on the location of the cancer within the stomach. Tumors located in the upper proximal portion of the stomach may be resected by a *subtotal esophagogastrectomy*. This operation consists of removal of the lower portion of the esophagus and resection of the cardia, fundus, and the body of the stomach. In addition, the supporting circulatory and lymphatic structures and the greater and lesser omenta are removed. The remaining esophagus is sutured to the duodenum or jejunum.

A total gastrectomy is usually performed for lesions located in the mid-portion of the stomach. The esophagus is then anastomosed to the jejunum. Lesions located in the antrum, or lower portion of the stomach, are treated by subtotal gastrectomy, using either a *Bilroth I* or *Bilroth II* procedure.

Immediate postoperative concerns include prevention of respiratory complications, infection, hemorrhage, and anastomotic leak. Patients who undergo gastric surgery may be affected by the *dumping syndrome* after the operation. This syndrome is caused by the sudden influx of hypertonic fluid into the jejunum when the stomach has been resected. This stimulus produces generalized vasodilation, resulting in hypotension, dizziness, nausea, pallor, pain, and sweating. Nurses need to counsel patients with dumping syndrome about diet and eating habits to minimize related symptoms. They should be instructed to eat foods low in carbohydrates and fat and high in protein. Fluids should be restricted 30 minutes before meals. Several small dry meals—up to six a day—can help to decrease the incidence of symptoms.

Patients with total or subtotal gastrectomies will eventually develop a vitamin B_{12} deficiency once their liver stores of vitamin B_{12} have been depleted. These patients will require lifelong monthly administration of intramuscular vitamin B_{12}.

Radiation therapy: Gastric and intestinal mucous membranes tolerate the effects of irradiation poorly. Nausea, esophagitis, and diarrhea are frequently observed following intestinal radiation. As a result, radiotherapy is rarely used as the sole treatment modality because of the difficulty in administering curative doses without unacceptable gastrointestinal toxicity.

More commonly, radiation therapy is combined with surgery or chemotherapy for patients with unresectable, partially unresectable, or recurrent disease. When combined with surgery, radiation may be given preoperatively, intraoperatively, or postoperatively. The sequencing of these two modalities remains controversial. Radiotherapy administered with 5-FU has been shown to be more effective than either radiotherapy or chemotherapy alone in prolonging survival.

Chemotherapy: The use of chemotherapy in the treatment of gastric cancer is primarily limited to patients with unresectable or metastatic disease, although adjuvant chemotherapy following surgical resection is being evaluated for its role in improving survival. Combination chemotherapy regimens appear to be more successful than single agents. When 5-FU is combined with doxorubicin and mitomycin C or with the nitrosoureas, survival time is slightly increased.

Palliative care: In advanced gastric cancer, nutritional maintenance becomes a serious problem. The resulting malnutrition and weight loss decrease the patient's ability to withstand the rigors of therapy, resist infection, and perform self-care activities. Patients with unresectable obstructing gastric cancer can obtain palliative nutrition through double lumen tubes placed by endoscopy. One lumen allows the obstructed gastric fluid to drain; the second is placed in the jejunum for tube feedings. The nurse can greatly support the individual during this difficult time when cure is no longer realistic and health care goals turn from treatment to promotion of comfort and maintenance of autonomy.

Bibliography

American Cancer Society. (1990). *Cancer facts and figures—1990.* Atlanta, GA; American Cancer Society.

Boyce, H. W. Jr. (1982). Approaches to management of cancer of the esophagus. *Hospital Practice, 17*(11), 109-112, 117-118, 121.

Casciato, D., & Lowitz, B. (1983). *Manual of bedside oncology.* Boston: Little, Brown & Co.

Frogge, M. (1987). Gastrointestinal malignancies: Esophagus, stomach, pancreas, and liver. In S. Groenwald (Ed.), *Cancer nursing principles and practice* (pp. 508-543). Boston: Jones and Bartlett Publisher, Inc.

Macdonald, J. S., Steele, G. Jr., & Gunderson, L. L. (1989). Cancer of the stomach. In V. T. DeVita Jr., S. Hellman, & S. A. Rosenberg (Eds.), *Cancer: Principles and practice of oncology* (pp. 765-799). Philadelphia: J. B. Lippincott Co.

Mackety, C. (1985). Esophageal cancer palliation with endoscopic lasers. *Today's OR Nurse, 7*(12), 34-39.

Marshall, C. (1984). Celestin tube. *Nursing Mirror, 159*(4), 50-1.

Rosenberg, J. C., Lichter, A. S., & Leichman, L. P. (1989). Cancer of the esophagus. In V. T. DeVita Jr., S. Hellman, & S. A. Rosenberg (Eds.), *Cancer: Principles and practice of oncology* (pp. 725-764). Philadelphia: J. B. Lippincott Co.

4 COLORECTAL CANCER

Carol Sun Redfield and Nancy Reilly

INCIDENCE

Cancer of the colon and rectum, often called colorectal cancer, is one of the most common malignancies in the United States. It affects both sexes equally and occurs approximately as often in blacks as in whites. Colorectal cancer, which is second only to lung cancer in mortality, causes an estimated 61,000 deaths in the United States each year.

Five-year survival for both colon and rectal cancers has improved in the past 20 years, but remains just over 50% for all stages of disease combined. When their disease is detected in an early, localized state, 87% of colon cancer patients and 79% of rectal cancer patients survive 5 years or more, compared with 58% and 46%, respectively, of patients with locally advanced or metastatic disease. The statistics support the need for screening and early detection programs.

RISK FACTORS

Advanced age is strongly associated with the development of colorectal cancer: the incidence increases after age 40, and more than 94% of all cases occur after age 50. Individuals at greater risk of developing colorectal cancer include those with a history of familial polyposis, familial cancer syndromes, inflammatory bowel disease, or villous adenomatous polyps.

Research indicates that diet may play a role in the development of this cancer, possibly affecting the interaction of carcinogens with the intestinal mucosa. Increased intake of dietary fats has been linked to greater incidence of colorectal cancer. High-fiber diets on the other hand, may work in several ways to decrease cancer risk— perhaps by protecting the intestinal mucosa from carcinogens that pass through the bowel.

DETECTION AND DIAGNOSIS

Figure 1 illustrates the relative distribution of cancers within the colon and rectum. Symptoms vary according to the location of the tumor. The most common symptoms are rectal bleeding, a

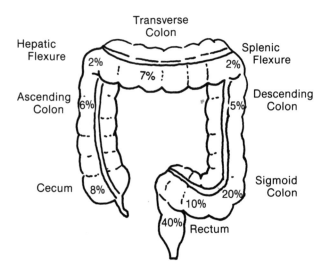

Figure 1. Cancer incidence. Two-thirds of all colorectal cancers occur in the rectosigmoid and the rectum. Many of these cancers are within reach of the examining finger, and 50% are within the reach of a sigmoidoscope.
Source: From "Nursing Management of the Patient with Colon and Rectal Cancer" by D. M. Otte, 1988, *Seminars in Oncology Nursing, 4*(4), p. 286. Reprinted with permission of Grune and Stratton.

change in bowel habits, abdominal pain or cramping, and unexplained weight loss or anemia. The American Cancer Society recommends reporting any of these symptoms to a physician, as well as the following procedures for asymptomatic individuals: annual digital rectal exams beginning at age 40, annual testing of stool for occult blood beginning at age 50, and sigmoidoscopy every 3 to 5 years on the advice of a physician starting at age 50. Because early detection can improve colorectal cancer survival rates, nurses play an important role in educating the public about the importance of early diagnosis.

The stool guaiac, or hemoccult, test is inexpensive and can be done either at the doctor's office or at home. This test is not specific for cancer, and therefore should be performed in conjunction with the annual rectal examination and sigmoidoscopy.

Sigmoidoscopy permits inspection and biopsy of suspicious tissues of the rectum and left side of the colon. There are two types of sigmoidoscopes: rigid and flexible. The rigid sigmoidoscope is an inexpensive and disposable 20 cm device that can provide visualization of up to 18 cm of the rectal mucosa. The flexible sigmoidoscope is a 35 to 65 cm device that can provide visualization of up to 2 to 3 times more of the colon than the rigid sigmoidoscope. If an experienced physician performs a *colonoscopy*, another colon examination procedure, the entire colon can be visualized. The sigmoidoscope and colonoscope can also be used to remove suspicious polyps.

A barium enema is often indicated to evaluate an unexplained abdominal mass, iron-deficiency anemia (with occult blood in stools), or overt rectal bleeding without an obvious site of active bleeding in the rectum or anus.

Carcinoembryonic antigen (CEA) is a tumor marker measured in a blood sample that may indicate the presence of colorectal cancer. Because CEA is not specific for colorectal cancers, it is more commonly used to evaluate response to treatment or disease recurrence.

Evaluation of the extent of disease may also require a chest film, liver scan, computerized axial tomography (CT) scan of the abdomen and pelvis, and laparotomy. Pretreatment evaluation will also include obtaining a history of polyps, colorectal cancer, and other cancers.

PATHOPHYSIOLOGY

Most colorectal cancers are adenocarcinomas. They begin in the bowel mucosa and spread through the bowel wall to the peritoneal surface. The liver is the most common site of distant metastases, followed by the lung. Prognosis depends on the extent of invasion of the bowel wall and the number of disease-affected lymph nodes.

Several staging systems are used in colorectal cancers. Most are variations of the Dukes' classification, which categorizes this disease according to the depth of anatomic spread and presence or absence of lymph node metastasis. In the Dukes' Systems (1932), "A" refers to tumor limited to the submucosa, "B" refers to tumor invasion into or through the bowel wall but with negative nodes, and "C" refers to tumor with lymph node metastasis. A modification of the Dukes' system is the more detailed Astler-Coller System (1954). Table 1 outlines the commonly used staging systems.

TREATMENT

Surgery

Historically, surgery has been the primary treatment for colorectal cancers. In potentially curable colon cancers, the extent of bowel dissection is determined by the biology of local tumor growth and

Table 1. Stage Classification and Stage Grouping in Carcinoma of the colorectum

AJCC 1982*	UICC 1978 (3rd ed)	Dukes (1932, 1935)†	Astler-Coller‡
Stage 0 Carcinoma in situ TIS N_0 M_0	Stage 0 TIS, N_0, M_0		Stage 0 0
Stage I IA Tumor confined to mucosa or submucosa T_1, N_0, M_0 1B Tumor involves muscularis propria but not beyond T_2, N_0, M_0	Stage I 1A T_1, N_0, M_0 1B T_2, N_0, M_0	A A	Stage I A A B1
Stage II Involvement of all layers of bowel wall with or without invasion of immediately adjacent structures T_3, N_0, M_0	Stage II T_3, T_4, N_0, M_0 (T_{3a} with fistula) (T_{3b} without fistula)	B	Stage II B2
Stage III Any degree of bowel wall with regional node metastasis Any T, N_{1-3}, M_0 Extends beyond contiguous tissue or immediately adjacent organs with with no regional lymph node metastasis T_4, N_0, M_0	Stage III Any T, N_1, M_0	C (1932) C1 (1935) C2 (1935)	Stage III C1 C2
Stage IV Any invasion of bowel wall with or without regional lymph node metastasis but with evidence of distant metastasis Any T, any N, M_1	Stage IV Any T, any N, M_1	Type 4 (so-called D)	Stage IV D

*From American Joint Committee on Cancer: Manual for Staging of Cancer, (2nd Ed.) (p. 73), by OH Behrs and MH Myers (Eds), 1983, Philadelphia, JB Lippincott Co.

†Dukes: A, Limited to bowel wall; B, Spread to extramural tissue; C, Involvement of regional nodes (C1: Near primary lesions; C2: Proximal node involved at point of ligation); Type 4 (so-called D), Distant metastasis.

‡Astler-Coller: A, Limited to mucosa; B1, Same as AJCC Stage 1B (T_{2a}); B2, Same as AJCC Stage 1B (T_{2b}); C1, Limited to wall with involved nodes; C2, Through all layers of wall with involved nodes.

Source: From Cancer Treatment, (p. 283), 2nd Ed. From C.M. Haskall, Philadelphia: W. B. Saunders. Reprinted with permission of the publisher.

Table 2. Summary of Site-Specific Surgical Approaches in Colorectal Cancer

Tumor Location	Usual Procedure
Cecum/Ascending Colon	Right hemicolectomy with anastomosis.
Hepatic Flexure	Extended right hemicolectomy with anastomosis.
Transverse Colon	Usually resection of all colon proximal to the descending colon. A more limited transverse colectomy may also be done.
Splenic Flexure	As with transverse colon lesions, an extensive resection of all proximal colon generally is preferred. Care is taken to avoid an unnecessary splenectomy as this can adversely affect survival.
Descending Colon	A left hemicolectomy with high ligature of the inferior mesenteric artery and vein.
Sigmoid	Wide sigmoid resection.
Rectum—upper third	Anterior or low anterior resection. Bowel continuity is restorable.
—middle third	Abdominal perineal resection with permanent colostomy or sphincter-saving resection.
—lower third	Abdominal perineal resection with permanent colostomy.

Source: From "Colorectal Cancer," by A. M. Cohen, B. Shank, and M. A. Friedman, 1989, In V. T. DeVita, S. Hellman, and S. A. Rosenberg, (Eds.), *Cancer: Principles and Practice of Oncology,* (pp. 920–923). Philadelphia: J. B. Lippincott Co. Adapted with permission of publisher.

the extent of lymphadenectomy. Lymph nodes are dissected for both staging and therapeutic reasons. Surgery is usually fairly site-specific. General guidelines for operative resection are summarized in Table 2. Poor survival rates among patients with locally extensive or metastatic disease treated only with surgery have prompted studies combining surgery with other treatment modalities.

Ostomies: A permanent colostomy is seldom needed for cancers of the colon or upper one-third of the rectum, because improved surgical techniques permit end-to-end anastomosis of the remaining intestine at a lower level than previously possible. In some cases, the physician will create a temporary colostomy during surgery to divert fecal flow until the anastomosis site has adequately healed. Patients and families often have grave concerns about the possibility of a colostomy. They need to know that the majority of colorectal cancers can be treated without an ostomy.

An enterostomal therapy (ET) nurse is often available to work with patients requiring colostomies. The ET nurse works closely with the staff to assess the patient's emotional disposition and plan for a smooth transition from diagnosis to rehabilitation. Preoperatively, the ET nurse explains to the patient what can be expected with a colostomy. This nurse also discusses the placement of the stoma site with the surgeon, since placement has a large impact on overall colostomy management. Other issues the ET nurse addresses include: patient acceptance; handling elimination (via pouch system or irrigation); obtaining ostomy equipment; dietary management; and special problems related to consistency of the stool, passage of flatus, and odor control.

Surgical Complications: The most common complication of bowel surgery is infection. For this reason, thorough preoperative evacuation of stool and prophylactic administration of antibiotics pre and postoperatively are important to prevent infection.

Obstruction and perforation are serious complications of colorectal cancer. These can occur as a manifestation of initial or recurring disease or as a result of adhesions from surgery. In addition, certain surgical procedures involving pelvic structures can cause sexual dysfunction. For example, partial to complete sexual dysfunction in males is commonplace after abdominal perineal resection. The wide dissection necessary involves the nerves governing sexual function. Retrograde ejaculation occurs after pelvic surgery. In females, dysfunction after surgery is less common but may occur from post-surgical scarring or contractures. For further information on other aspects of sexual function related to radiation or chemotherapy, see Unit IV, Chapter 5. The health care team should discuss possible complications with patients before surgery.

Radiation Therapy

The disease site may be externally irradiated before, during, or after surgery, depending on the extent of disease. The sequencing of surgery and radiation in combination therapy remains controversial. Preoperatively, radiotherapy may reduce the size of the tumor and improve resectability. Theorectically, preoperative administration also reduces the number of cancer cells that can spread locally or to distant sites during surgery.

The major advantage of postoperative radiotherapy is that surgical staging can be incorporated into treatment planning. After surgery, the tumor bed and involved lymph nodes or the whole abdomen is irradiated to decrease local recurrences from residual microscopic disease.

Patients with locally advanced rectal cancers or recurrent disease may receive intra-operative radiotherapy. This technique permits delivery of a larger dose (sometimes referred to as a boost) directly to the tumor bed while minimizing the dose to normal tissues. Radiotherapy is often the primary modality for cases in which surgery poses an unsuitable risk or is refused. Radiation may also be employed palliatively to relieve pain, obstruction, and hemorrhage.

Chemotherapy

Chemotherapy is generally reserved for patients with advanced inoperable or recurrent disease, but adjuvant chemotherapy may be used for patients with resectable tumors who are at risk for recurrent disease. This approach has improved disease-free survival in several large studies. Researchers are also studying perioperative portal-vein infusion of chemotherapy because of the high risk of disseminating tumor cells into the hepatic circulation during surgery. Another investigational approach used in the management of metastatic disease is intra-arterial chemotherapy administration to patients with liver metastases. Patients require hospitalization for 1-2 days for arterial catheter placement and drug administration.

NURSING CONSIDERATIONS

Common problems that patients encounter during and after treatment for colorectal cancer include: altered eating and elimination habits, chronic diarrhea, abdominal cramps, adhesions from surgery or radiation, pain from adhesions or bone metastases, neutropenia, and fatigue. The nurse's roles in caring for these patients range from symptom management to lifestyle counseling.

Nurses can acquaint patients who have a new colostomy or ileostomy with the numerous sources of assistance available to them. A referral to the home health nurse may ease the transition from hospital to home. Nurses play a vital role in coordinating these resources during the patient's recovery from surgery.

Often the most difficult aspect for the colostomy patient to deal with is altered body image. Preoperative patient education—particularly showing the patient photographs of an actual stoma—will help reduce the patient's potential "shock" upon seeing the stoma for the first time.

After surgery, the patient is gradually taught the mechanics of the colostomy pouching system, starting with the simplest task and progressing to independent colostomy care. Today, many patients are offered colostomy irrigation as an alternative to wearing a pouch. Table 3 lists possible ostomy problems and suggestions for their management.

The nurse should reassure the patient that having a colostomy need not substantially alter individual lifestyle. Most communities have a local chapter of the United Ostomy Association, which, in cooperation with the American Cancer Society, offers an Ostomy Visitor Program. Among the services of the program is an ostomy visitor who provides a positive experience for the new ostomy patient and introduces him or her to a peer support group that can be an invaluable source of assistance and information.

Table 3. Management of Common Colostomy, Ileostomy, or Urostomy Problems

Problem	Cause or Sign	Treatment	Manufacturer

Odor
a) Fecal
	Food
	Oral medicines
	Active disease
		Topical, in appliance
		  a) Banish, 10 drops in pouch PRN
		  b) Odour-guard
		Oral medication
		  a) Bismuth subgallate 250 mg four
		     id
		  b) Bismuth subcarbonate 0.6 gm
		     four id
		  c) Derifil, one tid
			United Surgical
			
			Marlen
			
			Parthenon
			
			Lilly
			
			Rystan

b) Urinary	Poor hygiene Infection	Avoid rubber pouch Soak appliance in vinegar/water 1:4	

Crystals	Encrustation of
	stoma, skin, or
	appliance
	Bleeding stoma
		Acidification of urine
		  a) 8 to 16 oz cranberry juice daily
		  b) Ascorbic acid 1.0 gm four id
		  c) Acetic acid in pouch, solution 1:8	

Skin Irritation	Appliance leaks or fits badly or improperly	Large karaya gum ring of Colly-seel Stomahesive Temporary appliance New proper permanent appliance	Mason Labs Squibb United Surgical Marlen, Torbot, etc.
	Allergy to adhesive or material	Patch test to find cause of allergy	
	Flush stoma	Deep convex appliance Consider revision or stoma at a new site	Permatype
Fistula	Deep infection	Revision or stoma at a new site	
Ulcer of Peri- stomal Skin	Rigid appliance disc	Colly-seel and temporary appliance Flexible mounting ring of appliance	Hollister
Cut Stoma	Sliding or small appliance	Colly-seel and temporary appliance, then proper appliance Nonallergic tape to help hold ap- pliance in place	
Hyperkeratosis	Peristomal skin over-exposed to urine	Apply pressure to area with a firm mounting ring measured to exact stoma size	

Source: From *Managing Colostomies* (pp. 8–9.) by J.L. Rowbotham, 1982, Atlanta, GA: American Cancer Society, No. 3422-PE. Reprinted with permission of publisher.

Patients who will receive radiation therapy and/or chemotherapy after surgery should learn how these therapies will affect their dietary and elimination habits. They will need to be taught to manage their energy expenditure. Colostomy patients may need to alter their colostomy care routines during treatment.

Follow-up

The detection of asymptomatic recurrence is an important aspect of patient follow-up. The preferences of the individual physician guide the extent and frequency of follow-up, but a reasonable approach would include a history and physical examination, fecal occult stool, and sigmoidoscopy every 3 to 4 months for 3 years and then every 6 months for 2 years. New primary colorectal cancers can occur in about 5% of patients; patients who have had colorectal cancer may also be at greater risk for the development of certain other cancers, including ovarian, cervical, or breast cancer in females. When providing information to patients after surgery, the nurse should emphasize the value of close follow-up for the detection of asymptomatic recurrence.

Bibliography

Boarini, J. (1990). Gastro-intestinal cancer: Colon, rectum, and anus. In S. L. Groenwald, M. H. Frogge, M. Goodman, & C. H. Yarbro (Eds.), *Cancer nursing principles and practice* (pp. 792-805). Boston: Jones and Bartlett Publishers.

Bouwman, D. L., & Weaver, D. W. (1988). Colon cancer: Surgical therapy. *Gastro-Enterology Clinics of North America, 17*(4), 859-872.

Broadwell. D. C., & Jackson, B. S. (1982). *Principles of ostomy care.* St. Louis: C. V. Mosby Company.

Cohen, A. M. Kaufman, S. D., & Kadish, S. P. (1986). Cancer of the colon and rectum. In Cady, B. (Ed.), *Cancer manual* (7th Ed.), (pp. 212-221). Boston: American Cancer Society.

Cohen, A. M., Shank, B., & Friedman, M. A. (1989). Colorectal cancer. In V. T. DeVita, S. Hellman & S. A. Rosenberg (Eds.), *Cancer: Principles and practice of oncology* (pp. 895-964). Philadelphia: J. B. Lippincott Co.

Dobkin, K. A., & Broadwell, D. C. (1986). Nursing and considerations for the patient undergoing colostomy surgery. *Seminars in Oncology Nursing, 2*(4), 249-255.

Doughty, D. B. (1986). Colorectal cancer: Etiology and pathophysiology. *Seminars in Oncology Nursing, 2*(4), 235-241.

Otte, D. M. (1988). Nursing management of the patient with colon and rectal cancer. *Seminars in Oncology Nursing, 4*(4), 285-292.

Silverstein, E., Boring, C. C., & Squires, T. (1990). Cancer statistics, 1990. *Cancer, 40*(1), 9-26.

Silverstein, F. (1980, April). *Flexible sigmoidoscopy.* Presented at the general oncology update for physicians and nurses, University of Washington, Seattle, WA.

Sischy, B., & Gunderson, L. L. (1986). The evolving role of radiation therapy in the management of colorectal cancer. *Cancer, 36*(6), 351-359.

Wicks, L. J. (1986). Treatment modalities for colorectal cancer. *Seminars in Oncology Nursing, 2*(4), 242-248.

Witt, M. E., McDonald-Lynch, A., & Grimmer, D. (1987). Adjuvant radiotherapy to the colorectum: Nursing implications. *Oncology Nursing Forum, 14*(3), 17-21.

5 CANCERS OF THE PANCREAS, HEPATOBILIARY, AND ENDOCRINE SYSTEMS

Katherine Talmage Alkire

CANCER OF THE DIGESTIVE GLANDS

Cancers of the pancreas, liver, and gallbladder occur with limited frequency in the United States, but are becoming increasingly prevalent in some foreign countries. Cancer of the pancreas, for example, has increased approximately fourfold in Japan and three-fold in Asia over the past 50 years. Because symptoms of these neoplasms—vague complaints of abdominal pain, weight loss, gastric distress, or cachexia—are nonspecific, they are often diagnosed in advanced stages, when prognosis is usually poor.

Cancer of the Pancreas

Incidence and Risk Factors: Cancer of the pancreas accounts for 2-3% of all cancers, but is the fourth most frequent cause of cancer deaths. Pancreatic cancer is more common among males than females, with the peak incidence occurring at age 60.

The etiology of the disease remains unclear. Cigarette smoking has been associated with an increased incidence of pancreatic cancer. Long-term exposure to certain chemical carcinogens, such as dry cleaning chemicals, or gasoline or metallurgic fumes, also appears to increase the risk of this cancer. Research has yielded conflicting data on the causative roles of alcohol and coffee. Although an increased incidence is observed in patients with chronic pancreatitis and diabetes mellitus, it has been suggested that the onset of pancreatic insufficiency may occur months before the cancer becomes clinically apparent.

Clinical Manifestations and Diagnosis: There are few early signs and symptoms of pancreatic cancer, and this complicates diagnosis. Many patients wait until symptoms become worse before visiting a physician. By the time the diagnosis is made, the cancer has spread; almost half of pancreatic cancer patients have metastatic disease when diagnosed. Seventy percent of all pancreatic cancers appear in the head of the gland. Early diagnosis of a tumor in the head of the pancreas is sometimes possible because of jaundice and pruritus that result from biliary obstruction. Pain is usually the complaint that motivates patients to seek a physician's care. Pain may occur well before other signs and symptoms. Almost all patients with pancreatic cancer will have pain at some point in their disease, caused by pressure from the tumor or by infiltration of the splenic nerves. Patients with cancer in the body or tail of the pancreas frequently experience back or abdominal pain. This pain may lessen after meals or when patients assume the fetal position. Other symptoms of pancreatic cancer include anorexia, weight loss, abdominal distention, diarrhea, and nausea.

Diagnosis is made by physical and radiologic examination. Patients may exhibit obstructive jaundice. Physical exam will frequently reveal an enlarged liver, palpable gallbladder, and a mass in the upper abdomen. Computerized tomography (CT) scan and ultrasound are used to determine the extent of tumor invasion. *Endoscope retrograde cholangiopancreatogram* (ERCP) is used to localize the tumor or document blockage of pancreatic ducts. In patients with metastatic or unresectable disease who are not candidates for surgery, a CT-guided needle biopsy of the pancreas may be performed to confirm the malignancy.

Treatment: Surgical resection is performed only when disease is localized and the potential for cure exists. Most commonly, a Whipple procedure (*pancreatoduodenectomy*) will be performed. Surgery is not done if disease has spread beyond the pancreas. Palliative bypasses (such as *cholecystojejunostomy*) are performed when obstruction is present and cure is not possible.

Patients who have had curative surgery must take supplemental pancreatic enzymes orally before eating for the remainder of their lives. Total pancreatectomy will render the patient an insulin-dependent diabetic. Patients need instruction about enzyme use and diabetic care.

Radiation can be used postoperatively to eradicate remaining disease or for palliation. Radioactive implants and intraoperative radiation may also be used to deliver higher doses of radiation directly to the tumor. Depending on the dose and extent of the field involved, gastrointestinal distress frequently accompanies radiation.

Inoperable carcinomas can sometimes be temporarily palliated with combined radiotherapy and chemotherapy—usually 5-fluorouracil (5-FU) and mitomycin C or doxorubicin and streptozocin. Combination chemotherapy has produced better results than single-agent therapy, although the 5-year survival rate for patients with extensive disease is less than 9%. Many patients with adenocarcinoma of the pancreas die within a year of diagnosis.

An islet cell neoplasm is a rare form of cancer that arises from the endocrine parenchyma. These neoplasms, which can occur in any portion of the pancreas, are usually small, well circumscribed, and rarely extend beyond the pancreas. Surgical resection followed by adjuvant chemotherapy is the standard treatment regimen for islet cell carcinomas.

Cancer of the Liver

Incidence and Risk Ractors: Cancer of the liver is a rare malignancy in the United States, but in parts of Asia and Africa it is one of the most common malignancies. In the United States the average age of onset is 60 to 70 years; the disease occurs more frequently in males than females.

There is a strong association between chronic hepatitis B infection and the development of hepatocellular carcinoma. People with cirrhosis also have an increased risk of liver cancer. Other possible hepatocarcinogens include aflatoxin, nitrosamines, oral estrogen compounds, and numerous other chemicals.

Clinical Manifestations and Diagnosis: Signs of liver cancer include weakness, anorexia, fever of unknown origin, abdominal fullness or bloating, and dull upper quadrant abdominal pain. The clinical presentation will vary depending on the presence or absence of cirrhosis. Patients with cirrhosis exhibit rapid onset of symptoms; in the absence of cirrhosis, signs are much more subtle. As the tumor grows, pain may radiate to the back. Patients must be assessed carefully, as weight loss is often obscured by ascites. The liver is generally tender to palpation, and jaundice and portal hypertension may be present.

Diagnosis is made using radioisotope scans, CT scans, or hepatic arteriography. Many patients will have advanced disease at diagnosis. Cancer of the liver spreads throughout the organ and invades the portal vein and lymphatics. The most common sites of distant metastases are the lungs and brain.

Treatment: Surgical resection is attempted if no nodal involvement or distant spread is found. Even with resection, recurrence of liver cancer is common, and 5-year survival is rare. Patients may be treated with chemotherapy infused directly into the hepatic circulation. With this type of treatment, a catheter is surgically placed in the hepatic artery and the chemotherapeutic agent is continuously infused. The most commonly used agents are 5-FU, doxorubicin, and methotrexate. Side effects of this technique include toxic hepatitis (which subsides after discontinuation of therapy), and catheter displacement or occlusion.

Radioimmunotherapy is an experimental form of treatment used for some types of liver cancer. A radioactive isotope is attached to a radiolabeled antibody against ferritin, a specific protein found in human liver tumors. The isotope is given intravenously and concentrates in the liver, where it radiates the tumor internally. No immediate treatment side effects have been noted, but thrombocytopenia and neutropenia occur 4 to 6 weeks after treatment.

The prognosis for liver carcinoma patients is poor. Untreated patients usually die in 3 to 4 months; treated patients may live 6 to 18 months if they respond to therapy. Long-term survival is seen occasionally after successful subtotal hepatectomy for noninvasive carcinoma. Because the normal metabolic and storage functions of the liver are impaired, patients are at risk for nutritional and bleeding complications.

Cancer of the Gallbladder

Incidence and Risk Factors: Carcinoma of the gallbladder accounts for 0.2 to 0.4% of all malignancies. It is seen more frequently in women than in men, with the incidence increasing in those over age 55. Because the disease is usually advanced at diagnosis, the prognosis is poor, with 5-year survival rates of less than 5%.

Cholelithiasis has been linked to the development of cancer of the gallbladder. Approximately 60 to 90% of these patients have a history of biliary calculi.

Clinical Manifestations and Diagnosis: Symptoms of the disease mimic acute and chronic cholecystitis, with right quadrant abdominal pain, anorexia, weight loss, nausea, vomiting, and fever as the chief complaints. About 50% of patients exhibit jaundice and gallbladder enlargement.

Because radiologic and laboratory tests lack specificity, the diagnosis is generally confirmed by laparotomy. Direct extension to the liver is common; other metastatic sites include the lymph nodes, lungs, bone, and the adrenal glands.

Treatment: Treatment for cancer of the gallbladder includes cholecystectomy with subtotal hepatectomy if distant metastases are absent. Most patients have local recurrences. Radiation and/ or chemotherapy may be used for local control, but palliation of obstructive jaundice remains the primary treatment goal.

CANCER OF THE ENDOCRINE GLANDS

Endocrine cancers include malignancies located in the thyroid, adrenal, and pituitary glands, and pancreatic islets. The prognosis for these tumors is highly variable. Endocrine cancers cause morbidity by compressing nearby anatomic structures or by secreting excess amounts of the hormones they normally secrete.

Thyroid Cancer

Cancer of the thyroid gland accounts for approximately 1.1% of all malignancies. Its incidence in women is more than twice that in men, and it can occur at any age.

Radiation to the head and neck region for benign conditions (such as acne and tonsillitis) during childhood or adolescence is the only well-documented factor in the etiology of thyroid cancer. There is generally a prolonged latency period between radiation exposure and the development of thyroid cancer (over 20 years) with risk increasing as the latency period increases. Patients with an endemic goiter are also thought to be at increased risk for this malignancy.

The four main types of primary thyroid carcinoma are *papillary, follicular, medullary,* and *anaplastic* or undifferentiated. Most papillary and follicular types are slow-growing and associated with a very favorable prognosis. Medullary carcinomas occur less frequently, and generally follow an indolent course. Anaplastic carcinomas are rapidly growing neoplasms; patients usually die within months of diagnosis, regardless of therapy. Patients may have a genetic predisposition to medullary and papillary thryoid carcinomas.

Clinical presentation varies according to the type of malignancy. An asymptomatic thyroid mass and cervical lymphadenopathy are common signs. Less frequently, patients may exhibit hoarseness or signs of tracheal or esophageal compression.

The most important means of diagnosing thyroid cancer is fine-needle aspiration biopsy of the suspicious nodule. Radionuclide scans can also provide information about whether the mass is able to concentrate iodine in the same way as the normal thyroid gland.

Surgery is the treatment of choice. A near total or total thyroidectomy is performed on most patients. Complications of surgery include: hemorrhage; damage to the parathyroid glands, leading to temporary or permanent hypoparathyroidism; and temporary or permanent vocal cord paralysis. Patients are given exogenous thyroid hormone to prevent hypothyroidism postoperatively.

Following surgery, many patients with papillary and follicular thyroid cancers are given radioactive iodine orally; this concentrates in the thyroid bed to destroy any residual thyroid tissue or tumor. This treatment is not used for medullary or anaplastic tumors because they do not concentrate this radioisotope. Side effects of this treatment include inflammation of the salivary glands, nausea, vomiting, fatigue, and bone marrow suppression.

Chemotherapy is used only for the treatment of advanced thyroid cancers. Results are not encouraging.

Cancer of the Adrenal Glands

Adrenal malignancies are rare. Tumors can arise in either the outer cortex or inner medullary portions of the gland and may be functional or nonfunctional. Functional tumors produce excess amounts of the hormones normally secreted by the adrenals. Diagnostic tests include measurement of hormone levels, and CT scans or magnetic resonance imaging (MRI). Nonfunctional tumors do not produce hormones, but the tumor mass may produce other symptoms.

Adrenocortical Tumors: Adrencortical tumors can secrete glucocorticoids, mineralocorticoids, androgens, estrogens, and progestins. The clinical symptoms associated with excess secretion of adrenocortical hormones are listed in Table 1.

**Table 1. Clinical Manifestations of
Excess Secretion of Adrenocortical Hormones**

Hormones	Clinical Effects
Cortisol	Glucose intolerance, moon face, truncal obesity, hypertension, osteoporosis, renal calculi, psychiatric problems
Sex hormones (testosterone, estrogen, progesterone)	*Females:* Male pattern baldness, hirsutism, deepening voice, breast atrophy, decreased libido, oligomenorrhea *Males:* Gynecomastia, breast tenderness, testicular atrophy, decreased libido
Aldosterone	Hypernatremia, hypokalemia, hypertension, neuromuscular weakness and paresthesias, EKG and renal function abnormalities

Surgery is the primary treatment for adrenocortical carcinoma. Most patients will have locally advanced or metastatic disease at the time of surgery. As a result, the spleen, kidney, and part of the pancreas are often removed during surgery in an attempt to debulk the tumor before the start of additional therapy. Glucocorticoids are given before and after surgery to prevent adrenal insufficiency; this replacement therapy continues until the unaffected adrenal gland begins to function again.

The drug, o,p'-DDD (mitotane), which causes necrosis of the adrenal cortex, is given postoperatively to patients with residual disease. This drug is a derivative of DDT. Side effects are severe and include: nausea, vomiting, anorexia, lethargy, and profound depression. Aminoglutethamide, which blocks corticosteroid secretion, may also be given. Treatment results are generally poor, with less than 30% of patients surviving 5 years.

Cancer of the Adrenal Medulla: The most common tumor of the adrenal medulla is the *pheochromocytoma*, which produces large amounts of the catecholamines, epinephrine and norepinephrine. Pheochromocytomas are extremely rare.

Excess catecholamines produce symptoms such as hypertension, sweating, palpitations, nausea and vomiting, headache, and anxiety.

Any accessible primary or metastatic tumor mass is removed surgically. Patients are treated preoperatively with adrenergic blocking agents to prevent a sudden, potentially fatal release of catecholamines during surgery. Metastatic disease may be treated with antihormonal agents to decrease adrenal steroid production.

Pituitary Tumors

Pituitary tumors account for approximately 10% of all intracranial neoplasms. They may be hormonally active or inactive lesions. Hormonally active tumors can secrete any of the pituitary hormones, but most commonly secrete growth hormone, ACTH, or prolactin. The syndromes resulting from this excess secretion are described in Table 2. Other symptoms include headache due to increased intracranial pressure, visual defects from optic nerve compression, and, less frequently, cerebrospinal fluid leakage.

**Table 2. Clinical Manifestations
of Excess Secretion of Pituitary Hormones**

Hormone	Clinical Effects
Prolactin	*Females:* amenorrhea, infertility, galactorrhea *Males:* decreased libido, impotence
Growth hormone	Acromegaly, gigantism
Adrenocorticotropic hormone	Cushing's disease
Thyroid-stimulating hormone	Hyperthyroidism
Follicle-stimulating hormone/luteinizing hormone	May be clinically asymptomatic and detected by elevated hormone levels

Diagnostic tests include measurement of pituitary hormone levels, CT and MRI scans, and occasionally, arteriography. These tests aim to determine the extent of the pituitary mass and its ability to produce hormones.

For hypersecreting or fast-growing tumors, surgery to debulk and decompress vital structures is indicated. Most tumors are resected by the transsphenoidal route or through the nose. Complications of surgery are meningitis, cerebrospinal fluid leakage, and diabetes insipidus. Postoperatively, hormone levels are measured to assess the extent to which the hormone-producing tumor tissue was removed.

Radiation may be used for incompletely resected tumors; however, this therapy is less effective against hypersecreting tumors because it takes months to years to lower hormone levels to normal levels.

Drugs may also be used to control excess hormone secretion, and are frequently given preoperatively to reduce tumor size. Bromocriptine, a dopamine agonist, reduces prolactin levels. If used alone, it must be continued indefinitely, because discontinuation will result in rapid tumor regrowth. Another agent used is SMS 201-995, an investigational drug that suppresses growth hormone secretion.

The prognosis for pituitary tumors is dependent on the effective control of excess hormone secretion and on the reversibility of preoperative neurologic defects caused by the expanding tumor. After surgery, hormone levels return to normal in 65-85% of patients. These results can be improved slightly with the addition of postoperative irradiation.

Bibliography

Brennan, M. F. (1987). Adrenocortical carcinoma. *CA—A Cancer Journal for Clinicians, 37*(6), 348-365.

Ceric, I. (1985). Pituitary tumors. *Neurologic Clinics, 3*, 751-766.

DeVita, V. T., Hellman, J., & Rosenberg, S. (1989). *Cancer: Principles and practices of oncology*, (pp. 800-874 and 1269-1344). Philadelphia: J. B. Lippincott and Co.

Harvey, A. M., Jones, R. J., McKusick, V. A., Owens, A. H., & Ross, R. S. (1988). *The principles and practice of medicine* (pp. 831-836, and 869-917). Norwalk, CT: Appleton-Century Crofts Inc.

Oberfield, R. A., Steele, G., Jr., Gollan, J. L., & Sherman, D. (1989). Liver cancer. *CA—A Cancer Journal for Clinicians, 39*(4), 206-218.

6 URINARY TRACT CANCERS

Julena Lind

BLADDER CANCER

Incidence and Risk Factors

Bladder cancer accounts for approximately 4-5% of all cancers in the United States. The incidence of bladder cancer in men is three times that in women, and the age-adjusted bladder cancer rate in white men is almost twice that in black men.

Possible etiologic factors include: cigarette smoking; exposure to chemicals called arylamines (used in the textile and rubber industries); and exposure to *Schistosoma haemotobium*, a parasite commonly encountered in Asia, Africa, and South America.

Pathology

Most bladder cancers are carcinomas of the transitional epithelium of the bladder's mucosal lining. Although 90% of the cases are localized at diagnosis, up to 80% will recur.

Tumors are graded according to degree of cellular abnormality, with the most atypical cells designated as high-grade tumors. Staging of this cancer is based on the depth of invasion into the bladder muscle and surrounding structures. The most common bladder staging systems used in the United States are the Jewett-Strong System (modified by Marshall) and the TNM system (Figure 1).

The 5-year survival rate is 76% for whites and 55% for blacks. Invasive bladder tumors spread rapidly to the regional lymph nodes and then into adjacent structures.

Clinical Presentation and Diagnosis

Patients with bladder cancer usually present with gross hematuria. Other manifestations include bladder irritability (dysuria, frequency, or urgency) and symptoms of urethral obstruction. Obstruction of the ureters causes flank pain and results in hydronephrosis. Advanced tumors may compress the pelvic lymph nodes, resulting in rectal obstruction, pelvic pain, and lower extremity edema.

An excretory urogram (intravenous pyelogram, IVP) is initially performed to identify the cause of clinical symptoms. The diagnosis

BLADDER CANCER
STAGING

1964 Jewett-Strong	1952 Jewett	1952 Marshall		1974, TNM Clinical	Patho-logical
		O {	No tumor definitive speciment	T-0	P-O
			Carcinoma-in-situ	TIS	PIS
			Papillary tumor s̄ invasion		
A	A {	A	Invasion lamina propria }	T$_{-1}$	P$_{-1}$
B	{ B$_{-1}$	B$_{-1}$	Superficial } Muscle invasion	T$_{-2}$	P$_{-2}$
	B$_{-2}$	B$_{-2}$	Deep	T$_{-3A}$	
C	C	C	Invasion perivesical fat	T$_{-3B}$	} P$_{-3}$
		D$_{-1}$	Invasion contiguous viscera	T$_{4A-B}$	P$_{-4}$
			Pelvic nodes		N$_{1-3}$
		D$_{-2}$	Distant metastases		M$_{-1}$
			Nodes above aortic bifurcation		N$_{-4}$

Figure 1. Bladder Cancer Staging systems.

Source: From "Bladder Cancer" by J. B. deKernion, 1990, p. 750. C. M. Haskell, (Ed.), *Cancer Treatment,* 3rd edition, Philadelphia: W. B. Saunders Co. Reprinted with permission of the publisher.

is then confirmed by cystoscopy and biopsy of the suspicious lesion and a staging work-up is performed.

Treatment

Surgery: The extent of surgery is dependent on the pathological stage of the disease. If the lesion penetrates no deeper than the mucosa, every attempt is made to salvage the bladder. Early disease (Stages 0 to A) is generally treated by intravesical chemotherapy and transurethral resection. Locally invasive disease (Stages B to C) can usually be managed only by radical cystectomy and urinary diversion. However, when there are only solitary lesions in the dome of the bladder, and random mucosal biopsies of distant bladder sites are normal, a partial cystectomy can be performed. Pelvic lymph node dissection is frequently performed during the cystectomy to stage the disease and to attempt to prevent local pelvic recurrence and metastasis. When urinary diversion is anticipated, the enterostomal therapist can assist in preoperative teaching and in marking for stomal placement.

The urinary diversion associated with radical cystectomy may be an intestinal conduit such as an *ileal conduit,* or a *continent urinary reservoir.* Figure 2 shows an ileal conduit; Figure 3 depicts one type of continent urinary reservoir called a Kock pouch, which is constructed with a piece of ileum. *Ureterosigmoidostomy,* a procedure in which the ureters are implanted in the sigmoid colon and urine is then excreted through the rectum, is rarely performed today.

Wound infections, enteric fistulae, urine leaks, ureteral obstruction, bowel obstruction, and pelvic abscesses may occur for the first month after an ileal conduit is created. Later complications include stomal stenosis, peristomal hernias, chronic pyelonephritis, ureteroileal obstruction, intestinal obstruction, calculi, and hyperchloremic acidosis.

Superficial recurrences are managed by repeated transurethral resections and intravesical chemotherapy. About 50% of patients with high-stage, high-grade tumors will eventually relapse following cystectomy. Surgery is seldom performed to palliate symptoms in these patients.

Postoperative nursing care includes monitoring the urinary diversion for urine secretion immediately following surgery. The urinary stoma, which protrudes approximately one-half inch above the skin, should be fitted with a urinary appliance. The color of the stoma should be checked frequently for several days after surgery. Normal color is deep pink to dark red, and a dusky appearance could indicate stomal necrosis.

Mucus will be present in all urinary diversions constructed from bowel segments because the intestine normally produces mucus. Excessive mucus can clog the urinary appliance. This problem can be minimized by increasing the patient's fluid intake to 3 liters per day. Nurses should teach patients adequate skin care and pouching of the stoma. Other topics include handling equipment, early identification of kidney infections, community- and hospital-based resources, and body image issues. Generally, the nurse should not begin teaching these procedures until patients' physical discomfort has subsided and their physiologic state has returned more or less to normal.

With a continent ileal reservoir, there is no need for an external appliance, and catheterization of the pouch duplicates normal bladder function. These patients will need to learn self-catheterization techniques. Enterostomal therapists can provide valuable technical information and advice on urinary diversion management that will permit patients to live as normally as possible.

In cystectomy, operative damage to nerves responsible for erectile function renders most male patients physiologically unable to have or maintain an erection, but some patients are still able to achieve

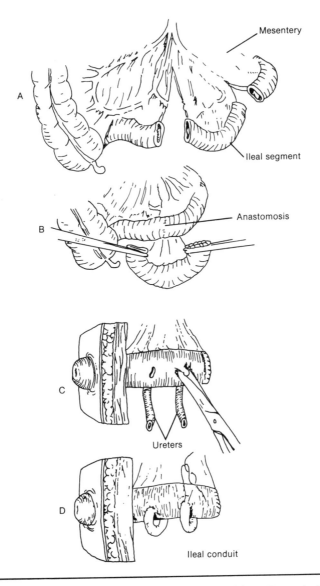

Figure 2. Ileal conduit. *A*, A segment of ileum is isolated from the gastrointestinal tract with its mesenteric blood flow. *B*, The gastrointestinal tract is reanastomosed. One end is sutured closed, and the other end will be used to form an abdominal stoma. *C*, The ureters, which are located retroperitoneally, are brought into the abdominal cavity. Incisions are made in the conduit for ureteral implantation. *D*, The abdominal stoma is matured, and the ureters are anastomosed to the ileum segment in an end-to-side fashion.

orgasm. Because the prostate and seminal vesicles are removed, men experience dry orgasms without emission of semen. Penile implants may be useful for some patients. Women who undergo cystectomy may experience some physiologic problems during intercourse as a result of a shortened vagina.

Radiation Therapy: Definitive radiotherapy is generally reserved for bladder cancer patients who are not candidates for surgery. However, in settings outside the United States, radiotherapy is frequently used as the primary therapy for invasive bladder cancer. Complications of radiotherapy include radiation enteritis or colitis and skin reactions.

Chemotherapy: For superficial, low-grade disease, chemotherapy is applied *intravesically* (directly into the bladder) to concentrate the drug at the tumor site and eliminate any residual tumor mass after resection. Thiotepa is the drug most commonly used; however, mitomycin C, doxorubicin, and the immunotherapeutic agent BCG (*Bacillus Calmette Guerin*) have also been used.

Systemic chemotherapy may also be used to manage advanced bladder cancer; complete response rates of 30-50% have been

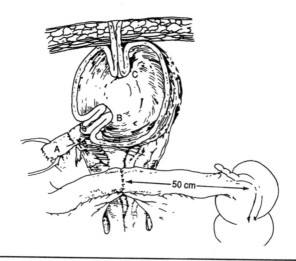

Figure 3. The continent ileal reservoir. *A*, The original ileal conduit with implanted ureters. *B*, The reflux-preventing nipple valve. *C*, The continence-maintaining nipple valve.

Source: From "The Kock Continent Ileal Reservoir for Supravesical Urinary Diversion" by A. Gerber, 1983, *American Journal of Surgery, 146,* p. 16. Reprinted with permission of The The American Journal of Surgery.

reported. Single agent chemotherapy has demonstrated limited success, with cisplatin proving the most effective agent. Many patients with advanced cancer receiving combination treatment with cisplatin, doxorubicin, and cyclophosphamide have exhibited a complete or partial response.

CANCER OF THE KIDNEY

Incidence and Risk Factors

Renal cell carcinoma, which occurs in the parenchyma of the kidney, is the most common type of renal cancer, accounting for approximately 3% of adult malignancies. Carcinoma of the renal pelvis is rare, comprising only 5% of all kidney tumors. Only renal cell cancer will be discussed here.

Renal cell carcinoma is more common in males than females and is rare in people under age 35. Cigarette smoking is the most definitive risk factor for the development of renal cell carcinoma, with approximately 25 to 30% of cases directly attributable to smoking.

Although prolonged estrogen administration can induce kidney tumors in animals, the relationship between hormone ingestion and the development of these carcinomas in humans remains unclear.

Other risk factors for renal cell carcinoma are the use of phenacetin-containing analgesics and exposure to asbestos, cadmium, or gasoline. Patients who develop cystic disease while on chronic hemodialysis may also be at a greater risk for renal cell cancer.

Patterns of Spread

Renal cell carcinoma spreads locally to the medullary portion of the kidney, to the renal vein, and sometimes into the vena cava. The most common sites of distant metastasis are the lungs, bones, brain, and liver. About 30% of patients present with metastasis at diagnosis.

Clinical Manifestations and Diagnosis

Over 40% of patients with renal cell cancer exhibit gross hematuria. Patients may also present with a dull, aching flank pain or a palpable abdominal mass. Other presenting symptoms include fever, weight loss, anemia, and hypercalcemia.

Diagnosing and staging tests for renal cell cancer include: kidney/ureters/bladder radiograph (KUB), excretory urogram (IVP), renal ultrasound, CT, magnetic resonance imaging (MRI) and renal angiography.

Treatment

Surgery: Radical nephrectomy is the treatment of choice for localized renal cell cancer that may extend into the renal vein and vena cava. Nephrectomy is not usually performed in patients with disseminated disease. Bleeding, pain, and fever related to tumor growth can usually be better controlled by angioinfarction. In this procedure, the renal artery is embolized, thereby eliminating the blood supply to the kidney and causing organ infarction.

Regional retroperitoneal lymph node dissection is often performed along with radical nephrectomy, although its impact on survival is not clear.

Postoperative nursing interventions include prevention of atelectasis, pneumonia, and infection at the incision site; assessment of remaining kidney function; and monitoring for bleeding and paralytic ileus.

Pain can be quite severe after nephrectomy. Patients may experience incisional pain and, as a result of the position on the operating table, muscular discomfort as well. Before the operation, it may be useful to explain the surgical positioning and resulting discomfort. Postoperatively, relief can be provided with moist heat, massage, and pillows to support the patient's back while he or she is lying on one side.

Radiation and Chemotherapy: The use of radiotherapy for renal cell tumors is controversial, but pre- and postoperative radiotherapy may be combined with nephrectomy. Chemotherapy has not been effective in the treatment of renal cell carcinoma.

Immunotherapy: Preliminary studies suggest that renal cell carcinoma is particularly responsive to adoptive immunotherapy using *lymphokine activated killer* (LAK) cells with recombinant *interleukin-2* (IL-2). However, this treatment is complicated, toxic, and expensive. While LAK cell infusions alone are well tolerated, high-dose IL-2 has caused many complications, including malaise, fever, hepatic dysfunction, thrombocytopenia, somnolence, disorientation, and pulmonary edema. Respiratory distress, coma, and myocardial infarctions have also been reported. Nursing interventions for this investigational immunotherapy include extensive patient education and support and intensive monitoring of the severe side effects.

Alpha interferon has also been evaluated for the treatment of advanced renal cell carcinoma; it shows modest activity, with overall response rates of 15 to 20%. See Unit III, Chapter 4 for further information on biotherapy.

Bibliography

Belldegrun, A., Uppenkamp, I., & Rosenberg, S. A. (1988). Anti-tumor reactivity of human lymphokine activated killer (LAK) cells against fresh and cultured preparations of renal cell cancer. *Journal of Urology, 139*, 150-155.

Broadwell, D. C., & Jackson, B. S. (Eds.). (1982). *Principles of ostomy care.* St. Louis: C. V. Mosby.

deKernion, J. B. (1986). Renal cell carcinoma. *Journal of Urology, 136,* 882.

Lind, J., & Nakao, S. L. (1987). Urologic and male genital malignancies. In S. Groenwald (Ed.), *Cancer nursing principles and practice* (pp. 700-745). Boston, MA: Jones & Bartlett.

Paulson, D. F. (1987). Treatment strategies in renal carcinoma. *Seminars in Nephrology, 7*(2), 140-151.

Pritchett, T. R., Lieskovsky, G., & Skinner, D. G. (1988). Manifestations and treatment of renal parenchymal tumors. In D. G. Skinner & G. Lieskovsky (Eds.), *Diagnosis and management of genitourinary cancer* (pp. 337-361). Philadelphia: W. B. Saunders.

Ross, R. K., Paganini-Hill, A., & Henderson, B. E. (1988). Epidemiology of bladder cancer. In D. G. Skinner & G. Lieskovsky (Eds.), *Diagnosis and management of genitourinary cancer* (pp. 23-31). Philadelphia: W. B. Saunders.

Silverberg, E., Boring, C. C., & Squires, T. S. (1990). Cancer statistics, 1990. *CA— A Journal for Clinicians, 40*(1), 9-288.

Skinner, D. G., & Lieskovsky, G. (1988). Management of invasive and high grade bladder cancer. In D. G. Skinner & G. Lieskovsky (Eds.), *Diagnosis and management of genitourinary cancer.* (pp. 604-703). Philadelphia: W. B. Saunders.

vonEschenbach, A., & Rodriguez, D. (Eds.). (1981). *Sexual rehabilitation of the urologic cancer patient.* Boston: G. K. Hall.

7 CANCER OF THE BREAST

Rebecca Hunter Dorcas

The management of breast cancer has become increasingly complex, offering new challenges in nursing care of patients and their families as they cope with decision making, physical changes, psychosocial impact, and rehabilitation needs.

INCIDENCE

The American Cancer Society estimates that in the United States during 1990, over 150,000 women will be diagnosed with breast cancer, and nearly 40,000 will die from this disease. In the United States breast cancer accounts for 29% of all cancers in women; one woman out of ten will develop breast cancer sometime during her life. Although earlier detection results in higher cure rates, breast cancer remains the leading cause of cancer death of adult women under 54 years of age and the second most common cause after age 54. Among women of all ages, breast cancer is second only to lung cancer as the leading cause of cancer deaths in women. Less than 1% of all breast cancer cases occur in men. The course of disease and its clinical management are very similar to that in women.

SCREENING AND DETECTION

With modern technology, breast cancer can be detected at a very early stage of development when the chance of cure is highest. The key to cure is early detection and prompt treatment. Physical examination, mammography, and breast self-examination comprise an early detection approach. The nurse in any health care setting is in a key position to determine a woman's need for information on breast cancer detection guidelines and to provide instruction on *breast self-examination* (BSE).

Women over age 20 should practice BSE monthly. BSE is best done one week after menstruation starts, or on the same day each month for the post-menopausal woman. The BSE techniques recommended by the American Cancer Society are illustrated in Figure 1. Asymptomatic women should have their breasts examined by a trained health professional every 3 years from ages 20 to 40 and annually thereafter.

There are many good reasons for doing the breast self-exam (BSE) each month. One reason is that breast cancer is most easily treated and cured when it is found early. Another is that if you do BSE every month, it will increase your skill and confidence when doing the exam. When you get to know how your breasts normally feel, you will quickly be able to feel any change. Another reason, it is easy to do.

The best time to do BSE is about a week after your period, when breasts are not tender or swollen. If you do not hae regular periods or sometimes skip a month, do BSE on the same day every month.

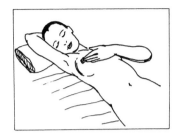

Remember: BSE could save your breast—and save your life. Most breast lumps are found by women themselves, but, in fact, most lumps in the breast are not cancer. Be safe, be sure.

1. Lie down and put a pillow under your right shoulder. Place your right arm behind your head.
2. Use the finger pads of your three middle fingers on your left hand to feel for lumps or thickening. Your finger pads are the top third of each finger.
3. Press firmly enough to know how your breast feels. If you're not sure how hard to press, ask your health care provider. Or try to copy the way your health care provider uses the finger pads during a breast exam. Learn what your breast feels like most of the time. A firm ridge in the lower curve of each breast is normal.
4. Move around the breast in a set way. You can choose either the circle (A), the up and down line (B), or the wedge (C). Do it the same way every time. It will help you to make sure that you've gone over the entire breast area, and to remember how your breast feels each month.
5. Now examine your left breast using right hand finger pads.
6. If you find any changes, see your doctor right away.

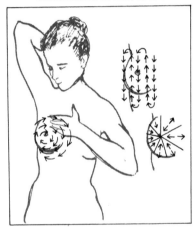

You might want to check your breasts while standing in front of a mirror right after you do your BSE each month. See if there are any changes in the way your breasts look: dimpling of the skin, or changes in the nipple, redness or swelling. You might also want to do an extra BSE while you're in the shower. Your soapy hands will glide over the wet skin making it easy to check how your breasts feel.

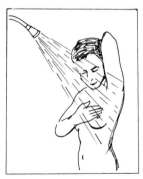

Figure 1. The nurse has an important role in teaching and promoting the regular practice of breast self examination. These instructions describe the most commonly taught techniques.
Source: From *How To Do Breast Self-Examination.* No. 2674. Atlanta, American Cancer Society.

Symptoms or physical findings the nurse should report to the physician are: a breast or axillary lump or thickening; nipple scaling, retraction, thickening, or discharge; skin dimpling or erythema; edema; ulceration; or distended veins in an irregular pattern. Breast pain is seldom a symptom of early breast cancer.

Mammography is a special x-ray technique used to examine the breast. The American Cancer Society recommends that asymptomatic women have a baseline mammogram between the ages of 35 and 39, mammograms every 1 to 2 years between ages 40 to 49, and annually thereafter. Women with a family history of breast cancer may have more frequent mammography. The typical radiation exposure is very low, approximately 0.02 cGy/exposure. The risk from this exposure to the breast after age 35 is considered negligible.

The major advantage of mammography is that breast cancer can be found before it can be palpated. Nevertheless, women need to know that BSE and physical examination by a trained professional continue to be important, because mammography does not detect about 10-14% of breast cancers found on physical examination.

RISK FACTORS

All women are at risk for breast cancer. Women at a higher risk for developing breast cancer are those with a strong family history of breast cancer, a personal history of breast cancer, early menarche or late menopause, or a first full-term pregnancy after age 30. The risk of developing breast cancer also increases with age being most common after age 50. Long-term estrogen therapy, a high fat diet, and alcohol use have been reported as possible risk factors, but the extent of their relationship to the onset of breast cancer remains unclear.

DIAGNOSIS

The diagnosis of breast cancer can only be made by pathological examination of breast tissue. A lump in the breast usually warrants biopsy even when the mammogram is described as being normal. Breast tissue may be obtained by needle aspiration biopsy or surgical biopsy.

Needle aspiration is used by some physicians to help differentiate between cysts and solid tumors. Cysts frequently disappear after aspiration and the removal of fluid. Cytological or pathological examinations of material removed in aspiration can be used to identify cancer. Ultrasound may help determine whether the lump is solid or cystic.

Surgical biopsy is generally performed under general or local anesthesia in an ambulatory surgical center. Excisional biopsy, the most commonly performed procedure, is used when lumps are small. In these cases, the entire tumor and a margin of normal tissue are excised. If the tumor is large, incisional biopsy may be done to remove a small amount of tissue for pathological examination. Tissue obtained from surgical biopsy is evaluated by frozen section, which permits a diagnosis within 15 minutes and may be followed by definitive surgery; but most surgeons wait for a permanent section, which takes about 24 to 48 hours. The latter approach allows the patient time to discuss treatment options with the physician and is the common approach today.

Breast cancer tissue should also be assayed for estrogen and progesterone receptors. These *hormone receptor assays* aid in predicting whether certain hormones influence the growth of the cancer. Women with positive hormone receptor assays are more likely to respond to hormone therapy and also have a better overall prognosis.

STAGING AND TYPES OF BREAST CANCER

Staging is a method of grouping patients by the extent of disease to determine the choice of treatment, predict prognosis, and compare the results of different treatment approaches. The more advanced the disease, the poorer the prognosis. The staging system recommended by the American Joint Committee on Cancer is defined in Figure 2.

The most common route of spread of breast cancer is to the axillary lymph nodes (Figure 3). About 50% of breast cancer patients already have positive (disease-affected) axillary nodes when the tumor is palpable. The more axillary nodes that are involved, the greater the risk of *micrometastases* (clinically undetectable tumor cells) elsewhere and relapse or recurrence.

The common sites of breast cancer metastases are local recurrence or distant spread to bone, liver, lung, and brain. Some complications of metastatic disease include spinal cord compression, pathologic bone fractures, pleural effusion, and tracheal obstruction (see Unit IV, Chapter 4).

Breast cancers are divided according to cell type, with types varying in incidence, patterns of growth and metastases, and survival. Infiltrating ductal carcinoma is the most common type of breast cancer accounting for about 70% of tumors. The rare inflammatory breast cancers (1-4% of breast cancer cases) are associated with the poorest prognosis. *Carcinoma in situ* (CIS) is a non-invasive cancer that has an excellent prognosis and can often be detected by mammography when nothing significant is palpable.

BREAST CANCER STAGE GROUPING

	Tumor	Nodes	Metastasis
Stage O	Tis	N0	M0
State I	T1	N0	M0
Stage IIA	T0	N1	M0
	T1	N1	M0
	T2	N0	M0
Stage IIB	T2	N1	M0
	T3	N0	M0
Stage IIIA	T0	N2	M0
	T1	N2	M0
	T2	N2	M0
	T3	N2	M0
	T3	N1,N2	M0
Stage IIIB	T4	Any N	M0
	Any T	N3	M0
Stage IV	Any	Any N	M1

DEFINITION OF TNM (Primary Tumor (T))

Definitions for classifying the primary tumor (T) are the same for clinical and for pathologic classification. The *telescoping* method of classification can be applied. If the measurement is made by physical examination, the examiner will use the major headings (T1, T2, or T3). If other measurements, such as mammographic or pathologic, are used, the telescoped subsets of T1 can be used.

TX Primary tumor cannot be assessed.
T0 No evidence of primary tumor
Tis Carcinoma *in situ*. Intraductal carcinoma, lobular carcinoma *in situ*, or Paget's disease of the nipple with no tumor.
T1 Tumor 2 cm or less in greatest dimension
T1a 0.5 cm or less in greatest dimension
T1b More than 0.5 cm but not more than 1 cm in greatest dimension
T1c More than 1 cm but not more than 2 cm in greatest dimension.

T2 Tumors more than 2 cm but not more than 5 cm. in greatest dimension.
T3 Tumor more than 5 cm in greatest dimension
T4 Tumor of any size with direct extension to chest wall or skin.
T4a Extension to chest wall
T4b Edema (including peau d'orange) or ulceration of the skin of the breast or satellite skin nodules confined to the same breast.
T4c Both (T4a and T4b)
T4d Inflammatory carcinoma (see definition of inflammatory carcinoma in Table 1).

REGIONAL LYMPH NODES (N)

NX Regional lymph nodes cannot be assessed (e.g., previously removed)
N0 No regional lymph node metastasis
N1 Metastasis to movable ipsilateral axillary lymph node(s)
N2 Metastasis to ipsilateral axillary lymph node(s) fixed to one another or to other structures.
N3 Metastasis to ipsilateral internal mammary lymph node(s)

DISTANT METASTASIS (M)

MX Presence of distant metastasis cannot be assessed
M0 No distant metstasis
M1 Distant metastasis (includes metastasis to ipsilateral supraclaviclar lymph node(s))

Figure 2. Staging Classification for Breast Cancer
Source: From *Manual for Staging of Cancer* (3rd ed.). (pp. 146–147) by O.H. Beahrs, P.E. Henson, R.V.P. Hutter, & M. H. Myers (Eds.), 1988, Philadelphia: J.B. Lippincott 1988.

TREATMENT

Treatment recommendations differ depending on the type and stage of disease at the time of diagnosis. Today women have treatment options. Several states, such as California, Pennsylvania,

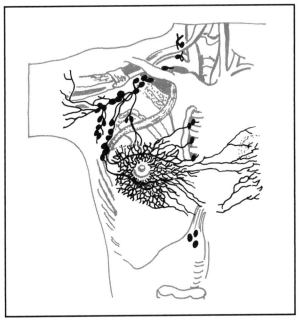

Figure 3. The lymphatic spread of breast cancer.
Source: From *A Cancer Source Book for Nurses.* (p. 73), 1981,
Atlanta: American Cancer Society. Reprinted with permission of
publisher.

and Florida have laws that require that a woman be informed of such options. The nurse's role in supporting patients in the decision-making process is very important. Stage I or II disease is generally treated by breast conservation surgery and irradiation, or modified radical mastectomy with or without breast reconstruction. Mastectomy and irradiation are local treatments and obviously will not affect cancer cells that have already metastasized. *Adjuvant chemotherapy* may also be given to patients with early-stage disease who are at a higher risk for developing metastatic disease. At present there is some disagreement about whether all patients with breast cancer should receive adjuvant chemotherapy.

Patients with locally advanced breast cancers (stage III) have a poorer prognosis and are not candidates for curative surgery. However, good local control may be achieved with a combination of surgery, chemotherapy, and irradiation. Chemotherapy should be considered because many patients with stage III disease are at risk for developing distant metastases.

Treatment approaches for patients with locally recurrent or metastatic disease vary depending on the site and extent of disease. In many cases, local and systemic therapy are combined to provide long-term survival. Because patients with metastatic disease rarely exhibit a lasting response to standard treatments, researchers are investigating the use of high-dose chemotherapy regimens followed by autologous bone marrow transplant to see if better results can be obtained.

Surgery

Breast conservation surgery consists of a wide excision of the tumor and a partial axillary lymph node dissection. The terms "lumpectomy," or "segmental resection," "tylectomy," and "partial mastectomy," are frequently used to describe the extent of the local surgery. Surgery may be followed by radiation therapy. Recent studies of patients with small tumors and no evidence of multifocal disease or extensive intraductal cancer show no difference in survival between breast conservation surgery followed by radiation therapy and modified radical mastectomy. One disadvantage of breast conservation is that the costs may be greater because of radiation therapy. Some women experience psychosocial concerns related to their disease. A woman may struggle with the questions: "Did I do the right thing?" and "Do I want a breast that had cancer in it?"

Modified radical mastectomy is a removal of the entire breast plus an axillary node dissection. The disadvantages of a modified radical mastectomy are cosmetic deformity and the potential for psychosocial problems affecting body image and self-concept.

Breast conservation surgery may be performed as an outpatient procedure or may require an overnight stay. Patients are generally hospitalized for 2 to 5 days following a modified radical mastectomy. The trend toward shorter hospital stays for these procedures means that many patients will be discharged with a surgical drain in place. Patient education needs to include this care component. The potential consequences and implications of primary therapy for breast cancer are summarized in Table 1.

Impaired shoulder mobility may occur if exercises are not begun soon after surgery. Exercises help reduce lymphedema and prevent limitation of joint motion. Patients start with limited exercises of the lower arm, such as squeezing a rubber ball. These begin as soon as the surgeon decides that the wound is healing adequately, often within 24 hours of surgery. Shoulder exercises may begin 7 days after surgery or when surgical drains are removed. The specific exercises the surgeon orders may vary with the surgical

Table 1. Potential Consequences and Implications of Primary Therapy for Breast Cancer

Modified Radical Mastectomy	Shared Symptomatology	Partial Mastectomy, Axillary Node Dissection, & Irradiation
Loss of body part	Cancer diagnosis	Breast fibrosis
Altered body image	Sensory loss	Hyperpigmentation
Prosthesis	Hand and arm care	Rib fractures
Reconstructive surgery	Post-op complications: seroma, hematoma, wound infection	Breast edema
Chest wall tightness	Lymphedema	Changes in skin sensitivity
Skinflap necrosis	Arm weakness	Myositis
	Pain	Prolonged duration of primary therapy
	Psychologic distress	
	Impaired arm mobility	
	Fatigue	
	Adjuvant chemotherapy	

Source: From *"Primary breast cancer: physical consequences and rehabilitation."* M. K. T. Knobf. *Seminars in Oncology Nursing,* 1(3), (p. 220.) Reprinted with permission of W.B. Saunders.

procedure but some of the arm and shoulder exercises frequently taught to patients are shown in Figure 4.

Other operative complications that can occur include seromas, hematomas, nerve injury, and lymphedema. A *seroma* is the accumulation of serous or serosanguinous fluid in the dead space of the axillary fossa or chest wall. The fluid is readily aspirated or drained. Seromas can delay healing and foster infection. Hematomas occur when blood accumulates in the interstitial space and can be aspirated when liquified or be reabsorbed over time without intervention.

Nerve injury may occur despite surgical efforts to avoid trauma. Patients may complain of sensations of pain, tingling, numbness, heaviness, or increased skin sensitivity on the arm or chest. These sensations change over time and usually disappear during or after 1 year. Less often, muscle atrophy may occur secondary to nerve injury and result in decresed arm or shoulder function.

The trend toward less radical surgery has reduced the incidence of lymphedema of the arm. Transient arm swelling lasting a few weeks after surgery is not unusual. Patients should report arm numbness, paresthesias, heaviness, and pain. Management of lymphedema includes arm elevation at night , mild exercise, and an elastic support sleeve that is put on in the morning. If necessary, a pneumatic compression sleeve or pump can be used. Teaching measures to prevent infection in the affected arm is also important.

After a mastectomy a temporary breast prosthesis can be worn for a cosmetic appearance. In 4 to 6 weeks, the woman can be

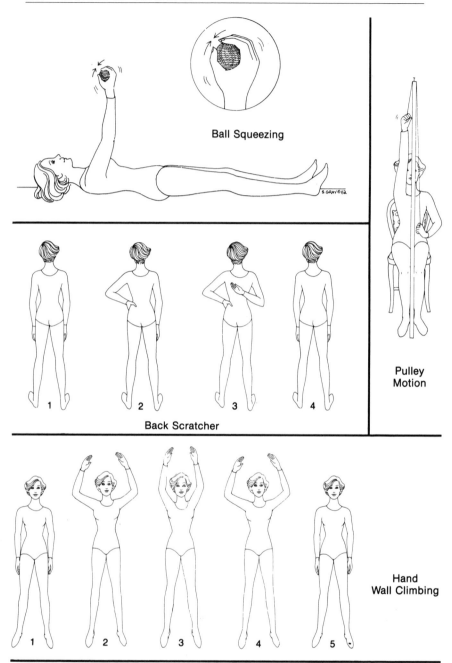

Figure 4. Arm and shoulder exercises commonly prescribed for patients following breast cancer surgery.

Source: From *Reach to Recovery Exercises After Mastectomy Patient Guide.* 1983. Atlanta, American Cancer Society. No. 4624-PS. Reprinted with permission of publisher.

fitted for a permanent prosthesis. Today's prostheses come in a variety of shapes, sizes, and colors. A good fit is important to self-image, posture, balance, and clothing fit.

Reconstruction has become an option for more women due to improved surgical techniques. Reconstruction restores symmetry, obviates the need for prostheses, and improves the patient's self-image. It is important for a woman to discuss the option of breast reconstruction with her surgeon before a mastectomy, since the surgeon may want to consult a plastic surgeon about the location of the mastectomy incisions or to perform reconstruction at the time of the mastectomy.

Reconstruction can be done right after the mastectomy or any time after healing has occurred. Implant reconstruction is the most common, requiring 1 to 3 days of hospitalization. Implants are commonly placed under the pectoralis muscle. The surgery creates a new breast mound. Nipple/areola reconstruction is an additional option. Other procedures using tissue and skin from the lower abdomen, back, or buttocks may be used to reconstruct the breast.

Radiation Therapy

Since clinically undetectable breast cancer cells may be left following local excision of the cancer, radiation therapy is given for local tumor control. Women with large tumors or evidence of tumor cells in the margins of the excised tissue will also benefit from radiation to reduce the chance of local recurrence. Chest wall recurrence following mastectomy can be treated with radiation therapy.

Radiation therapy can also be used preoperatively to shrink large breast tumors and make them more easily resectable. Palliative radiation therapy is commonly used to relieve the pain of bone metastasis and for the symptomatic management of metastases to other sites, such as the brain.

Fatigue, skin reactions, changes in sensation and color and texture of the skin, and breast swelling are common during and immediately following a course of radiation therapy to the breast.

Chemotherapy and Hormonal Therapy

Chemotherapy alone, hormonal therapy alone, or a combination of the two can be used to palliate the effects of metastatic disease. Recommendations for adjuvant chemotherapy and/or adjuvant hormone therapy are usually based on the number of positive axillary nodes, menopausal status, and the estrogen receptor assay. The use of adjuvant chemotherapy for all node-positive, premenopausal patients was recommended by the National Institutes of Health Consensus Development Panel (1985). For postmenopausal women with positive nodes, the panel recommended Tamoxifen therapy. A 1989 consensus panel recommended that physicians consider adjuvant chemotherapy for node-negative women as well, but this recommendation is controversial because studies have yet to demonstrate the survival benefit of this approach.

The chemotherapeutic drugs most commonly used are alkylating agents, antimetabolites, antitumor antibiotics, and vinca alkaloids. Hormone manipulation is achieved primarily through hormone blockers and infrequently by surgical removal of sex hormone-producing glands (oophorectomy, adrenalectomy, or hypophysectomy). Tamoxifen, an anti-estrogen, is the most widely used hormonal agent. Appendix II provides a review of the hormonal agents that can be used in the management of breast cancer.

Side effects vary with specific drugs and may include fatigue, weight gain, nausea, vomiting, alopecia, disturbances in appetite and taste, neuropathies, diarrhea, bone marrow suppression, and menopausal symptoms.

Hair loss and weight gain or loss can affect a patient's body image. Premenopausal women commonly experience premature menopause, with symptoms of decreased vaginal lubrication, hot flashes, irregular menses, or amenorrhea.

Patients with distant metastases require systemic treatment with cytotoxic chemotherapy or hormonal manipulation. At this stage the goal of therapy is to provide the best possible quality of life.

NURSING CONSIDERATIONS

The period following the discovery of a breast tumor is very stressful for the patient. The breast may represent femininity, sexuality, love, nurturance, and maternal feelings for a woman and is, therefore, often an important part of her self-image. Feelings of anxiety, anger, and depression are not uncommon. The woman may view the possible loss of a breast as an assault. The woman is also dealing with the fact that she has cancer and the threat that the diagnosis has to life itself.

Women undergoing a mastectomy may have feelings of mutilation, a decrease in self-image, and problems in sexual and family relationships. These feelings also have an impact on the spouse or significant other and the family. Feelings of despair, helplessness, shock, guilt, and personal vulnerability are common (See Unit IV, Chapter 5.).

Key sources of support at this time are physicians, nurses, family, and friends. Additionally, through the American Cancer Society's Reach to Recovery program, women living successfully after treatment for breast cancer volunteer to visit other patients. After training, they offer support and provide advice on the various aspects of living with a mastectomy. Because of the variety of new approaches for managing breast cancer, the program has selected volunteers available who have had breast-conservation surgery, radiation therapy, chemotherapy, and reconstruction. The volunteer never gives medical advice, but serves as a role model of a recovered breast cancer patient, providing information about her own positive experience. Other patient education and support groups, such as "I Can Cope" and "CanSurmount," may also be useful.

Nursing care for the patient who has had a mastectomy includes rehabilitation for physical restoration of shoulder and arm function, emotional support, prevention of complications, adjustment to social and sexual activities, aid in the return to vocational and occupational goals, and cosmetic rehabilitation through prosthesis or breast reconstruction information.

Unfortunately, metastases may be present at the time of diagnosis, but more commonly occur after an apparent disease-free interval. The recurrence of breast cancer produces a significant emotional reaction that may include anxiety, depression, and disorganization as the patient and family are once again confronted with issues of new treatment decisions and possibly death. Because prolonged survival can be achieved in many cases of recurrence, patients require periodic follow up after the first definitive treatment.

Bibliography

Beahrs, O. H., Henson, D. E., Hutter, R. V. P. & Myers, M. H. (Eds.). (1988). *Manual for staging of cancer* (3rd ed.). Philadelphia: J.B. Lippincott, pp 146–147.

Bostwick, J. (1989). Breast reconstruction following mastectomy. *CA, 39*, 40–49.

d'Angelo, T., & Gorrell, C. R. (1989). Breast reconstruction using tissue expanders. *Oncology Nursing Forum, 16*(1), 23–27.

Greifzu, S. (1986). Breast cancer: The risks and the options. *RN,* (Oct.) 23–42.

Holland, J.C., & Mastrovito, R. (1980). Psychologic adaptation to breast cancer. *Cancer, 46,* l045–1052.

Knobf, M. K. (1985). Primary breast cancer: Physical consequences and rehabilitation. *Seminars in Oncology Nursing, 1*(3), 214–224.

Knobf, M. K. (1986). Physical and psychologic distress associated with adjuvant chemotherapy in women with breast cancer. *Journal of Clinical Oncology, 4*, 678–684.

Seminars in Oncology Nursing (1985) *1*, 3, Entire Issue.

Schwarz-Appelbaum, J., Dedrick, J., Jusenius, K., & Kirchner, C. W. (1984). Nursing care plans: Sexuality and treatment of breast cancer. *Oncology Nursing Forum, 11*(6), 16–24.

Swain, S. M., & Lippman, M. E. (1989). Systemic therapy of locally advanced breast cancer: Review and guidelines. *Oncology, 3*, 39–45.

8 GYNECOLOGIC MALIGNANCIES

Mary Beth Tombes

Cancers of the female genital tract account for about 15% of all new cancers diagnosed in women. Although gynecologic cancers are the fourth leading cause of female cancer deaths in the United States, most are highly curable when detected early.

ENDOMETRIAL CANCER

Incidence and Etiology

Cancer of the endometrium is the most common gynecologic malignancy, usually occurring in women between the ages of 55 and 70. Factors associated with an increased risk of endometrial cancer include obesity, hypertension, diabetes, a history of infertility, failure to ovulate, and prolonged estrogen therapy.

Clinical Manifestations

Vaginal bleeding during or after menopause can be a cardinal sign of endometrial cancer. Persistent, irregular premenopausal bleeding, especially in obese women, may also indicate a malignancy and deserves further evaluation.

Screening and Diagnosis

The American Cancer Society recommends that a uterine tissue sample be obtained from all high-risk women at menopause. A fractional dilatation and curettage is performed to confirm a diagnosis of endometrial cancer. Seventy-five percent of patients with this disease are diagnosed in the early stages. The staging classification of endometrial cancers is based on uterine size, cervical involvement, and tumor cell differentiation (Table 1).

Treatment

Surgical intervention usually consists of a *total abdominal hysterectomy and bilateral salpingo-oophorectomy* (TAH-BSO) with or without removal of the surrounding lymph nodes. In most cases, some form of radiation therapy is recommended for all but earliest stage disease. In patients with advanced or recurrent disease, a

**Table 1. International Federation of Gynecology and Obstetrics
(FIGO) Staging for Endometrial Cancer**

Stage	Description
Stage 0	Carcinoma *in situ*
Stage I	Carcinoma confined to corpus Cases are subgrouped with regard to histologic type: Grade 1, highly differentiated adenomatous carcinoma Grade 2, moderately differentiated adenomatous carcinoma Grade 3, undifferentiated carcinoma
Stage IA	Length of uterine cavity is 8 cm or less
Stage IB	Length of uterine cavity is more than 8 cm
Stage II	Carcinoma involves corpus and cervix
Stage III	Carcinoma has extended outside uterus but not outside true pelvis
Stage IV	Carcinoma has extended outside true pelvis or has involved mucosae of bladder or rectum
Stage IVA	Spread to adjacent organs
Stage IVB	Spread to distant organs

Source: From "Tumors of the Female Reproductive Tract" by J.B. Beecham, B.F. Hel Kamp, and P. Rubin. 1983, pp. 428–481. In P. Rubin (Ed.), *Clinical Oncology: A Multidisciplinary Approach.* Atlanta: American Cancer Society. Reprinted with permission of the publisher.

regimen of chemotherapy and/or hormonal agents may be combined with other treatment modalities.

Five-year survival ranges from approximately 90% of patients with stage I disease to less than 10% of patients with stage IV.

OVARIAN CANCER

Incidence and Etiology

Ovarian cancer is the second most common gynecologic malignancy and accounts for over half of all deaths from female reproductive tract cancers. The incidence of ovarian cancer peaks between the ages of 40 and 70. Risk increases with advancing age. Other factors that may influence the development of ovarian cancer include: nulliparity; a history of breast, endometrial, or colorectal cancer; a family history of ovarian cancer; infertility; early menopause; exposure to asbestos or talc; and a high-fat diet.

Clinical Manifestations

Because their early-stage symptoms are non-specific, most patients do not seek medical attention until the disease is advanced. Persistent, vague gastrointestinal complaints, abdominal discomfort, indigestion, early satiety, or mild anorexia in a woman 40 years or older should be evaluated to rule out ovarian cancer. Ascites, pain, and a pelvic mass usually signal advanced disease.

Diagnosis

Not all ovarian tumors are palpable. Early lesions remain difficult to detect by computerized tomography (CT), sonogram, or magnetic resonance imaging (MRI). An exploratory laparotomy is performed for diagnostic and staging purposes. Staging involves intraoperative examination of peritoneal surfaces and pelvic and abdominal organs. Generally, stage I disease is limited to the ovaries; stage II involves spread to surrounding pelvic organs; stage III indicates extension to other abdominal organs below the diaphragm, and stage IV refers to disease that has metastasized above the diaphragm.

Treatment

A total abdominal hysterectomy and bilateral salpingo-oophorectomy with tumor debulking are performed for all stages of ovarian cancer. Either chemotherapy or radiotherapy is used postoperatively depending on the extent of disease. External beam radiation is given to early-stage patients with little or no residual tumor. Complications of radiation include radiation enteritis, which causes diarrhea, nausea and vomiting, and weight loss. Patients may also develop bowel obstructions caused by adhesions from surgery or radiation.

Chemotherapy is commonly used in patients with advanced disease. Cyclophosphamide, cisplatin, hexamethylmelamine, and doxorubicin are chemotherapeutic drugs with demonstrated antitumor activity.

Investigational approaches to the treatment of ovarian cancer include the instillation of chemotherapeutic, biological, or radioactive agents through peritoneal catheters—a procedure similar to peritoneal dialysis. This approach is generally limited to patients with small amounts of residual disease in the peritoneal cavity following surgery.

Many patients have a "second-look" laparotomy when therapy is completed to evaluate treatment response and the need for further therapy.

CERVICAL CANCER

Incidence and Etiology

Carcinoma of the cervix is the third most prevalent gynecologic cancer. Since the widespread introduction of the *Papanicolaou*

Table 2. Classification and Comparative Nomenclature of Cervical Smears

Class I	Normal smear No abnormal cells.	
Class II	Atypical cells present below the level of cervical neoplasia.	
Class III	Smear contains abnormal cells consistent with dysplasia.	Mild dysplasia = CIN 1 Moderate dysplasia = CIN 2
Class IV	Smear contains abnormal cells consistent with carcinoma *in situ*	Severe dysplasia and Carcinoma *in situ* = CIN 3
Class V	Smear contains abnormal cells consistent with carcinoma of squamous cell origin.	
Key: CIN = cervical intraepithelial neoplasia		

Source: From "Cervical Intraepithelial Neoplasia (Dysplasia and Carcinoma In Situ) and Early Invasive Cervical Carcinoma," J.R. Nelson, Jr., H.E. Averette, and R.M. Richart, 1989, *CA—A Journal for Clinicians,* 39 159. Reprinted, with permission of the publisher.

(Pap) smear as a standard screening tool, the diagnosis of cervical cancer at the invasive stage has steadily decreased, while the diagnosis of highly curable, *pre-invasive carcinoma in situ* (CIS) has increased. CIS is more common in women 30 to 40 years old, while invasive carcinoma is more frequent in women over age 40.

Factors associated with a higher incidence of cervical cancer include early age at first sexual intercourse, early pregnancy, low socioeconomic status, history of any sexually transmitted disease, or history of multiple sex partners. In addition, women whose mothers used the drug *diethylstibestrol* (DES) during their pregnancy have been shown to be at higher risk for some types of cervical cancer. Viral infection may also play as important role in the development of the disease.

Screening and Detection

Since early cervical cancer may be asymptomatic, the Pap smear plays an important role in its early detection. Pap smears are highly accurate and permit detection of precancerous changes in cervical cells. Eradication of such lesions can prevent the development of invasive cancer. The classification of Pap smears is shown in Table 2.

Given the curable nature of early cervical cancer, the American Cancer Society recommends that all women age 18 and over, and those under 18 who are sexually active, have an annual Pap smear and pelvic examination. After three negative annual exams, the Pap smear may be performed less frequently at the discretion of the

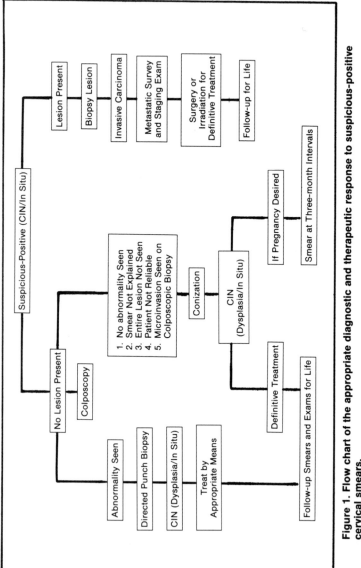

Figure 1. Flow chart of the appropriate diagnostic and therapeutic response to suspicious-positive cervical smears.

Source: From "Cervical Intraepithelial Neoplasia (Dysplasia and Carcinoma In Situ) and Early Invasive Cervical Carcinoma" by J. H. Nelson, Jr., H. E. Averette, and R. M. Richart, 1989, *CA—A Journal for Clinicians, 39, 36,* p. 161. Reprinted with permission of the American Cancer Society.

physician. Women with risk factors for cervical cancer should continue to have an annual Pap smear.

Clinical Manifestations

Symptoms of advanced cervical cancer include painful intercourse, postcoital, coital, or intermenstrual bleeding; and a watery, foul-smelling discharge.

Diagnosis

Patients with abnormal Pap smears undergo colposcopy, which is an excellent means of visualizing the cervical canal and identifying abnormal areas to be biopsied. In some cases, *conization*, a resection of a cone-shaped portion of cervical tissue, may be necessary to obtain adequate tissue for diagnosis. Figure 1 outlines the recommendations for the evaluation of suspicious or positive cervical smears.

Treatment

Choice of therapy is dictated by the stage of the disease (Table 3) and the grade of cervical dysplasia. For patients with pre-invasive cervical cancer (stage 0) who want to retain their fertility, a therapeutic conization is the treatment of choice, but these patients must be followed closely because of the risk of recurrent disease with such minimal intervention. Close follow-up is also necessary for patients treated with laser surgery, cryosurgery, or electrocautery.

Patients with stage IA disease may be treated with a hysterectomy or intracavitary radiation. For stages IB and IIA disease, either radical hysterectomy and pelvic lymphadenectomy or full pelvic irradiation is equally effective. Radiation therapy alone is the treatment of choice for patients with disease more advanced than Stage IIA. Combinations of external beam and intracavitary radiation may be used in this group.

Total pelvic exenteration (TPE) is indicated in very few cases because of the high morbidity associated with this procedure. Total pelvic exenteration includes removal of the bladder, uterus, cervix, vagina, and urethra, with the formation of ureteral and intestinal diversions.

Patients with recurrent disease or nodal metastases may be treated with chemotherapy, but its usefulness may be limited by lack of effective agents and because of the decreased blood supply to pelvic tumors. In advanced cervical cancers, chemotherapy has produced only short-term responses.

Table 3. Clinical Stages of Cervical Cancer

Stage 0 Carcinoma in situ, intraepithelial carcinoma.
Stage I The carcinoma is strictly confined to the cervix (extension to the corpus should be disregarded).
Stage IA Preclinical carcinomas of the cervix—that is, those diagnosed by microscopy.
Stage IA1 Minimal microscopically evident stromal invasion.
Stage IA2 Lesions detected microscopically that can be measured. The upper limit of the measurement should not show a depth of invasion of more than 5 mm taken from the base of the epithelium, either surface or glandular, from which it originates, and a second dimension, the horizontal spread, must not exceed 7 mm. Larger lesions should be staged as IB.
Stage IB Lesions of greater dimension than Stage IA2 whether seen clinically or not; preformed space involvement should not alter the staging, but should be specifically recorded to determine whether it should affect treatment decisions in the future.
Stage II The carcinoma extends beyond the cervix, but has not extended to the pelvic wall. The carcinoma involves the vagina, but not as far as the lower third.
Stage IIA No obvious parametrial involvement.
Stage IIB Obvious parametrial involvement.
Stage III The carcinoma has extended to the pelvic wall. On rectal examination, there is no cancer-free space between the tumor and the pelvic wall. The tumor involves the lower third of the vagina. All cases with a hydronephrosis or nonfunctioning kidney are included.
Stage IIIA No extension to the pelvic wall. Tumor involves the lower third of the vagina.
Stage IIIB Extension to the pelvic wall and/or hydronephrosis or nonfunctioning kidney.
Stage IV The carcinoma has extended beyond the true pelvis or has clinically involved the mucosa of the bladder or rectum. A bullous edema as such does not permit a case to be allotted to Stage IV.
Stage IVA Spread of the growth to adjacent organs.
Stage IVB Spread to distant organs.

Source: From "Cervical Intraepithelial Neoplasia (Dysplasia and Carcinoma In Situ) and Early Invasive Cervical Carcinoma," J.R. Nelson, Jr., H.E. Averette, and R.M. Richart, 1989, *CA—A Journal for Clinicians,* 39 168. Reprinted, with permission of the publisher.

VULVAR CANCER

Incidence and Etiology

Invasive vulvar cancers represent less than 4% of all gynecologic malignancies. The majority of invasive vulvar malignancies are diagnosed after menopause, but pre-invasive disease may be diagnosed in females under the age of 50. Venereal disase and a history of chronic vulvitis are conditions associated with these malignancies.

Vulvar cancers are most frequently found on the labia. The clitoris is the site of less than 15% of all vulvar cancers.

Clinical Manifestations

Patients with vulvar malignancies may present with pruritus, bleeding, pain, an ulcerated lesion, a mass, or an unusual pigmentation.

Diagnosis

A punch biopsy of the suspicious lesion is performed to obtain tissue for diagnosis. In some cases, colposcopy may be used to improve visualization of the lesion. In 40% of vulvar cancer patients, the disease has spread to the inguinal lymph nodes at diagnosis. Table 4 shows staging classification for vulvar cancer.

Treatment

The goal of vulvar cancer treatment is complete eradication of tumor with minimal disfigurement and maintenance of optimal sexual function. Some patients with stage 0 disease may be treated with topical 5-fluorouracil (5-FU) alone. Most patients are treated surgically with wide local excision and a *skinning vulvectomy* followed by skin grafting. Both treatments produce good cosmetic results and maintain clitoral sensitivity and overall sexual function. However, prolonged bedrest is required after a skinning vulvectomy to preserve the skin graft.

Radical vulvectomy is performed in most patients with stage I-III disease. In this procedure the labia, subcutaneous tissue, and clitoris are removed, and parts of the distal urethra, vagina, or anus may be resected. Patients with involved lymph nodes will also require bilateral groin node dissections.

Stage IV disease may require radical vulvectomy and pelvic exenteration. Patients with metastases may be treated palliatively with combined radiation and chemotherapy. The use of vulvar

Table 4. International Federation of Gynecology and Obstetrics (FIGO) Staging Classification of Carcinoma of the Vulva

Stage No.	Description
Stage 0	Carcinoma *in situ*
Stage I	Tumor confined to vulva; 2 cm or less in largest diameter
Stage II	Tumor confined to vulva; greater than 2 cm in diameter
Stage III	Tumor of any size with adjacent spread to urethra, vagina, peritoneum or anus; palpable movable nodes in either or both groins; or both
Stage IV	Tumor of any size infiltrating bladder or rectal mucosa; or fixed to bone, or other distant metastases; or both

Source: From "Treatment Modalities for Gynecological Cancers," C. Robertson, 1986, *Seminars in Oncology Nursing, 2,* p. 279. Reprinted, with permission of W.B. Saunders.

radiation is limited because of the potential for severe vulvar tissue reaction.

A common complication of vulvectomies is impaired wound healing. Keeping the surgical wounds scrupulously clean, dry, and debrided can minimize this complication and speed healing. Lower extremity lymphedema can also occur when pelvic or inguinal lymph nodes are removed.

VAGINAL CANCER

Incidence and Etiology

Vaginal cancer is a rare malignancy diagnosed most frequently in women aged 50 to 70. A higher incidence of this cancer has been observed in patients with a prolapsed uterus or vagina, previous vaginal radiation, or history of maternal DES exposure during early pregnancy.

Clinical Manifestations

Patients with pre-invasive forms of the disease are frequently asymptomatic. As the cancer progresses, patients may experience abnormal vaginal bleeding (postmenopausal, post-coital, or intermenstrual), changes in patterns of urination, or a foul-smelling vaginal discharge.

Screening and Diagnosis

Pap smears can detect vaginal cancers in the pre-invasive stage. Any lesions detected during speculum examination should be biopsied. Since the vagina is a common site of spread from the ovary, endometrium, cervix, or bowel, it is important to determine if the lesion is a primary cancer or a metastatic lesion.

Treatment

Pre-invasive lesions of the vagina may be treated with topical chemotherapy or laser therapy. Radiation therapy is the treatment of choice for the majority of invasive vaginal cancers. *Brachytherapy* (an implanted radioactive source) is the most common type of vaginal radiation, although external beam radiation therapy may be added for large tumors. Surgery is not usually performed because of the excellent results achieved with radiation therapy alone. Recurrent disease is treated surgically with local excision, vaginectomy, or pelvic exenteration.

For isolated cases of extensive vaginal cancer, treatment may consist of radiation plus partial or total vaginectomy. The vagina may be reconstructed with skin grafts to maintain sexual function. Although the vagina may remain intact when the cancer is treated with radiation therapy, the tissue may atrophy, limiting lubrication and sexual pleasure. Vaginal reconstruction can restore function but not vaginally induced pleasure.

FALLOPIAN TUBE CANCER

Incidence and Etiology

Fallopian tube cancer, the rarest of gynecologic malignancies, is seen most often in women aged 50 to 70. Factors associated with fallopian tube cancer include nulliparity, infertility, and chronic tubal infections (salpingitis).

Clinical Manifestations

Abnormal vaginal bleeding, abdominal pain, or a vaginal discharge may signal cancer of the fallopian tube, although these symptoms are also seen in the more common gynecologic malignancies.

Screening and Diagnosis

Early detection of a tubal malignancy is rare; most malignancies are diagnosed only by exploratory laparotomy. Cancer of the fallopian tube is staged similarly to ovarian cancer (see Table 5),

Table 5. International Federation of Gynecology and Obstetrics (FIGO) Staging for Fallopian Tube Cancer

Stage No.	Description
Stage 0	Carcinoma *in situ*
Stage I	Tumor extending into submucosa or muscularis, but not penetrating to serosal surface of fallopian tube
Stage II	Tumor extending to serosa of fallopian tube
Stage III	Direct extension of tumor to ovary or endometrium
Stage IV	Extension of tumor beyond reproductive organs

Source: From "Treatment Modalities for Gynecological Cancers," C. Robertson, 1986, *Seminars in Oncology Nursing,* 2, p. 279. Reprinted, with permission of W.B. Saunders.

and assessment for peritoneal spread is equally crucial in tubal cancer cases. Patients with early-stage disease have a much better prognosis than those with advanced disease.

Treatment

Tubal malignancies are treated primarily with surgical removal of the tumor via total abdominal hysterectomy and bilateral salpingo-oophorectomy. If the patient wishes to remain fertile, a unilateral salpingo-oophorectomy may sometimes be performed. Adjuvant radiation therapy is used for some stages of disease. Because tubal malignancies are rare, little information is available on the value of chemotherapy. Regimens used in treating fallopian tube cancers are similar to those used in treating ovarian cancer.

GESTATIONAL TROPHOBLASTIC DISEASE

Gestational trophoblastic disease occurs when the cells of trophoblastic tissue from a developing placenta change abnormally. There are three types of gestational trophoblastic tumors: hydatidiform mole, invasive mole, and choriocarcinoma. Although the disease is most frequently seen in women 25 to 29 years of age (because the incidence of pregnancy is highest in this group), the risk is highest in women over 40.

A *hydatidiform mole,* or molar pregnancy, is a benign tumor that develops in the uterine cavity. Embryonic tissue is present in partial moles and absent in complete moles. Approximately one-half of all gestational trophoblastic diseases develop after molar pregnancy. Fifteen to twenty percent of hydatidiform moles will progress to malignant gestational trophoblastic disease, either in the form of a persistent hydatidiform mole or choriocarcinoma.

Complete moles, which occur more frequently than partial moles, are more likely to progress to malignancy.

An *invasive mole* is similar to an hydatidiform mole except that the tumor invades the endometrial lining and penetrates the musculature of the uterus. Both hydatidiform and invasive molar tissue resemble a "bunch of grapes" inside the uterus.

Choriocarcinoma occurs most frequently after treatment for hydatidiform mole, but it can occur after any gestational event—ectopic pregnancy, abortion, or full-term pregnancy. Choriocarcinoma is a highly aggressive form of gestational trophoblastic disease that frequently presents as metastatic disease. Until recently, it was considered uniformly fatal within a few months; now it is considered highly curable with appropriate treatment and follow-up.

Clinical Manifestations

Symptoms are similar to those seen in pregnancy. Gestational trophoblastic disease should be suspected when a supposedly pregnant woman has vaginal bleeding, unusually severe nausea and vomiting, and a uterus larger or smaller than expected for her length of gestation. Normal indications of fetal activity (heart sounds, movement) are absent in a molar pregnancy.

Diagnosis

Ultrasound confirms the presence of a molar pregnancy. An elevated serum or urine *human chorionic gonadotropin* (HCG) level is not diagnostic, because HCG is secreted by normal placental cells in pregnancy as well as by tissue from gestational trophoblastic diseases.

Treatment

Once a suspected gestational trophoblastic disease is confirmed by ultrasound, dilatation and curettage is performed. The patient's serum HCG level is monitored at 1- to 2-week intervals following evacuation of the mole. When the HCG level returns to normal, it is measured every 1 to 2 months for 1 year. If, at any time during follow-up, the HCG level plateaus or begins to rise, therapy for malignant gestational trophoblastic disease is started immediately. At that time, patients are evaluated for local involvement and metastatic disease. Oral contraceptives are strongly recommended to prevent conception during follow-up, because there is no way to distinguish conception from recurrent disease through measurement of HCG.

Chemotherapy is the primary mode of treatment for malignant gestational trophoblastic disease once a molar pregnancy has been removed. Treatment depends on whether the patient fits a low- or high-risk profile. High-risk factors include a very high HCG level, symptoms lasting longer than 4 months, liver or brain metastases, prior unsuccessful treatment, and disease that develops after a full-term pregnancy. For low-risk disease, single-agent chemotherapy with or without an abdominal hysterectomy is recommended. Chemotherapy is continued until the HCG level drops to normal. Once a normal HCG level is attained, therapy is discontinued and the level is monitored for 1 year. If the level plateaus or rises, combination chemotherapy is initiated.

Aggressive combination chemotherapy is the initial therapy for all high-risk patients. Radiation therapy may also be indicated if brain metastases are present.

Even with successful evacuation and surveillance following a molar pregnancy, disease-free patients may be concerned about recurrence with subsequent conception. If the patient receives chemotherapy, she will require information about potential sterility and teratogenicity in order to make decisions about future family planning. Although there may be some minimal risk of recurrence after hydatidiform mole, most women are not dissuaded from conceiving.

NURSING CONSIDERATIONS

Nursing care needs of women with gynecological cancer will vary according to the cancer site, stage, and the treatment modalities used. Diagnostic and staging procedures can be frightening and embarrassing. Many patients will be reassured by careful explanations of procedures and efforts to safeguard their privacy.

Wound management is often a major concern, especially in patients undergoing radical vulvectomy, which carries a high risk of infection. The presence of urinary catheters and surgical drains adds to the risk of infection. The perineal area should be kept clean and dry to promote healing. As patients are able, nurses can encourage patient participation in infection prevention and wound care.

Elimination difficulties are common. Patients are frequently discharged with urinary catheters in place and will need detailed instructions for care and/or removal. The enterostomal therapy (ET) nurse is a valuable resource when the patient has fistulas, ostomies, or wounds that are difficult to manage. The ET nurse can develop an individual plan of care to meet specific patient needs and can also assist with patient and family teaching.

The diagnosis and treatment of gynecological cancer can affect a woman's self-concept, body image, sexuality, and sexual functioning. These subjects are discussed in Unit III, Chapters 5 and 6. Women in the later stages of disease may need assistance in maintaining nutritional status (see Unit IV, Chapter 3), managing pain (see Unit IV, Chapter 2), or managing symptoms (see Unit IV, Chapter 1).

Bibliography

Frank-Stromborg, M. (1986). The role of the nurse in cancer detection and screening. *Seminars in Oncology Nursing, 2*(3), 191–199.

Gusberg, S. B., Shingleton, H. M., & Deppe, G. (1988). *Female genital cancer.* New York: Churchill Livingstone.

Kaempfer, S. H., & Major, P. (1986). Fertility considerations in the gynecology oncology patient. *Oncology Nursing Forum, 13*(1), 23–27.

Lamb, M. A. (1985). Sexual dysfunction in the gynecologic oncology patient. *Seminars in Oncology Nursing, 1*(1), 9–17.

Lamb, M. A., & Chu, J. (1988). Invasive cancer of the vulva. *AORN Journal 47*(4), 928–936.

Lovejoy, N. (1987). Precancerous lesions of the cervix: Personal risk factors. *Cancer Nursing, 10*(1), 2–14.

Miller, N. J., & Pazdur, M. (1987). Gynecologic malignancies. (In) S. Groenwald (Ed.). *Cancer nursing: Principles and practice.* pp 558–592. Boston: Jones and Bartlett Publishers, Inc.

Nelson, J. H., Averette, H. E., & Richart, R. M. (1989). Cervical intraepithelial neoplasia (dysplasia and carcinoma *in situ*) and early invasive cervical carcinoma. *Ca-a Cancer Journal for Clinicians, 39*(3), 157–178.

Robertson, C. (1986). Treatment modalities for gynecological cancers. *Seminars in Oncology Nursing, 2*(4), 275–280.

Smith, D. B. (1986). Gynecological cancers: Etiology and pathophysiology. *Seminars in Oncology Nursing, 2*(4), 270–274.

Walczak, J. R. (Guest Ed.). (1990). Gynecologic cancers. *Seminars in Oncology Nursing, 6*(3): entire issue.

9 CANCERS OF THE MALE GENITAL ORGANS

Mark Redmond

PROSTATE CANCER

Prostate cancer is one of the most common cancers in men in the United States second only to skin cancer. Along with colon and rectal cancer, it is the second leading cause of cancer deaths in men. The incidence is highest in black men. Approximately 60% of prostate cancers are detected while still localized; 5-year survival for these patients is 84%. Increasing age is the most obvious risk factor, as almost all clinically detectable cases occur in men over the age of 50; but the disease may also be associated with positive family history, dietary fat, and occupational exposure to cadmium.

Clinical Manifestations

Many patients with localized disease are asymptomatic. In these cases the malignancy is often found on routine digital rectal examination or during pathologic examination of prostate tissue following *transurethral resection of the prostate* (TURP) for presumed benign hypertrophy. As the tumor grows, patients may present with changes in urinary patterns: frequency, hesitancy, nocturia, and narrowing of stream. Since prostate cancer frequently metastasizes to the bone, patients with metastasis may present with bone or joint pain and, occasionally, pathologic bone fractures.

Screening/Diagnosis

Rectal examination remains the most effective screening tool for the early detection of prostate cancer. The American Cancer Society recommends annual digital rectal examination for all men over 40 years old.

Serum levels of *prostate-specific antigen* (PSA), an antigen produced only by the prostate gland, are generally elevated in patients who have increased volume of prostatic tissue. Because this test cannot differentiate between benign and malignant conditions, it cannot be used as the sole screening tool for prostate cancer, but may be used in conjunction with other tests to definitively diagnose the disease. PSA is most commonly monitored as a tumor marker that indicates progressive disease following radical treatment.

The use of transrectal ultrasound to screen large numbers of patients has not been particularly effective, but this technique may be useful to screen men at high risk and to stage patients with localized disease. The diagnosis of prostate cancer is confirmed by transrectal, transurethral, or perineal biopsy of the prostate gland.

Treatment

The treatment of prostate cancer depends upon the stage of the disease (Figure 1) and the age of the patient. In patients over age 60 with stage A_1 prostate cancer found incidentally by the TURP procedure, immediate treatment is not indicated because it may take years for the occult malignancy to become clinically evident. These patients should be followed at 6-month intervals; this early disease is generally indolent and may never progress or require additional treatment. Surgery is recommended for most younger patients with stage A_1 disease and for patients with stage B disease. Radiation therapy is also used in some settings to cure these early-stage cancers. Multimodality approaches combining surgery or radiation with hormonal therapy or chemotherapy are used for patients with stages C and D disease.

Surgery: Generally, a radical prostatectomy is performed as a curative procedure for localized disease. The surgeon may approach the prostate gland via the perineum or the lower abdomen above the pubic bone. Postoperatively, patients will have hematuria and require an indwelling urinary drainage catheter. Hematuria resolves within 5 to 7 days. Other complications of this procedure include impotence and urinary incontinence.

A nerve-sparing radical prostatectomy may be performed on patients with stage A_2 or B disease. This approach preserves potency in approximately 75% of patients. Erectile functioning, if it has been retained, may take up to a year to return. Therefore, patients are advised to wait at least 6 months before considering surgical correction of impotence by implanation of a penile prosthesis.

Approximately 5% of patients will experience urinary incontinence that persists beyond the immediate postoperative period. In some cases, this can be an emotionally devastating condition resulting in the patient's social withdrawal and isolation. An enterostomal therapist may be helpful in recommending appliances or pads if medical management fails to resolve this problem.

Radiation Therapy: Radiation therapy alone can also be used curatively for patients with localized disease. It can be delivered

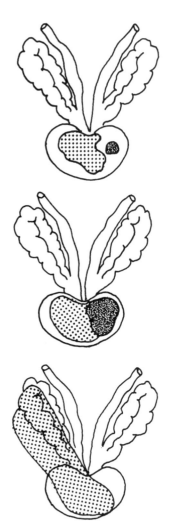

Stage A — Confined to prostate (tumor nondetectable on rectal examination)
A$_1$ — focal
A$_2$ — diffuse

Stage B — Confined to prostate (tumor evident on rectal exam)
B$_1$ — nodule up to 2 cm; palpable involvement of an entire lobe
B$_2$ — larger than 2 cm; palpable involvement of both lobes

Stage C — Extraprostatic tumor extension without metastases (palpable extraprostatic tumor)

Stage D — Local findings as in stages A, B, or C plus metastases
D$_1$ — regional lymph node metastases only
D$_2$ — detectable distant organ metastases

Figure 1. Staging of prostate cancer.
Source: From "Surgery versus Radiation for Localized Prostate Cancer" by M. M. Lieber, 1987, *Oncology* 1(1), pp. 61-68. Reprinted with permission of Dominus Publishing Co.

interstitially with surgically implanted seeds or via external beam irradiation. Select patients with stage A_2 or B disease treated with irradiation may also be candidates for bilateral *lymphadenectomy* (removal of ilioinguinal and pelvic lymph nodes) to eliminate the risk of pelvic nodal metastasis. This procedure is generally used only for patients who have a high risk of nodal involvement, because the combination of external beam radiation and lymphadenectomy often results in lymphedema of the legs, scrotum, and penis.

Another acute local complication of radiation therapy is rectal irritation, which results in abdominal cramping, diarrhea, and rectal pain. Antidiarrheals or soothing suppositories and enemas can be used to control these symptoms. Urinary tract symptoms such as bladder spasms, dysuria, and frequency can be treated with antispasmodics. Irradiation to the pelvis can result in rectal stenosis or urethral stricture in rare cases. Radiation-induced skin reactions can be managed with careful skin hygiene and soothing lotions or ointments as ordered.

Approximately 25-30% of patients undergoing external beam irradiation become impotent, but only 10-15% of those with interstitial implants experience this problem. Unlike the impotence caused by prostate surgery, radiation therapy produces a gradual loss of erectile function that usually occurs within the first year after treatment.

Hormonal Therapy: Because the growth of prostatic cancers is androgen-dependent, hormonal therapy is used to counteract the growth-stimulating effects of these male hormones. This type of therapy is the most common treatment for patients with disseminated disease. For patients at this stage, the goals of therapy are disease control and palliation of symptoms rather than cure. Hormonal therapy includes estrogen administration, orchiectomy, and administration of gonadotropin-releasing hormone analogues and "antiandrogens." The agents most commonly used and their toxicities are listed in Appendix II.

Treatment selection is dependent on certain clinical and psychological factors. *Orchiectomy*, or surgical castration, removes the source of the androgens but is psychologically distressing for many patients. Patients commonly grieve for the real and symbolic loss associated with this procedure. Surgical implantation of testicular prostheses may alleviate the patient's body image concerns.

The standard type of estrogen for this therapy is *diethylstilbestrol* (DES). Because of the increased risk of cardiovascular toxicity associated with the use of estrogens in men, this therapy may be contraindicated in patients with pre-existing cardiovascular disease. Other side effects include penile atrophy and decreased libido, although erectile function may be retained. *Gynecomastia*, the enlargement of the breasts in males, is common, and can be a painful and embarrassing condition. This side effect can be prevented by radiating both breasts before estrogen therapy.

Synthetic hormones that mimic the action of *gonadotropin-releasing hormone* (GnRH analogues) are also used to suppress the production of testosterone. These drugs can be combined with anti-androgens, such as flutamide, to totally block androgen production. Thus far, these drugs have shown fewer serious side effects than estrogen.

Chemotherapy: Chemotherapy is generally reserved for patients with advanced disease who no longer respond to hormonal manipulation. The most frequently used agents are cyclophosphamide, doxorubicin, 5-fluorouracil (5-FU), and methotrexate. Results are generally poor.

Palliation: Bone pain due to skeletal metastases is the most significant problem in the patient with advanced prostate cancer. Pathologic fractures are not uncommon, and patients with spinal metastases are at an increased risk for developing spinal cord compression (refer to Unit IV, Chapter 4). Radiation of sites of bone metastases can provide symptomatic relief.

PENILE CANCER

Cancer of the penis is a rare disease in the United States. One predisposing factor is poor hygiene in the uncircumcised male. Most cases occur in patients over age 50.

Patients generally present with a painless ulcer or growth on the penis, although the lesion may be obscured by an unretractable foreskin. In this case, its presence may be signalled by a persistent discharge.

The diagnosis of penile cancer can be emotionally devastating to the patient. The realistic fear of surgical amputation of the penis may outweigh the threat of mortality; this may be a factor in a patient's delay in seeking medical attention for his condition.

Treatment

Surgery: If the lesion is small and confined to the skin, it may be surgically excised. Patients must be followed closely for evidence of recurrence.

When deeper tissues or structures of the penis are involved, a partial or total penectomy is performed. Lymphadenectomy may also be performed if regional lymph node involvement is suspected.

Complications of lymphadenectomy include skin flap necrosis and infection at the incision site. Edema of the lower extremities may also occur when these lymph nodes are removed. Lymphedema can be reduced by fitting the patient with elastic leg stockings and by keeping him on strict bedrest with legs elevated after surgery.

Radiation Therapy: Radiation therapy may be used in an attempt to preserve the structure and function of the penis. Nodal irradiation is also delivered to the inguinal and pelvic nodes to improve local control.

This therapy usually causes moist skin desquamation. Guidelines for skin care are included in Unit III, Chapter 2. Infected lesions require immediate treatment. Patients should report any changes in urinary patterns that may indicate a urinary tract infection or a urethral stricture.

Patients will require surgery if local control is not achieved with radiation alone.

Chemotherapy: Chemotherapy has been used for palliation of penile cancers. Investigations comparing the efficacy of different chemotherapeutic regimens have been limited because of the rarity of this disease.

TESTICULAR CANCER

Testicular cancer is a relatively rare disease that occurs most frequently in men between the ages of 15 and 40. Although the disease is uncommon, it is the most common cancer in men of this age group. Advances in treatment have made cure possible for 80-90% of patients.

Patients with a history of cryptorchidism, or undescended testes, are at greater risk for this cancer, even after surgical correction of this condition.

Clinical Presentation

Patients frequently present with a painless enlargement of one of the testicles or a testicular lump or nodule. Some patients report a sensation of heaviness or dragging in the lower abdomen or scrotum. In some cases, presenting symptoms may be due to advanced disease involving the lung or abdomen.

Classification

The majority of testicular tumors arise from germinal cells. These germ cell neoplasms are broadly classified as *seminomas* and *nonseminomatous* (NS) tumors, with seminomas accounting for 60% of these malignancies. Figure 2 depicts the cell derivation of testicular tumors. Some patients will have combination tumors. The staging system for testicular tumors is shown in Table 1.

Screening/Diagnosis

The American Cancer Society recommends monthly testicular

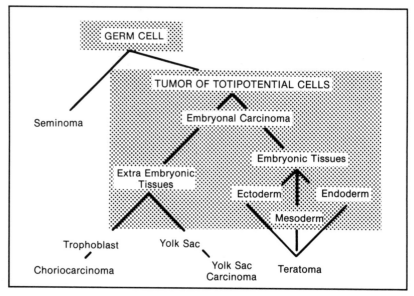

Figure 2. A representation of the unified theory for the derivation of testicular tumors.
Source: From "Pathology of Germ Cell Tumors of Testis: A Progress Report" by F. K. Mostofi, 1980, *Cancer (Suppl) 45*, pp. 1735–1754. Reprinted with permission of J.B. Lippincott Co.

self-examination and can provide pamphlets for nurses to use to educate their patients and the public.

The diagnostic work-up for a suspected testicular tumor may include a computerized axial tomography (CT) scan of the pelvis and abdomen, chest x-ray, and blood tests. The latter are performed to check for the presence of tumor markers, such as alpha-fetoprotein (AFP) and human chorionic gonadotropin (HCG), that are sometimes detected in patients with testicular cancer. A positive test for AFP can confirm the presence of nonseminomatous disease, since this tumor marker is rarely elevated in pure seminomas.

Treatment

Surgery: Radical orchiectomy is performed on the involved testis to determine the histologic type of the tumor. No further surgery is indicated in patients with pure seminomas.

Patients with mixed tumors or those with elevated AFP levels are treated as if they had nonseminomatous tumors. Until recently,

Table 1. Staging Classification for Testicular Tumors

	Seminomas	Nonseminomas
Stage I	Tumor confined to testis	Tumor confined to testis
Stage II	Nodal metastases below the diaphragm A. Minimal retroperitoneal disease B. Bulky metastases	Nodal metastases below the diaphragm A. < 5 positive nodes B. > 5 positive nodes
Stage III	Tumor involving lymph nodes above the diaphragm	Metastases above the diaphragm or in other viscera
Stage IV	Extranodal metastases	—

a radical retroperitoneal lymph node dissection was performed on all NS tumor patients to surgically stage the disease. This procedure results in infertility in most patients, partly because retrograde ejaculation (ejaculation into the bladder) occurs and seminal emission during orgasm is reduced or absent. A radical lymphadenectomy can also damage many of the perineal nerves essential to erectile function.

Most testicular cancer patients are young adults, so fertility issues are of great concern and should be discussed with patients before treatment. For some men, the potential loss of fertility may be a larger threat to their self-esteem than the orchiectomy itself. Unilateral orchiectomy does not affect fertility, because the remaining testis usually produces sufficient quantities of sperm and testosterone for conception.

Radiation Therapy: Radiotherapy is seldom used in the treatment of NS tumors because surgery and chemotherapy produce excellent results. But seminomas are radio-sensitive tumors, so patients with stage I and II disease receive radiation therapy to the pelvis and lower abdomen after a radical orchiectomy. Complications of irradiation include skin reactions and bladder irritation. Sperm production may be diminished or absent for months to years after treatment; however, patients should be advised to use birth control during radiation therapy, since the risk of birth defects in fetuses conceived during treatment is not known.

Chemotherapy: Combination chemotherapy regimens have been used to treat NS tumors with excellent results. Patients with stage III NS disease are treated initially with chemotherapy. Most regimens include cisplatin, VP-16, and bleomycin. Chemotherapy is also used for patients with advanced seminomas or those unresponsive to radiotherapy.

Chemotherapy has produced high cure rates in patients with advanced and recurrent NS disease. Patients with no obvious disease after an orchiectomy and careful staging should be followed closely; if they relapse, some can be treated with chemotherapy. This surveillance approach is designed to preserve fertility in a higher proportion of men. Surgical resection of residual masses may be recommended after the chemotherapy regimen is completed.

Administration of cisplatin is associated with severe nausea and vomiting, neurotoxicity, and nephrotoxicity. Cisplatin-related renal toxicity can be prevented with vigorous pre- and post-treatment hydration. Cisplatin-induced nausea and vomiting are treated with antiemetics (see Unit IV, Chapter 1). Toxicities associated with other chemotherapeutic agents used for testicular cancer are listed in Appendix I. It is important to prevent or ameliorate symptoms, since patients experiencing severe side effects from chemotherapy may not comply with treatment.

Chemotherapy may also affect fertility. All patients become azoospermic during treatment, but approximately 50% recover normal sperm production within 3 years of treatment. Young men may wish to consider sperm banking before treatment, although time constraints and the expense of sperm banking, as well as the location of storage facilities, may preclude this option. Because many patients with testicular cancer already have low sperm counts at diagnosis, it may not be possible to obtain an adequate specimen for preservation.

Bibliography

Bachers, E. S. (1985). Sexual dysfunction after treatment for genitourinary cancers. *Seminars in Oncology Nursing, 1,* 18–24.

Drago, J. R. (1989). The role of new modalities in the early detection and diagnosis of prostate cancer. *Ca—A Cancer Journal for Clinicians, 39*(6), 326–335.

Einhorn, L. H., Crawford, E. D., Shipley, W. U., Loehrer, P. J., & Williams, S. D. (1989). Cancer of the testes. In V. T. DeVita, S. Hellman, & S. A. Rosenberg (Eds.), *Cancer: Principles and practice of oncology* (pp. 1071–1098). Philadelphia: J. B. Lippincott Company.

Eschenbach, A. C. von. (1980). Sexual dysfunction following therapy for cancer of the prostate, testis, and penis. *Frontiers of Radiation Therapy and Oncology, 14,* 42–50.

Higgs, D. J. (1990). The patient with testicular cancer: Nursing management of chemotherapy. *Oncology Nursing Forum, 17*(2), 243–249.

Huben, R. P., & Murphy, G. P. (1986). Prostate cancer: An update. *Ca—A Cancer Journal for Clinicians, 36,* 274–292.

Fair, W. R., Perez, C. A., & Anderson, T. (1989). Cancer of the urethra and penis. In V. T. DeVita, S. Hellman, & S. A. Rosenberg (Eds.), *Cancer: Principles and practice of oncology* (pp. 1059-1070). Philadelphia: J. B. Lippincott Company.

Perez, C. A., Fair, W. R., & Ihde, D. C. (1989). Cancer of the prostate. In V. T. DeVita, S. Hellman, & S. A. Rosenberg (Eds.), *Cancer: Principles and practice of oncology* (pp. 1023-1058). Philadelphia: J. B. Lippincott Company.

Persky, L., & deKernion, J. (1986). Carcinoma of the penis. *Ca—A Cancer Journal for Clinicians, 36*, 258-273.

Sandella, J. A. (1983). Cancer prevention and detection: Testicular cancer. *Cancer Nursing, 6*, 468-486.

Schover, L. R., Eschenbach, A. C. von, Smith, D. B., & Gonzalez, J. (1984). Sexual rehabilitation of urologic cancer patients: A practical approach. *Ca—A Cancer Journal for Clinicians, 34*, 66-74.

10 CANCERS OF THE CENTRAL NERVOUS SYSTEM

Marybeth Chase

INCIDENCE

Cancers of the central nervous system (CNS) account for approximately 1.5% of all malignancies. The peak incidence of these tumors occurs between birth and age 6 and after age 45. Brain tumors cause only about 2.2% of cancer deaths, but are the second leading cause of cancer-related deaths in children below the age of 15, and the fourth leading cause of cancer-related deaths in persons age 15-34.

The incidence and location of CNS tumors differ in children and adults. Eighty percent of all CNS tumors are intracranial. Spinal cord tumors account for less than 15% of all CNS tumors and rarely occur in children. More than 60% of tumors in adults are supratentorial, or located in the cerebral hemispheres, while the majority of pediatric tumors are infratentorial, involving primarily the cerebellum and brain stem. Metastatic brain tumors account for 20-40% of all CNS neoplasms.

CLASSIFICATION

CNS tumors are classified according to their cell of origin within the central nervous system (Table 1). Each type of tumor listed can occur in the brain or spinal cord. Although some CNS tumors may be classified as benign, all should be considered potentially lethal because of their location in relation to other vital structures.

Tumors arising from astrocytes, or *gliomas*, are graded according to their malignant behavior, ranging from grade I benign *astrocytomas* to the most malignant astrocytoma, the grade IV *glioblastoma multiforme*. Approximately 50% of all intracranial tumors are gliomas, and 30% of these are glioblastoma multiforme.

Schwannomas and *meningiomas* are the most common tumors of the spinal cord, accounting for one-half of all neoplasms in this area. Other tumor types occur much less frequently. Primary CNS lymphomas occur more frequently in patients who have received immunosuppressive therapy for transplantation. These are malignant tumors that invade locally, and may develop subarach-

Table 1. Classification of Primary Intracranial Tumors by Cell of Origin

Normal Cell	Tumor
Astrocyte	Astrocytoma, astroblastoma, glioblastoma, spongioblastoma
Ependymocyte	Ependymoma, ependymoblastoma
Oligodendrocyte	Oligodendroglioma
Microgliocyte	Reticulum cell sarcoma or microglioma
Arachnoidal fibroblasts	Meningioma
Nerve cell or neuroblast	Ganglioneuroma, neuroblastoma, retinoblastoma
External granular cell or neuroblast	Medulloblastoma
Schwann cell	Schwannoma (neurinoma)
Melanocyte	Melanotic carcinoma
Choroid epithelial cell	Choroid plexus papilloma or carcinoma
Pituitary	Adenoma
Endothelial cell or "stromal" cell	Hemangioblastoma
Primitive germ cells	Germinoma, pinealoma, teratomas, cholesteatoma
Pineal parenchymal cells	Pinealcytoma
Notochordal remnants	Chordoma

Source: From *Cancer: Principles and Practice of Oncology.* (3rd Ed.) (p. 1558) by V. T. DeVita, Jr., S. Hellman, and S. A. Rosenberg, (Eds.), 1989, Philadelphia: J.B. Lippincott and Co. Reprinted with permission of publisher.

noid seeding. Pituitary tumors are discussed in the chapter on endocrine malignancies (Unit V, Chapter 5).

ETIOLOGY

No risk factors have been identified for the development of CNS neoplasms, but there is an increased incidence of CNS tumors noted in people with certain genetically transmitted disorders, such as neurofibromatosis, tuberous sclerosis, and familial polyposis.

CLINICAL PRESENTATION

Symptoms of CNS neoplasms result from the diffuse effects of increased intracranial pressure or focal neurological effects. Patients with increased intracranial pressure may experience headache, nausea and vomiting, personality changes, or slowed psychomotor functioning. A headache that is often worse in the morning and somewhat better later in the day is a common presenting symptom. Headache, seizures, mental change, and hemiparesis are seen in the majority of patients. Focal signs, such as seizures, visual disturbances, dysphasias, paresthesias, and ataxia may be helpful in localizing the lesion. Expanding intracranial tumors can ultimately cause brain stem herniation, resulting in respiratory arrest and

Table 2. Neurologic Alterations Associated with
Specific Areas of Brain Involvement

Brain Area Involved	Associated Impairment
Frontal Lobe	Disturbed mental status Personality/behavior alterations Changes in emotional responsiveness Speech disturbances Impaired sphincter control Contralateral paralysis
Temporal Lobe	Psychomotor seizures Visual field changes Memory impairment Dominant hemisphere; aphasia, dysphagia Nondominant hemisphere: nonverbal auditory per- ceptual disturbances, musical impairment
Parietal Lobe	Focal seizures Hypesthesia Paresthesia Dyslexia Hormonymous hemianopsia Nondominant hemisphere: perceptual alterations, visual-spatial disturbances, body scheme dis- turbances, impaired cognitive processes, alter- ation in emotional sensitivities
Occipital Lobe	Visual disturbances Hallucinations
Cerebellum	Disturbed equilibrium Impaired coordination
Brainstem	Cranial nerve palsies (temporary or permanent)

Source: From "Increased Intercranial Pressure" by Karen Kane, 1985, (p. 403). In *Handbook of Oncology Nursing.* B. L. Johnson and J. Gross (Eds.) New York: Delmar Publishers, Inc. Reprinted with permission of Delmar Publishing.

death. Table 2 highlights neurologic alterations associated with specific areas of brain involvement.

Symptoms of spinal cord neoplasms are related to the location of the tumor. Pain is the most common presenting symptom. Motor, sensory, and reflex functions need to be evaluated. Involvement of the spinal nerve roots produces pain at the level of the lesion. Patients may also exhibit weakness, spasticity, or sensory impairment below the involved segment of the spinal cord. External urethral and anal sphincters are often impaired.

Clinical manifestations of CNS neoplasms may be more difficult to evaluate in the pediatric population because children are less able to relate and report symptoms. Parents, teachers, and other caretakers of the child may notice changes or problems before the child is aware of change.

DIAGNOSIS

Computerized tomography (CT) scans, particularly with contrast, and *magnetic resonance imaging* (MRI) are the most valuable tests to evaluate the extent of the tumor. These studies have largely replaced other, more invasive tests in the imaging of CNS neoplasms, although cerebral angiography may be indicated for tumors surrounding cerebral blood vessels. This latter procedure also reveals the vascular supply to tumors. Visual field testing can also be helpful in localizing the lesion. Lumbar puncture is generally not indicated for patients with increased intracranial pressure because of the risk of brain stem herniation. This procedure is used to rule out meningeal involvement, particularly in periventricular tumors and CNS lymphoma.

TREATMENT

The prognosis for patients with CNS tumors varies according to the type and grade of tumor. For example, grade I astrocytomas are 90-100% curable, while less than 10% of patients with grade IV astrocytomas (glioblastoma multiforme) survive for 2 years. The most important prognostic factor in grades III and IV is the size of the tumor at diagnosis. The patient's pre- and postoperative neurological status will also influence the individual's ability to resume normal daily activities.

Dexamethasone (Decadron®) is usually administered once the tumor is diagnosed to decrease cerebral edema. It may also be temporarily increased during treatment to combat additional edema that can result from cytotoxic therapy—particularly radiation therapy. If complete resection of the tumor is not possible, patients may be maintained on steroids. Patients may also need anticonvulsants to prevent or control seizure activity. These drugs are started before surgery and are continued as long as indicated.

Surgery

Surgery is the initial treatment for CNS tumors. Biopsies are usually performed to establish diagnosis, and surgery is also used to prevent further neurological deterioration caused by intracranial pressure. In addition, the tumor is often debulked surgically because both radiation and chemotherapy are most effective when the residual tumor burden is as small as possible. Complete resection of CNS tumors is often difficult or impossible because of potential damage to normal tissue and proximity to vital structures. Intracranial tumors are rarely cured with surgery alone.

Craniotomy is performed in most patients to achieve adequate visualization of the tumor, and as much tumor as possible is removed without damaging surrounding normal brain tissue.

Stereotactic surgery employs a mechanical device guided by CT scan or MRI to gain access to discrete areas within the brain. It is used most commonly to obtain a tissue biopsy for pathologic examination. Stereotactic procedures may be indicated in patients with very small, centrally located or poorly demarcated lesions; those too ill for craniotomy; and those who would suffer a significant neurological deficit as a result of extensive resection during craniotomy. Patients with gliomas involving the brain stem may not be candidates for biopsy with or without resection because of the potential damage to vital normal tissues; these patients may begin nonsurgical treatment without a tissue diagnosis.

Radiation Therapy

Postoperative external beam irradiation improves survival for many patients with incompletely resected tumors or for patients whose tumors are not surgically accessible. The amount of radiation that can be delivered safely to this area is limited because of the tissue tolerance of nervous system tissue. A critical question the radiation therapist must consider is the size of the radiation field. Whenever possible, radiotherapy is delivered to a localized area of the brain to minimize the volume of tissue irradiated. In other patients, such as those with large tumors or those with a high risk of spread to the subarachnoid space, whole-brain or craniospinal irradiation may be indicated. Radiation doses for brain tumors are relatively high, ranging from 4500-6000 cGy given over a 6 to 8 week period. Toxicity is related to the volume of tissue irradiated and the total dose given.

Stereotactically or surgically inserted radioactive sources may also be used, sometimes as supplemental therapy. This localized radiation source delivers a high dose to a specific area. Several experimental studies are being undertaken to further define the role of radioactive seed placement in CNS tumor treatment.

When treatment begins, neurological symptoms may temporarily worsen due to radiation-induced edema. This is controlled with dexamethasone. Children have also exhibited impaired intellectual functioning as a late effect of cranial irradiation, especially when given in conjunction with chemotherapy. Children under age 3 are at the greatest risk for this complication.

Chemotherapy

Chemotherapy may be used in conjunction with surgery and radiation therapy for the treatment of gliomas, medulloblastomas, and other selected tumors. The major limitation of many standard chemotherapeutic agents is the drugs' inability to penetrate the blood-brain barrier in sufficient concentrations to be therapeutic. The remarkable heterogeneity of brain tumors also seems to limit the effectiveness of chemotherapy for CNS tumors. The *nitrosoureas* (BCNU, CCNU) are the most commonly used drugs, but methotrexate, vincristine, thiotepa, cisplatin, and prednisone may also be given depending on the type of tumor and method of administration.

Chemotherapy is usually given orally or intravenously. In some patients, an *Ommaya reservoir* may be inserted for administration of chemotherapeutic agents directly into the cerebrospinal fluid. This device consists of a reservoir or pouch connected to a catheter that is placed surgically into the ventricles. It can be accessed through the scalp and eliminates the need for repeated lumbar punctures. Chemotherapy may also be infused intra-arterially—via the carotid or vertebral artery—to deliver high concentrations of the drug directly to the tumor bed, but this approach remains experimental.

METASTATIC CNS TUMORS

Brain metastases occur in approximately 35% of all cancer patients, especially in those with advanced breast or lung cancer. The treatment selected for brain metastases depends on the nature of the primary tumor and the presence and location of metastases, but hormonal therapy, chemotherapy, radiation therapy, and surgery have been used to provide palliation.

NURSING CARE

A safe, supportive environment is essential to providing care for patients with CNS lesions. Monitoring changes in the patient's ability to perform activities of daily living, instituting seizure precautions, and teaching the patient and family members about medication side effects and signs of increased intracranial pressure are important nursing functions.

One of the major challenges of caring for the child or adult with a brain tumor lies in helping the patient and the family deal with compromised mental abilities. In addition, patients with cognitive, motor, and sensory losses resulting from brain tumors frequently experience difficulty performing activities of daily living. It is often useful to enumerate skill areas and behavior domains that remain unaffected, as well as specifying emerging deficits. A successful rehabilitation program can include many of the same procedures used by people adjusting to stroke or the declining mental agility associated with old age. A strategy that builds on strengths rather than stressing deficits is particularly useful with children.

Other nursing management problems arise from the side effects of specific treatment. Alopecia and skin changes, for example, are common radiation side effects that require careful assessment and should be incorporated into the patient's care plan (see also Unit III, Chapter 2 and Unit 4, Chapters 1 and 4). Steroids are commonly used for symptom management in metastatic brain disease. It is important that nurses monitor symptoms of acute adrenal insufficiency, gastrointestinal disturbance, and other common side effects of these compounds, and discuss these effects with the patient and family.

Bibliography

Burgess, K. E. (1983). Neurological disturbances in the patient with an intracranial neoplasm: Sources and implications for nursing care. *Journal of Neurosurgical Nursing, 15*(4), 237–242.

Esparza, D. M. (1982). Nursing care for the patient with an Ommaya reservoir. *Oncology Nursing Forum, 9*(4), 17–20.

Kane, K. K. (1985). Increased intercranial pressure. In B. L. Johnson & J. Gross, (Eds.), *Handbook of oncology nursing* (pp. 399–412). New York: John Wiley and Sons.

Wegmann, J. A., & Chuman, M. (1987). Intracranial malignancies. In S. Groenwald (Ed.), *Cancer nursing: Principles and practice* (pp. 634–653). Boston, MA: Jones and Bartlett Publishers.

Wilson, C. B., Fulton, D. S., & Seager, M. L. (1980). Supportive management of the patient with malignant brain tumor. *Journal of the American Medical Association, 244,* 1249–1251.

Zegeer, L. J. (1982). Nursing care of the patient with brain edema. *Journal of Neurosurgical Nursing, 14*(5), 168–245.

11 SKIN CANCERS

Anne Marie Maguire

INCIDENCE

Skin cancers account for 40% of all cancers. The major types of skin cancer are *basal cell* carcinoma, *squamous cell* carcinoma, *malignant melanoma*, and *Kaposi's sarcoma*. Of the more than 600,000 skin cancers diagnosed each year, two-thirds are basal cell carcinomas, accounting for 20% of all cancers in men and 10-15% in women. Approximately 22% of skin cancers are squamous cell carcinomas.

The most serious skin cancer is melanoma. Although melanomas account for only 3% of all skin cancers, they are responsible for about 75% of all skin cancer deaths. The American Cancer Society notes that the incidence of malignant melanoma is increasing at the rate of 4% per year. In the United States, 27,600 new cases were diagnosed in 1990, and approximately 6,300 people will die from this disease. If this trend continues, by the end of the century one in every 90 Americans will develop melanoma.

Although classical Kaposi's sarcoma was originally described in 1872 as a rare skin cancer in elderly men of Mediterranean, Middle Eastern, or Jewish origin, most cases of this cancer now are the epidemic form seen in patients with AIDS or in renal transplant patients receiving immunosuppressive drugs. Table 1 lists the incidence and characteristics of the major skin cancers.

RISK FACTORS

The primary risk factor for basal cell carcinomas, squamous cell carcinomas, or malignant melanoma is exposure to *ultraviolet light* (UVL). Risk is increased at certain times of the day when the majority of the sun's rays are being reflected by the earth's surface. Maximal exposure occurs between 11 a.m. and 3 p.m. (daylight saving time), with almost 100% of UVL being reflected at noon. The incidence of and mortality from skin cancers also increases in populations living closer to the equator. The UVL produced at tanning booths and by sun lamps causes the same types of skin changes, putting users of these products at increased risk for developing skin cancers.

**Table 1. Incidence, Clinical Characteristics, and
Common Sites of Principal Cutaneous Cancers**

Incidence	Clinical Characteristics	Common Sites
Basal Cell Carcinoma Most common form of skin cancer; occurs primarily in patients exposed to prolonged or intense sunlight, especially whites with light eyes, light hair, and fair complexions.	Nodulo-ulcerative basal cell cancer: Elevated lesions with umbilicated, ulcerated centers; raised waxy or "pearly" borders; moderately firm. Superficial basal cell cancer: Barely elevated plaques, usually with crusted and erythematous centers and raised, thread-like pearly borders; often multiple.	Nose, eyelids, cheeks, and trunk. Uncommon on palms and soles. Metastases are extremely rare.
Squamous Cell Carcinoma Less common than basal cell carcinoma; occurs primarily on areas exposed to actinic radiation and on vermilion border of lips.	Appearance varies from an elevated nodular mass to a punched-out ulcerated lesion to a fungating mass. Unlike basal cell carcinomas, squamous cell carcinomas are opaque.	75% occur on head, 15% on hands, and 10% elsewhere. Can metastasize to regional lymph nodes; in more advanced lesions, visceral (especially pulmonary) metastases can occur.
Malignant Melanoma Far less common than basal cell carcinoma or squamous cell carcinoma.	Usually irregularly pigmented (black, gray, white, blue, brown, red); usually more than six mm in diameter and asymmetric. May be flat or elevated, eroded or ulcerated; outline usually irregular, often with notch; frequently mildly symptomatic (e.g., pruritic). Characteristic clinical features can be easily remembered by thinking of ABCD: A = Asymmetry B = Border irregularity C = Color Variegation D = Diameter generally greater than 6 mm.	Any cutaneous area, although the trunk in men and the legs in women are common; less common in areas unexposed to sun. Metastasizes, often first to regional lymph nodes.

Source: From *The Diagnosis and Management of Common Skin Cancers* (p. 5.) by O. F. Roses, S. L. Gumport, M. N. Harris, and A. W. Kopf, 1989, Atlanta, GA: American Cancer Society. Reprinted with permission of publisher.

The incidence of skin cancers is higher in people exposed to the sun in their occupations, such as farmers, sailors, and fishermen; but people with intense, weekend exposure during recreational activities are also at risk. Patients with *xeroderma pigmentosum*, a genetically inherited disorder, are at increased risk because they are unable to repair UVL's damage to DNA. Other risk factors include: exposure to ionizing radiation, or chemical and viral carcinogens; chronic irritation or inflammation; and, defects in the immune system that affect its ability to fight UVL-induced skin cancers.

Melanomas occur 10 times more frequently in Caucasians than in other races, especially those with fair skin that burns and freckles easily, light eyes, and blond or red hair. Patients with *dysplastic nevi* or *congenital melanocytic nevi* who are members of melanoma-prone families have a much greater risk of developing malignant melanoma than the general population.

Dysplastic nevi are pigmented lesions 5-12 mm in diameter, larger than common nevi (freckles, moles, and beauty marks). Their borders are irregular, ill-defined, and have a macular and papular component. Colors range from tan to dark brown on a pink background. They are especially common on the trunk, but also appear on covered areas of the body (i.e., the scalp, breast, and buttocks). There may be more than 100 nevi on the body; they usually begin appearing in adolescence and continue through adulthood. Their presence increases the lifetime risk of melanoma to 5-10% versus 0.7% in the general population.

Congenital melanocytic nevi (birth marks) are present at birth, although they may not be immediately apparent. Large and medium nevi usually have grossly irregular surfaces, varying shades of brown colors, and, perhaps, hair. Small lesions have smooth surfaces, more uniform color, and lack hair. The 1% of newborns who have these lesions have approximately a 6% chance of developing melanoma.

PREVENTION AND EARLY DETECTION

The incidence, morbidity, and mortality from skin cancers can be reduced by eliminating exposure to known risk factors or diagnosing cancers at an early stage when surgical cure is possible.

The Skin Cancer Foundation has guidelines for reducing the damaging effects of UVL (Figure 1). In general, the use of sunscreens and protective clothing help prevent most skin cancers.

Routine self-examination of the skin is a strongly recommended means of detecting skin cancer, particularly melanoma, in early stages. Two pamphlets, *Early Detection of Malignant Melanoma: The Role of Physician Examination and Self-examination of the*

Prevention Guidelines

- Minimize sun exposure between 10 a.m. and 2 p.m. (11 a.m. to 3 p.m. daylight saving time) when the sun is strongest. Try to plan outdoor activities for the early morning or late afternoon.
- Wear a hat, long-sleeved shirts, and long pants when out in the sun. Choose tightly woven materials for greater protection from the sun's rays.
- Apply a sunscreen before exposure to the sun, and reapply frequently and liberally, at least every two hours, as long as you stay in the sun. The sunscreen should always be reapplied after swimming or perspiring heavily, since products differ in their degrees of water resistance. We recommend sunscreens with an SPF (sun protection factor) of 15 or more printed on the label.
- Use a sunscreen when in high altitudes, such as for mountain climbing and skiing. At high altitudes, there is less atmosphere to absorb the sun's rays, so the risk of burning is greater. The sun also is stronger near the equator where the sun's rays strike the earth most directly.
- Don't forget to use sunscreen on overcast days. The sun's rays are as damaging to skin on cloudy, hazy days as they are on sunny days.
- Individuals at high risk for skin cancer (outdoor workers, fair-skinned individuals, and persons who have already had skin cancer) should apply sunscreen daily.
- Photosensitivity—an increased sensitivity to sun exposure—is a possible side effect of certain medications, drugs and cosmetics, and of birth control pills. Consult your physician or pharmacist before going out in the sun if you're using such products. You may need to take extra precautions.
- If you develop an allergic reaction to a sunscreen, change sunscreens. One of the many products on the market today should be right for you. Beware of reflective surfaces! Sand, snow, concrete, and water can reflect more than half the sun's rays onto your skin. Sitting in the shade does not guarantee protection from sunburn.
- Avoid tanning parlors. The UV rays emitted by tanning booths are the same as those in sunlight.
- Keep young infants out of the sun. Begin using sunscreens on children at six months of age, and then allow sun exposure with moderation.
- Teach children sun protection early. Sun damage occurs with each unprotected sun exposure and accumulates over time.

Figure 1. Guidelines for the prevention of skin cancer.
Source: From "Prevention of Malignant Melanoma." by A. W. Kopf, 1985, *Dermatology Clinics*, Vol. 3(2), pp. 351–360. Reprinted by permission of W.B. Saunders.

Skin, and *Why You Should Know About Melanoma,* are American Cancer Society professional and public education materials that nurses can use as teaching guides. The pamphlets contain colored photographs of melanomas and dysplastic nevi and illustrate skin self-examination techniques (Figure 2). Nurses should encourage individuals, particularly those at high risk, to perform skin self-examination once a month and also have an annual skin examination by a physician or nurse practitioner.

When examining the skin, it is important to differentiate abnormal moles from common benign pigmented lesions. The ABCD rule in Table 1 is the easiest method for recalling the danger signs associated with malignant melanomas.

Other signs and symptoms of melanoma include a change in the size, color, or surface of a nevus, development of an irregular border, oozing, bleeding, itchiness, tenderness, or pain.

BASAL CELL CARCINOMA AND SQUAMOUS CELL CARCINOMA

Pathology

Basal cell carcinoma occurs primarily on sun-exposed areas of the body. It will frequently appear as a raised nodular lesion with a smooth, clear border and telangiectasia. Ulceration, bleeding, and pruritus are common. These lesions typically appear in middle-aged and elderly people. This carcinoma often recurs within the treatment scar, at the edge of a skin graft, or within the suture line. It rarely metastasizes.

Squamous cell carcinoma commonly arises in areas of sun-damaged skin or from a pre-existing skin lesion. It appears as a scaly, keratotic, slightly elevated nodule. It may be oval or circular in shape, and ulceration can occur. If untreated, it can become a fungating mass. It metastasizes to the proximal lymph glands and to distant organs such as the lungs, bone, and brain. Lesions that invade deep into the dermal layer are more likely to metastasize.

Treatment

Both basal cell and squamous cell carcinoma have a very favorable prognosis. Ninety to ninety-five percent of patients with basal cell carcinoma, and 75-80% of patients with squamous cell carcinoma can be cured with appropriate treatment. Surgery and radiation therapy produce comparable results.

Basal cell carcinomas and superficial squamous cell carcinomas may be treated with electrosurgery. This process involves curettage followed by electrodesiccation, which destroys lesions or seals off blood vessels by monopolar high-frequency electric current. During curettage, the actual tumor is removed. Electrodesiccation is then used to burn a safe margin of skin around the tumor site. Because cosmetic defects such as contractures can occur with this technique, its use may be limited in certain anatomic areas. Other complications include scarring, delayed wound healing, and occasional bleeding if dessicated tissue separates from the wound. Wound care involves soaking the wound with hydrogen peroxide two or three times a day, followed by soap and water rinse and application of an antibiotic ointment and Telfa™ dressing.

Excisional surgery may also be used. This procedure involves complete excision of the tumor and permits examination of the tumor margins for evidence of disease. Depending on the size of the tumor removed, flaps or full- or split-thickness skin grafts may be needed to achieve a cosmetically acceptable result.

Cryosurgery, or the use of liquid nitrogen to destroy tissue by freezing it, is frequently used to treat primary basal cell carcinomas,

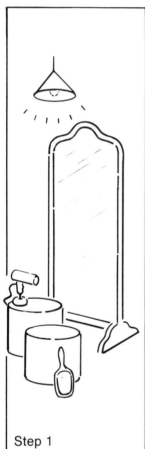

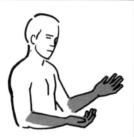

Step 2

Hold your hands with the palms face up, as shown in the drawing. Look at your palms, fingers, spaces between the fingers, and forearms. Then turn your hands over and examine the backs of your hands, fingers, spaces between the fingers, fingernails, and forearms.

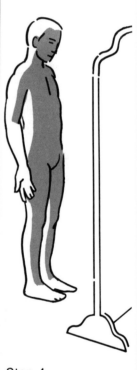

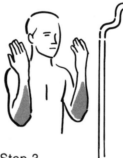

Step 4

Again using the full length mirror, observe the entire front of your body. In turn, look at your face, neck, and arms. Turn your palms to face the mirror and look at your upper arms. Then look at your chest and abdomen; pubic area; thighs and lower legs.

Step 1

Make sure the room is well-lighted, and that you have nearby a full-length mirror, a hand-held mirror, a hand-held blow dryer, and two chairs or stools. Undress completely.

Step 3

Now position yourself in front of the full-length mirror. Hold up your arms, bent at the elbows, with your palms facing you. In the mirror, look at the backs of your forearms and elbows.

Figure 2. Your Skin Self-Exam.

Source: From *Early Detection of Malignant Melanoma: The Role of Physician Examination and Self-Examination of the Skin* (pp. 20–23) by R. J. Friedman, D. S. Rigel, and A. W. Kopf, 1990, Atlanta, GA: American Cancer Society. Reprinted with permission of publisher.

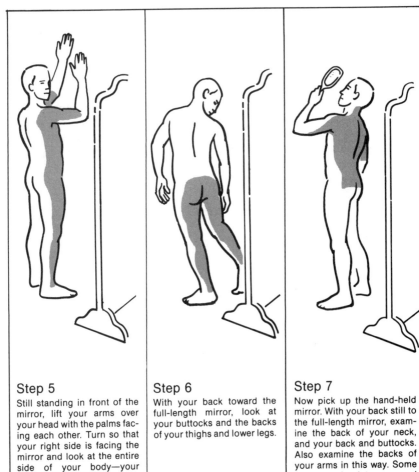

Step 5

Still standing in front of the mirror, lift your arms over your head with the palms facing each other. Turn so that your right side is facing the mirror and look at the entire side of your body—your hands and arms, underarms, sides of your trunk, thighs, and lower legs. Then turn, and repeat the process with your left side.

Step 6

With your back toward the full-length mirror, look at your buttocks and the backs of your thighs and lower legs.

Step 7

Now pick up the hand-held mirror. With your back still to the full-length mirror, examine the back of your neck, and your back and buttocks. Also examine the backs of your arms in this way. Some areas are hard to see, and you may find it helpful to ask your spouse or a friend to assist you.

Continued on next page

superficial squamous cell carcinomas, or patients who may not be good candidates for surgery. Although healing may be prolonged, wound contractures occur less often than with other types of surgery.

Aggressive and recurrent tumors are treated with *Mohs surgery,* in which the tumor is removed and each layer is microscopically examined to assure a complete resection of cancerous tissue while preserving normal tissue. This technique is frequently used for tumors located in cosmetically important areas such as the eyelid, nose, helix of the ear, and lips.

Because both basal cell and squamous cell carcinomas are radiosensitive, radiation therapy can be effective in select patients. Patients may be considered for radiation if they are elderly, medically debilitated, poor surgical risks, or have large lesions that might create a cosmetic defect if surgically removed. Radiotherapy is generally offered only to patients over age 45 because the radiated site can look progressively worse.

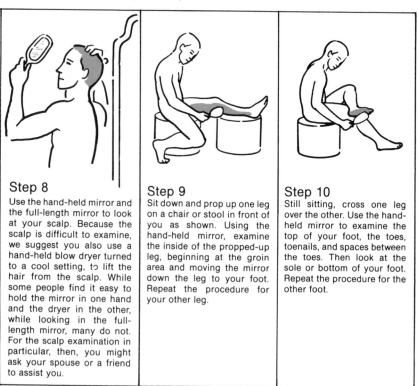

Step 8
Use the hand-held mirror and the full-length mirror to look at your scalp. Because the scalp is difficult to examine, we suggest you also use a hand-held blow dryer turned to a cool setting, to lift the hair from the scalp. While some people find it easy to hold the mirror in one hand and the dryer in the other, while looking in the full-length mirror, many do not. For the scalp examination in particular, then, you might ask your spouse or a friend to assist you.

Step 9
Sit down and prop up one leg on a chair or stool in front of you as shown. Using the hand-held mirror, examine the inside of the propped-up leg, beginning at the groin area and moving the mirror down the leg to your foot. Repeat the procedure for your other leg.

Step 10
Still sitting, cross one leg over the other. Use the hand-held mirror to examine the top of your foot, the toes, toenails, and spaces between the toes. Then look at the sole or bottom of your foot. Repeat the procedure for the other foot.

Figure 2. Your Skin Self-Exam—*continued*

The use of topical chemotherapy (5-fluorouracil) is limited to superficial basal cell carcinomas on the trunk or extremities, because the drug does not penetrate to tumor cells below the epidermis.

MALIGNANT MELANOMA

Pathology

Malignant melanoma originates in proliferative, single melanocytes in the lower epidermis. Lesions can arise on any epithelial surface (i.e., gall bladder, esophagus, meninges, vagina, or upper respiratory tract), but they usually occur on the skin. Growth can proceed radially or vertically. These cancers are found predominantly on the trunk, head, and neck of males, and on the lower and upper extremities of females. When blacks develop melanomas, they are commonly located on less pigmented skin areas, such as the palms of the hands, soles of the feet, and subungual areas.

Tumor thickness is the most important prognostic factor in early stages of the disease. Lesions less than 0.76 mm thick are almost 100% curable; lesions more than 3 mm thick are associated with only a 48% 10-year survival. Fewer than 20% of patients with metastatic disease survive 10 years or more. Melanoma metastasizes to lymph nodes, skin, lung, brain, liver, and bone.

Treatment

Excisional or incisional biopsy is performed to obtain tissue for pathologic examination. The primary therapy for malignant melanoma is wide excision surgery. Margins of normal tissue are usually excised at this time to prevent recurrence at the surgical borders. Biopsy and definitive surgery may be performed as a one- or two-stage procedure. Melanomas of the fingers and toes, regardless of thickness, are treated by amputation of the involved digit. Lymph nodes are dissected in most patients with regional nodal metastases.

Combination chemotherapy has been used for metastatic and recurrent disease with limited success. One to two percent of patients will exhibit a complete response, and 20-25% will achieve a partial, limited-duration response. The most commonly used drugs are dacarbazine (DTIC) and the nitrosoureas (carmustine, lomustine, and semustine).

Limb perfusion may be used for patients with multiple recurrences or local nodal metastases. In this procedure, the major artery and vein of the affected extremity are isolated with a tourniquet, and then temporarily oxygenated and perfused by a corporeal bypass machine. Extremely high doses of chemotherapy (6 to 10 times the usual systemic dose) are infused into the tumor. The tourniquet prevents systemic distribution of the drug. After 1 hour, the chemotherapy is stopped and the tourniquet is removed. The most common drugs used for limb perfusion are melphalan, thiotepa, dactinomycin, dacarbazine, carmustine, cisplatin, and doxorubicin.

Several immunologic and biologic agents—such as recombinant alpha interferon and interleukin-2—have shown some antitumor activity (see Unit II, Chapter 4). The role of these agents in the treatment of melanoma requires further investigation.

Since most melanomas are not radiosensitive, the use of radiation therapy is limited to the palliation of brain and bone metastases.

KAPOSI'S SARCOMA

Pathology

The classical form of Kaposi's sarcoma appears as dark-blue to reddish-purple spots or nodules on the arms (25%) or legs (75%). Patients exhibit edema and may have involved lymph nodes or viscera. In contrast, epidemic Kaposi's sarcoma is characterized by smaller pink to purple lesions on the trunk, head, and neck. Most patients have multiple lesions and edema secondary to lymph node blockage. Visceral lesions can occur on the gastrointestinal tract, lungs, liver, pancreas, gingiva, pharynx, tongue, soft palate, adrenal glands, spleen, testes, and larynx. GI lesions result in diarrhea. Pulmonary lesions cause dyspnea, orthopnea, and cough, which may be incorrectly attributed to pneumocystis carinii pneumonia. Many patients have additional symptoms that may be related to infection, including fever, weight loss, malaise, and anorexia.

Treatment

In epidemic Kaposi's sarcoma, radiation is primarily used for facial lesions or those that cause local problems, such as plantar lesions that limit mobility or pharyngeal lesions that cause dysphagia.

Vinblastine has been used with limited success for classic Kaposi's sarcoma patients who have generalized lesions or for whom radiation has failed. Treatment of epidemic Kaposi's sarcoma patients with chemotherapy has been complicated by opportunistic infections resulting from the drugs' immunosuppressive side effects.

Interferon is frequently given to treat epidemic Kaposi's sarcoma. Patients without opportunistic infections who receive high doses of interferon show some tumor response. Studies using interleukin-2, gamma interferon, and other biological response modifiers are planned and may offer hope to future patients.

Bibliography

American Cancer Society (1990). *Cancer facts and figures.* Atlanta, GA: Author.

Frank-Stromborg, M. (1986). The role of the nurse in cancer detection and screening. *Seminars in Oncology Nursing, 2*(3), 191–199.

Friedman, R. J., Rigel, D. S., & Kopf, A. W. (1990). *Early detection of malignant melanoma: The role of physician examination and self-examination of the skin* (No. 3334-PE). Atlanta, GA: American Cancer Society.

Kopf, A. W. (1985). Prevention of malignant melanoma. *Dermatologic Clinics, 3*(2), 351–360.

Lawler, P. E., & Schreiber, S. (1989). Cutaneous malignant melanoma: Nursing's role in prevention and early detection. *Oncology Nursing Forum, 16*(3), 345–352.

Muggia, F. M., & Lonberg, M. (1986). Kaposi's sarcoma and AIDS. *Medical Clinics of North America, 70*(1), 139–154.

Pathak, M. A. (1986). Sunscreens: Topical and systemic approaches for the prevention of acute and chronic sun-induced skin reactions. *Dermatologic Clinics, 4*(2), 321–334.

Seeger, J., Richman, S. P., & Allegra, J. C. (1986). Systemic therapy of malignant melanoma. *Medical Clinics of North America, 70*(1), 89–90.

Smith, T. J., Mihm, M. C., & Sober, A. J. (1986). Malignant melanoma. In B. Cady (Ed.), *Cancer manual* (7th ed.) (pp. 106–113). Boston: American Cancer Society.

Stegman, S. J. (1986). Basal cell carcinoma and squamous cell carcinoma recognition and treatment. *Medical Clinics of North America, 70*(1), 95–107.

Stewart, D. S. (1987). Indoor tanning: The nurse's role in preventing skin damage. *Cancer Nursing, 10*(2), 93–99.

White, M. J., & Polk, H. C. (1986). Therapy of primary cutaneous melanoma. *Medical Clinics of North America, 70*(1), 71–87.

Wick, M. M., Grande, D. J. & Lo, T. C. M. (1986). Cancer of skin. In B. Cady (Ed.), *Cancer manual* (7th ed.) (pp. 99–105). Boston: American Cancer Society.

12 CANCERS OF THE BONE

Jane Brewer Sloane

INCIDENCE

Malignant bone tumors are uncommon, comprising approximately 0.2% of all new cancer cases in the United States. The incidence of primary bone cancer is highest in children and adolescents, but cancer metastatic to bone is more common than primary bone malignancies in all age groups.

In the 1960s, when surgery alone was used for the treatment of primary bone cancer, only 15-20% of patients experienced long-term survival. The current outlook is much more optimistic: new surgical techniques and treatment regimens have eliminated the need for amputation in many cases, and overall survival rates have improved dramatically. When the treatment regimen includes pre- or postoperative chemotherapy, 50-80% of patients survive.

RISK FACTORS

Although the precise cause of bone cancer is not known, several factors are known to contribute to its development. Periods of rapid skeletal growth seem to be associated with at least some bone cancers, as the incidence of bone cancer is highest during the adolescent growth spurt. Individuals with conditions that stimulate increased bone metabolism, such as Paget's disease and hyperparathyroidism, are also at increased risk for bone cancer. Patients treated for other malignancies have exhibited secondary osteosarcomas and fibrosarcomas at sites of previous radiation exposure. No definitive relationship has been established between trauma and the development of bone cancers.

CLINICAL MANIFESTATIONS

Symptoms of bone cancer vary according to the type and location of the tumor, but pain is the prevailing complaint. Typically, the pain is unrelated to position or activity and is more intense at night. Some patients may also have a palpable mass. Less common symptoms include pathologic fractures and systemic complaints such as fever, weight loss, and general malaise. The lungs are the common site of metastasis; symptoms of pulmonary involvement range from cough and dyspnea to pleural effusion.

DIAGNOSIS

If a lesion found on x-ray is suspected to be malignant, the extent of disease is evaluated by bone scan, magnetic resonance imaging (MRI), or computerized axial tomography (CT) scan, and arteriography before surgical biopsy and resection. This information is used to determine whether a limb-salvage procedure or an amputation should be performed. Patients with a newly-diagnosed bone lesion, especially adults, should be evaluated for an undiagnosed primary tumor, since metastatic lesions to the bone are more common than primary cancers. Cancers of the breast, kidney, thyroid, and prostate are the most common sites of origin for bone metastases.

TYPES OF BONE CANCER

Osteosarcoma

The most common bone malignancy, *osteosarcoma*, primarily affects children and young adults. The majority of these tumors are located around the knee joint, either in the distal femur or proximal tibia. Osteosarcoma arises from *osteoblast cells*, those cells that multiply rapidly during periods of skeletal growth.

Many patients with osteosarcoma can be treated successfully with new surgical techniques that salvage the affected limb. With this approach, the segment of bone containing the tumor, as well as margins of unaffected bone on either side of the tumor, are surgically removed. Bone can be reconstructed using cadaver allografts or metal endoprostheses.

Not all patients are candidates for this approach. The major contraindications to limb salvage are major neurovascular involvement or the presence of pathologic fractures or infection before surgery. Also, young children whose linear growth is incomplete frequently will have better functional results with amputation and prostheses than with resection. The tumor can be controlled locally with surgery, but frequently metastasizes to the lungs if no other therapy is utilized.

Some patients who undergo an amputation may experience postoperative phantom pain, the perception of sensations in the amputated portion of the limb. While some degree of this sensation is common after amputation, severe or prolonged phantom pain occurs only in a very small percentage of amputees. Once the incision is healed, wearing a prosthesis or wrapping a piece of cloth around the stump and pulling on the ends may help alleviate phantom sensations by providing a tactile reminder of where the limb ends.

Combination chemotherapy has proven effective against osteosarcomas and is now a routine part of treatment. The use of chemotherapy before surgery has become widespread and permits intraoperative assessment of tumor response to the chemotherapy regimen. Modifications of the regimen can then be made postoperatively if tumor response has been inadequate.

High-dose methotrexate infusions, doxorubicin, cyclophosphamide, and cisplatin are among the most commonly used chemotherapeutic agents. Patients receiving infusions of high-dose methotrexate must be well hydrated and be given oral or intravenous sodium bicarbonate to keep the urine alkaline (a pH greater than 7) to promote excretion of the methotrexate. Side effects of methotrexate can be severe and include bone marrow depression, mucositis, nausea and vomiting, alopecia, and renal impairment. *Citrovorum factor* (leucovorin calcium) must be administered at specified intervals after the high-dose methotrexate infusion to "rescue" normal cells from the toxic effects of methotrexate. Further information on chemotherapy and chemotherapeutic agents is found in Unit III, Chapter 3 and in Appendix I.

Chondrosarcoma

Chondrosarcoma, the second most common bone tumor, arises from cartilage and is usually located in some portion of the pelvis or femur. Unlike osteosarcoma, this tumor occurs primarily in adults. Radical surgical resection with amputation is the treatment of choice for chondrosarcoma, although some patients with low-grade tumors are candidates for local resection and bone reconstruction. Five-year survival ranges from 55-75%, depending on whether any soft tissue or lymph nodes are involved. High-dose radiotherapy may be given to patients with unresectable disease, or used with surgery in patients with disease in the facial bones or skull. Chemotherapy is generally not used to manage this type of bone cancer.

Ewing's Sarcoma

Ewing's sarcoma is a rare small-cell bone tumor that occurs primarily in children and adolescents. In contrast to osteosarcoma, these tumors are more commonly found in the bones of the trunk than in long bones. Five-year survival ranges from 50-75%, although late relapse (more than 10 years after treatment) is not uncommon.

In the past, standard therapy for this radiosensitive tumor consisted of megavoltage radiation followed by chemotherapy. More recently, patient outcomes have been improved by a treatment regimen that included surgical excision of the tumor combined with pre- and postoperative chemotherapy. Radiation is still used in the management of surgically inaccessible tumors, or tumors whose removal would result in significant disability. See also Unit V, Chapter 15.

The chemotherapeutic agents most commonly used to treat Ewing's sarcoma are doxorubicin, dactinomycin, vincristine, and cyclophosphamide. Doxorubicin and dactinomycin administered following irradiation can potentiate local skin toxicity. Commonly called radiation recall, the reaction consists of erythema, vesicle formation, or wet desquamation in the area that had been irradiated.

Fibrosarcoma

Fibrosarcoma, a rare type of bone cancer primarily affecting adults, arises from the fibrous tissue of bone and is most often found in the femur or tibia. This radioresistant tumor is generally treated by surgical resection and reconstruction or amputation. Five-year survival is approximately 25%.

METASTATIC BONE CANCER

Cancer frequently metastasizes to the bone, causing pain and the risk of pathological fractures. Although many cancers can metastasize to the bone, the most common sources are primary tumors of the breast, lung, prostate, kidney, and thyroid. Metastasis to the bone indicates disseminated disease. A suspected lesion is evaluated by x-ray and bone scan. Treatment may include surgery, radiation therapy, and chemotherapy. Surgery may be performed for prosthetic arthroplasty or to place stabilization devices. External splinting or bracing may be used for spinal lesions. Radiotherapy may be used before surgery or for palliation of pain. It is also used following surgery to kill the tumor. Chemotherapy may be used to reduce the tumor mass; however, if used in conjunction with surgery, its administration will usually be delayed until wound healing is complete, as it can disrupt wound healing.

NURSING CONSIDERATIONS

Cancers of the bone occur in patients of widely different age groups. Because developmental stage and lifestyle alterations have a major impact on a patient's adjustment to the diagnosis and treatment of bone cancers, it is important that the nurse consider these variables when planning interventions and assessing responses.

When amputation is required, preoperative teaching about the procedure provides the patient and family with information needed to begin adjustment. A visit to the physical therapist will introduce the patient to the rehabilitation program. Patients may practice crutch walking before surgery, when balance is better and pain is not a factor. If time allows, meeting someone who has adapted successfully to amputation can have a positive effect on the patient's attitude. Nurses should also inform patients and their families that amputation invokes the kind of grief response that occurs after any loss. Assure the patient that feelings of denial, anger, and depression are normal and are often experienced before the loss is accepted.

Nearly all patients undergoing amputation will experience an alteration in body image and will grieve for the lost body part. This change may be especially difficult for adolescents, since this is a time of heightened concern about appearance and peer acceptance.

Amputees will also experience some degree of change in mobility and functional capacity. Lower extremity amputation affects both balance and mobility. These patients must relearn basic skills, including sitting, standing, and walking. The amputation of an upper extremity will also affect the patient's balance, but loss of manual dexterity probably has a greater impact on daily living.

Nurses should refer patients to the appropriate rehabilitation and prostheses experts immediately after surgery. Several types of prostheses are available. Many are designed for use in different sports, so physically active amputees should be encouraged to continue participating in athletics. Most lower-extremity amputees find that running is the most difficult skill to regain, and water sports are the easiest. Bone cancer patients with functional disabilities should be referred to vocational rehabilitation programs.

Patients undergoing limb-salvage procedures will also need significant rehabilitation. Following surgery, use of the limb is restricted so it can heal. For lower extremity procedures, weight bearing is gradually reintroduced. Until the prosthetic bone is stabilized and the surrounding muscles strengthened, crutches are required for ambulation.

Poor nutritional status due to chemotherapy-related nausea and vomiting, anorexia, and mucositis is a common problem for patients with osteosarcoma. Nurses should monitor eating habits and recommend nutritional support if nutritional status declines. Meticulous oral care, use of topical anesthetics for mucositis, and dietary alterations may help alleviate nutritional problems.

CONCLUSION

The addition of chemotherapy to standard bone cancer treatment regimens has substantially improved the outlook for many patients with these malignancies. As a result, minimizing disability and maximizing quality of life have become important goals of patient management. Nurses can work to achieve these goals by educating patients about their disease and its treatment, intervening early to help alleviate treatment side effects, and providing appropriate referrals for rehabilitation.

Bibliography

Bourne, B. A., & Kutcher, J. L. (1985). Amputation: Helping a patient face the loss of a limb. *RN, 48*, 38–44.

Eiber, F. R., Eckhardt, J., & Morton, D. L. (1984). Advances in the treatment of sarcomas of the extremity: Current status of limb salvage. *Cancer, 54*, 2695–2701.

Enneking, W. F., & Conrad, E. U. (1989). Common bone tumors. *Clinical Symposia, 41*(3), 1–32.

Kegel, B. (1985). Sports and recreation for those with lower limb amputation or impairment. *Journal of Rehabilitation Research and Development, 1* (Suppl.), 1–125.

Lasoff, E. M. (1985). When a teenager faces amputation. *RN, 48*, 44–45.

Malawer, M. M., Link, M. P., & Donaldson, S. S. (1989). Sarcomas of the bone. In V. T. DeVita, S. Hellman, & S. A. Rosenberg (Eds.), *Cancer: Principles and Practices of oncology.* 3rd edition (pp. 1418–1468). Philadelphia: J. B. Lippincott and Co.

Piasecki, P. A. (1990). Bone cancer, In S. Groenwald, M. H. Frogge, M. Goodman, & C. H. Yarbro (Eds.), *Cancer nursing: Principles and practice* (pp. 702–721). Boston: Jones and Bartlett Publishers, Inc.

Welch-McCaffrey, D. (1988). Metastatic bone cancer. *Cancer Nursing, 11*(2), 103–111.

13 LEUKEMIA

Cheryl R. Jedlow

INCIDENCE

Leukemia accounts for approximately 2.5% of all cancer cases in the United States. About 27,000 new cases are diagnosed each year, with incidence slightly higher in whites than in blacks and in males than in females. Acute leukemias occur at a rate of approximately 5:100,000 people. The incidence of chronic myelocytic leukemia is 1:100,000, with chronic lymphocytic leukemia occurring about twice as frequently.

ETIOLOGY

Leukemia is not a single disease entity, but several diseases involving the blood-forming tissues of the body—the spleen, lymphatic system, and bone marrow. The etiology of leukemia is not fully understood, but predisposing factors have been identified. Among these are certain genetic abnormalities, disorders of the immune system, excessive exposure to ionizing radiation, chemicals that suppress bone marrow function, and certain types of viruses.

PATHOPHYSIOLOGY

Leukemia is characterized by uncontrolled proliferation of hematopoietic cells. In most cases, the cells involved are white blood cells (WBC), but less frequently immature forms of red blood cells or platelets may predominate. *Pluripotent stem cells* in the bone marrow are the source of the various types of blood cells, as shown in Figure 1. At some point early in the development of stem cells, they become "committed" to differentiating into either red blood cells, platelets, or white blood cells. In leukemia, abnormal cells fill the bone marrow, spill into the circulating blood, and infiltrate many vital organs. Excessive production of leukemic cells in the bone marrow also inhibits normal blood cell growth and development.

Leukemias are classified as acute or chronic, depending on the maturity of the cells involved and the rapidity of symptom onset. In acute leukemias, *blasts*, or immature cells are overproduced. Because the development of these cells has been arrested at the

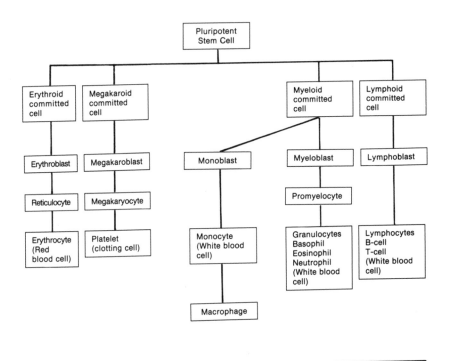

Figure 1. Cell line differentiation.

Source: From "Leukemia: The Treatment of Leukemia" by A. Freeley and H. Houlihan, 1981, *Cancer Nursing, 4*(3), Copyright 1981, Raven Press, New York. Adapted with permission of Raven Press.

blast stage, the cells are unable to perform the normal functions of a mature hematopoietic cell. In chronic leukemias, more mature but still ineffective cells proliferate. The onset of acute leukemias is sudden, and initial symptoms are frequently related to severe bone marrow suppression. In contrast, chronic leukemias evolve gradually, with a progressive worsening of symptoms over time.

Acute leukemias are further divided into *acute lymphocytic* (ALL) and *acute nonlymphocytic* (ANLL). Acute lymphocytic leukemia accounts for 85% of all leukemia in children and about 15% of leukemia in adults. Patients with ALL have an abnormal increase in immature lymphocytes in their blood and marrow. ALL immature lymphocytes are classified into three immune subtypes: T cell, B cell, and CALLA or non-T-cell/B-cell types. These subtypes are determined by the presence of T-cell antigens, B-cell antigens, or the CALLA (common ALL-antigens) on the cell surface of the lymphocyte. About 75% of patients have lymphoblasts that lack T-cell or B-cell markers, often referred to as null-cell leukemias because of the absence of cell surface markers. About 20% of adult patients with ALL have the T-cell type, and 5% have the B-cell type.

Acute nonlymphocytic leukemias are those in which the proliferating cells are not lymphoid cells. These leukemias are classified according to the hematopoietic cell that predominates in the blood or bone marrow: myelocytic, myelomonocytic, monocytic, erythroleukemia, promyelocytic, and megakaryocytic. Acute myelocytic leukemia (AML) is the most common type.

The two most common types of chronic leukemia are *chronic myelocytic* (CML) and *chronic lymphocytic* (CLL). Chronic myelocytic leukemia presents as an accumulation of abnormal granulocytes in the bone marrow or bloodstream. This is an adult form of leukemia, rarely seen in children. Median survival with remission is 36 to 44 months. Chronic lymphocytic leukemia, the most common form of chronic leukemia, is characterized by an increase of lymphocytes in the bone marrow and blood. The lymphocytes have B-cell features that resemble normal lymphocytes, but without their infection-fighting abilities. The average age of onset for CLL is 60 years old. *Hairy cell leukemia* (HCL) and *T-cell CLL* are rarer forms of chronic leukemia and are not discussed here.

CLINICAL MANIFESTATIONS

Fatigue, malaise, weight loss, and anorexia may be the earliest symptoms that prompt a patient to seek medical attention. Clinical signs and symptoms vary according to the type of leukemia, but anemia, thrombocytopenia, and granulocytopenia are also frequently present at diagnosis. Approximately one third of ANLL patients present with serious or life-threatening infections, but infection is unusual in ALL patients at diagnosis. Hemorrhage can occur when the platelet count drops below $50,000/mm^3$; petechiae (pinpoint hemorrhages on the surface of the skin) and abnormal bleeding from body orifices may also be observed. A clotting factor deficiency unique to promyelocytic leukemia can result in serious hemorrhage or *disseminated intravascular coagulation* (DIC). Patients with ALL, CML, and CLL frequently have enlarged lymph nodes and splenomegaly.

Acute nonlymphocytic leukemia patients with WBC counts greater than $200,000/mm^3$ are at increased risk for developing *leukostasis* in the small blood vessels of all major organs. With leukostasis, the WBCs clump together, plugging the capillary and causing it to rupture. When this occurs in the brain, patients are at risk for sudden death from intracranial hemorrhage. Other clinical complications of leukemia are summarized in Figure 2.

Bone Marrow Failure
Anemia Granulocytopenia Thrombocytopenia
Immunoparesis
Suppressor cell proliferation Helper cell reduction Reduction in functional B-cells
Infiltration
Leukemic meningitis Cranial nerve palsy Leukemic orchitis Hepatosplenomegaly Lymphadenopathy Leukemids (skin) Granulocytic sarcomas
Hyperleukocytosis
Central nervous system leukostasis/stroke Pulmonary leukostasis/adult respiratory distress syndrome
Metabolic

Blast cell turnover
   Hyperuricemia
   Hypercoagulation, disseminated intravascular coagulation
Hypercalcemia
Hyperkalemia
Weight loss
Nephromegaly
Lactate dehydrogenase elevation
Muramidasemia

Figure 2. Signs, symptoms, and laboratory abnormalities in leukemia.
Source: From "Current Therapy of Acute and Chronic Leukemia in Adults" by E. S. Henderson and T. Han, 1986, *CA: A Cancer Journal for Clinicians, 36*, p. 323. Reprinted with permission of the American Cancer Society.

DIAGNOSIS AND TREATMENT

Diagnosis is confirmed by examination of the peripheral blood and the bone marrow. Lumbar puncture is also performed to examine cerebrospinal fluid for signs of central nervous system involvement.

Acute Lymphocytic Leukemia

Approximately 75% of cases of acute lymphocytic leukemia (ALL) occur in children and about 25% in adults. Treatment recommendations differ slightly in children (see Unit V, Chapter 15). The goal of treatment for acute leukemias is the eradication of all leukemic cells, achievement of a normal bone marrow blast count (less than 5% of total cells), and reconstitution of the bone marrow with normal elements (i.e., WBC, RBC, and platelet counts within normal limits).

Chemotherapy is used to treat all forms of leukemia. *Induction chemotherapy* is the initial treatment given to achieve remission. For patients with ALL a common drug regimen is vincristine, prednisone and daunorubicin, with or without L-asparaginase. A complete remission has occurred when leukemia cells and all signs and symptoms are absent for at least 4 weeks, and normal functional status has returned.

Consolidation therapy, which frequently employs the same drugs successful in achieving remission, is given for several courses following complete remission to eliminate any undetected residual leukemic cells. Patients are then treated with *maintenance chemotherapy*.

Acute lymphocytic leukemia (ALL) patients are at risk for leukemic involvement of the central nervous system (CNS). Since most drugs do not cross the blood-brain barrier when given systemically, it is necessary to administer intrathecal methotrexate and/or cytarabine to prevent or treat CNS disease. This is accomplished either by lumbar puncture or through an Ommaya-type reservoir. Although CNS prophylaxis with cranial irradiation is routinely given to children in complete remission, its use in adults is controversial and may be reserved for those at a high risk for CNS relapse. When CNS relapse is documented, treatment includes intrathecal cytarabine and/or methotrexate alone or combined with cranial radiation.

Median survival for patients achieving complete remission is 2 to 4 years, but approximately one-third of adults will survive disease-free for 5 years or longer. Allogeneic bone marrow transplantation may also be performed in patients after induction therapy; results in children are comparable to those achieved in patients receiving post-remission chemotherapy. Transplants performed during remission are more successful than those performed after relapse. For more information on bone marrow transplantation see Unit III, Chapter 5.

Acute Nonlymphocytic Leukemias

Although the acute nonlymphocytic leukemias (ANLL) vary in biologic behavior and clinical presentation, they are generally responsive to the same therapies as are given for ALL. Standard induction therapy includes cytarabine and one of the anthracyclines, with or without other chemotherapeutic agents. Approximately 65% of adults achieve complete remission with this approach. Remission usually lasts from 1 to 1½ years, with about 25% of patients achieving long-term survival. CNS prophylaxis is not indicated in this group because meningeal involvement is uncommon at diagnosis. When CNS relapse is documented, the treatment is the same as with ALL.

Postremission treatment of ANLL remains controversial. Essentially, three different treatment strategies may be employed: long-term intensive maintenance therapy, intensive consolidation therapy without maintenance therapy, and allogeneic bone marrow transplantation without further therapy. Although treatment regimens frequently change, a currently recommended regimen for acute myelocytic leukemia, the most common ANLL, is summarized in Figure 3.

Remission Induction Chemotherapy
  Cytarabine 100-200 mg/m²/d for 7 days, plus daunorubicin 45-70 mg/m²/d for 3 days (mitoxantrone, amsacrine, or idarubicin may be substituted for daunorubicin)
Consolidation Chemotherapy
  2-4 courses involving high-dosage cytarabine or other intensive therapy similar to induction
Maintenance Chemotherapy
  Probably not indicated in patients receiving consolidation
Central Nervous System Prophylaxis
  Not indicated
Immunotherapy
  Not indicated
Bone Marrow Transplantation
  Allogeneic transplant from HLA-identical donor:
    Indicated for patients <30 years of age in first remission;
    Indicated at relapse or in second or greater remission for patients <50 years of age
  Autologous transplant or allogeneic transplant from HLA-nonidentical or unrelated donors:
    Indications uncertain, but probably effective for selected patients in second or greater remission

Figure 3. Therapy of acute myelogenous leukemia.
Source: From "Acute Myelogenous Leukemia: Biology and Treatment" by R. Champlin, 1988, *Mediguide to Oncology, 8*(4), p. 1-9. Reprinted with permission of Lawrence DellaCorte Publications Inc., NY.

Chronic Lymphocytic Leukemia

Chronic lymphocytic leukemia (CLL) occurs about twice as frequently as chronic myelocytic leukemia. The incidence is highest in people over 60 years old. In this type of leukemia, small B lymphocytes proliferate in the blood, bone marrow, lymph nodes, and spleen. Despite the presence of increased numbers of cells in the blood and bone marrow, many patients remain asymptomatic for years.

The stages of CLL are delineated in Figure 4. As the disease progresses, fatigue, lymphadenopathy, and hepatosplenomegaly become more prominent. In stage IV disease, patients may develop thrombocytopenia due to increased destruction of platelets by an enlarged spleen. Therapy is indicated when the patient exhibits fatigue, bulky lymphadenopathy, or progressive bone marrow involvement.

Initial treatment usually consists of oral chlorambucil or cyclophosphamide with or without prednisone. Treatment is continued until symptoms have been controlled, and is then stopped. For patients with isolated splenomegaly, low-dose splenic irradiation or splenectomy may be used to control excessive destruction of platelets and red blood cells; however, these interventions do not improve survival.

Patients unresponsive to standard treatments or presenting with dangerously high levels of WBCs may receive *leukopheresis* (re-

Stage		Survival Time (months from diagnosis)
0	Lymphocytosis only	150
I	With lymphadenopathy	101
II	With hepatosplenomegaly and with or without lymphadenopathy	71
III	With anemia and with or without hepatosplenomegaly and/or lymphadenopathy	19
IV	With thrombocytopenia and with or without anemia, hepatosplenomegaly, and/or lymphadenopathy	19

Figure 4. Staging system for CLL based on survival data.
Source: From "Current Therapy of Acute and Chronic Leukemia in Adults" by E. S. Henderson and T. Han, 1986, *CA: A Cancer Journal for Clinicians, 36*, p. 323. Reprinted with permission the American Cancer Society.

moval of large numbers of WBCs from the peripheral blood) to reduce the number of circulating lymphocytes. Symptoms may improve temporarily after this procedure. Investigational treatment of CLL currently include recombinant alpha interferon and Fludarabine.

Chronic Myelocytic Leukemia

Chronic myelocytic leukemia (CML) occurs predominantly in adults between ages 25 and 60. The development of CML is associated with a genetic abnormality of chromosomes 9 and 22, called the *Philadelphia chromosome* (Ph[1]). CML generally progresses in three phases: the chronic phase, the accelerated phase, and blast crisis. Patients generally present with vague symptoms including fever, malaise, early satiety, and left upper quadrant pain due to splenic enlargement. Median survival is 3 years from diagnosis.

Busulfan and hydroxyurea are the most commonly used chemotherapeutic agents for the chronic phase of CML. Doses are titrated to maintain a WBC count between 10,000-20,000/mm^3. Alpha interferon may be administered to prevent or delay progression of disease, but this approach remains experimental. Bone marrow transplants produce the best results when performed in the chronic phase. Allogeneic bone marrow transplantation offers the *only* chance for cure in these patients.

In the accelerated phase, patients gradually exhibit more symptoms and the WBCs become more difficult to control, ultimately requiring increasing doses of chemotherapy.

Blast crisis, the point at which the disease transforms into an acute leukemia, is the terminal stage of CML. Standard treatments for acute leukemias may be given, but results are poor and survival ranges between 2 and 6 months. High blast cell counts during this phase can cause leukostasis. Whole brain irradiation or leukopheresis may be used to rapidly reduce the WBC count.

Supportive Care

Disease symptoms can be compounded by treatment side effects. Because both the treatment and the disease itself can affect all major body systems, it is important for the nurse to be familiar with the drugs used and their potential toxicities. The patient and family should be taught about infection control and other aspects of care early in the course of treatment.

The hematologic effects of disease and treatment constitute the major problem in leukemia patients. Treatments that eradicate leukemic cells in the bone marrow also damage normal blood cells remaining in the bone marrow. Patients' blood counts should be monitored closely after treatment. Bone marrow suppression can last 4 weeks or longer after treatment. When the absolute neutrophil count decreases to less than 500/mm³, the risk of infection significantly increases. At this point, infection prevention measures are initiated to minimize exposure to both external and internal pathogenic microorganisms. Patients are placed in private rooms; some institutions still use reverse isolation procedures, but this is no longer recommended by the Centers for Disease Control.

Good handwashing technique must be practiced by anyone in close contact with leukemia patients. Good handwashing technique is the single most effective infection control strategy. The patient's skin, mouth, nostrils, and perineum should be inspected daily for signs of infection, since these areas may serve as entry portals for opportunistic microorganisms. Daily bathing with antimicrobial soaps is useful, with special attention to the axilla, groin, and perirectal area. A low microbial diet may also be ordered. The health-care team should use aseptic technique for all dressing changes and invasive procedures, examine intravenous sites for signs of infection, and change dressings according to institutional procedure. Because of the increased incidence of pneumonia in these patients, their daily care should include good pulmonary toilet to promote pulmonary ventilation, and ambulation to prevent atelectasis. The patient may wear a face mask if leaving the room.

Patients with very low WBC counts can develop infections without signs of inflammation, such as the presence of pus, since no WBCs are available. Health care staff should take vital signs with temperatures every 4 hours, and observe patients for chills. In febrile patients all potential sites of infection are cultured, a chest x-ray is done, and empiric antibiotic therapy is started as soon as cultures are obtained.

Patients with platelet counts of less than 50,000/mm³ should be placed on bleeding precautions. General measures include: inspecting the skin for petechiae, inspecting body orifices for evidence of abnormal bleeding, testing stool and urine for the presence of blood, avoiding intramuscular injections or catheterizations whenever possible, applying pressure to all venipuncture sites for 5 minutes or longer, avoiding aspirin-containing products, and use of electric razors instead of straight razors. Spontaneous bleeding can occur with platelet counts less than 20,000/mm³, increasing the risk of intrapulmonary and intracerebral hemorrhage.

All patients will require red blood cell and platelet transfusions during chemotherapy-induced bone marrow suppression to prevent hemorrhage and alleviate anemia symptoms. If a patient is an allogeneic bone marrow transplant candidate, blood products should be irradiated whenever possible before transfusion to decrease the patient's risk of graft-versus-host disease from donor lymphocytes.

Many of the chemotherapeutic agents used to treat leukemia cause mucositis. Damaged oral mucosa is particularly susceptible to pathogenic organisms, and good oral hygiene should be practiced regularly. Perineal hygiene routines should also be instituted.

Diarrhea, another common treatment side effect, can cause irritation or excoriation of the rectal area. This area should be kept clean. Sitz baths, good perianal care, and stool softeners may be ordered for patients with rectal abscesses or irritation. Perirectal abscess is a common problem that can be fatal.

Patients undergoing induction therapy for acute myelocytic leukemia, acute lymphocytic leukemia, and chronic myelocytic leukemia-blast crisis may experience tumor lysis syndrome. This complication and other treatment related side-effects are discussed in Unit IV.

Bibliography
Bowman, W. (1981). Childhood acute lymphocytic leukemia: Progress and problems in treatment. *Canadian Medical Association Journal 124*:129-142.
Champlin, R. (1988). Acute myelogenous leukemia: Biology and treatment. *Mediguide to Oncology, 8*(4): 1-9.
Champlin, R., & Golde, D. W. (1987). The leukemias. In Braunwatt, Isselbacher, Petersdorf, Wilson, & Fauci. (Eds.), *Harrison's principles of internal medicine.* (11th edition) (pp 1541-1550). New York: McGraw Hill Book Co.
Freeley, A., & Houlihan, H. (1981). Leukemia: The treatment of leukemia. *Cancer Nursing, 4*(3), 233-242.
Fox, L. S. (1981). Granulocytopenia in the adult cancer patient. *Cancer Nursing, 4*(6), 459-465.
Henderson, E. S., & Han, T. (1986). Current therapy of acute and chronic leukemia in adults. *Ca—A Journal for Clinicians, 36*(6), 322-350.
Moore, I. M., Kramer, J., & Albin, A. (1986). Late effects of central nervous system prophylactic leukemia therapy on cognitive functioning. *Oncology Nursing Forum, 13*(4), 45-51.
National Cancer Institute. (1985). Research report, leukemia. (DHHS Publication No. 85-329), Washington, D.C.: U. S. Department of Health and Human Services.
Newman, K. A. (1985). The leukemias. *Nursing Clinic of North America, 20*, 227-234.

14 THE LYMPHOMAS AND MULTIPLE MYELOMA

Margie Graff Anderson

The malignant lymphomas, first identified in 1832, are a group of immune system diseases caused by neoplastic proliferation of portions of the reticuloendothelial system such as the lymph nodes, bone marrow, spleen, and liver. Included in this group are Hodgkin's disease and non-Hodgkin's lymphoma. Multiple myeloma is also included in this chapter because it is a malignant disorder resulting from the proliferation of immunoglobulin-secreting plasma cells.

HODGKIN'S DISEASE

Incidence

Hodgkin's disease constitutes about 20% of malignant lymphomas. An estimated 7400 new cases of Hodgkin's disease are diagnosed annually, 50% of them in people between ages 20 and 40. Hodgkin's disease is slightly more common in males, who also have a slightly poorer prognosis.

Changes in treatments for Hodgkin's disease have significantly improved survival rates for these patients. Thirty-five years ago, average survival was only 30 months from onset of disease to death. Although variations in treatment regimens complicate the statistics, the current 5-year survival for Stage I and II disease is estimated to be as high as 80-90%, with 10-year survival ranging between 60-70%.

Etiology

Although the exact etiology of Hodgkin's disease is not known, it has been suggested that viruses play a role in its development. A slightly greater incidence of Hodgkin's disease has been observed in people who previously had infectious mononucleosis. Also, the defect in certain immune responses that occurs in Hodgkin's disease is similar to that seen in patients with other diseases caused by human retroviruses.

Pathology

The malignant cell of origin for Hodgkin's is not known, but it is thought to be derived from a B-lymphocyte, T-lymphocyte, or macrophage cell line. The presence of large, multinucleated Reed-Sternberg cells in the tumor is characteristic of Hodgkin's disease.

The disease is thought to originate from a single focus and, if left untreated, spreads in an orderly fashion from above the diaphragm through the entire lymphatic system. Patients with progressive Hodgkin's disease will also experience increasingly impaired immune responses.

Hodgkin's disease is divided into four different categories: lymphocyte-predominant, mixed cellularity, lymphocyte-depleted, and nodular sclerosing. The lymphocyte-predominant and nodular sclerosing types usually have a more favorable prognosis than the other two types.

Clinical Presentation

Patients typically present with painless lymph node enlargement with or without symptoms of fever, sweating, pruritus, and weight loss. Lymphadenopathy is most commonly found in the neck and supraclavicular areas. Hodgkin's disease may also be detected by routine chest x-ray, because approximately 50% of patients have mediastinal involvement. Frequently, the spleen, liver, and retroperitoneal lymph nodes are involved, although patients may not exhibit clinical signs of involvement at diagnosis.

Diagnosis

Diagnosis is confirmed by lymph node and bone marrow biopsy. Chest x-ray and computerized tomography (CT) scan may be used in staging the disease. Patients should also be questioned about the presence or absence of systemic symptoms—specifically fever, night sweats, pruritus, 10% weight loss, and alcohol-induced lymphatic pain, because these may indicate the disease stage. Occasionally, a *lymphangiogram* may be needed to document the presence of disease in the abdomen or retroperitoneal area. If the extent of disease cannot be determined by other diagnostic tests and confirmation of abdominal disease would alter the choice of therapy, a staging laparotomy may be performed.

It is important to determine the extent or stage of disease because treatment recommendations vary. The widely used Ann Arbor Staging System is shown in Table 1.

Treatment

Surgery: In Hodgkin's disease, surgery is used only to stage the disease. Laparotomy and splenectomy are done in select patients to determine the extent of subdiaphragmatic disease.

Table 1. Hodgkin's Disease: Ann Arbor Modification of Rye Staging System (1971)

Stage	Description
I	Involvement of a single lymph-node region (I) or of a single extralymphatic organ or site (I_E).
II	Involvement of two or more lymph-node regions on the same side of the diaphragm (II), or localized involvement of an extralymphatic organ or site and of one or more lymph-node regions on the same side of the diaphragm (II_E).
III	Involvement of two or more lymph-node regions on the same side of the diaphragm (III), which may also be accompanied by localized involvement of an extralymphatic organ or site (III_E) or by involvement of the spleen (III_S) or both (III_{SE}).
IV	Diffuse or disseminated involvement of one or more extralymphatic organs or tissues with or without associated lymph-node enlargement. Reasons for classifying the patient as stage IV should be identified.

Note. In Hodgkin's disease, all patients are subclassified A or B to indicate the absence or presence, respectively, of unexplained weight loss of more than 10 percent body weight, unexplained fever with temperatures above 38°C, and nightsweats.
Source: From "The Non-Hodgkin's Lymphomas" by J. E. Ullman and R. E. Jacobs, 1985, *CA—A Cancer Journal for Clinicians, 35*(2), p. 68. Reprinted with permission of The American Cancer Society.

Radiation Therapy: Radiation therapy alone is recommended for most patients with stage I and II disease. The radiation therapy fields, designed to treat all involved lymph nodes with the same radiation dose, are illustrated in Figure 1. Radiotherapy may also be given to chains of clinically uninvolved nodes to preclude the spread of disease along its predictable routes. Unless there is evidence of disease in the pericardium or hilum, the heart and lungs will be shielded during treatment.

Complications of radiotherapy for Hodgkin's disease are related to the dose given and volume of tissue irradiated. These include radiation pneumonitis, pericarditis, and hypothyroidism.

Chemotherapy: Intensive chemotherapy is used in most patients with stage III and IV Hodgkin's disease, and in select patients with earlier-stage disease. Combinations of at least four chemotherapeutic drugs are needed to achieve a cure. The most commonly used combination is *MOPP*: nitrogen mustard, vincristine, procarbazine, and prednisone. This regimen has induced complete remission in over 80% of cases. Cycles of MOPP may be alternated with other combination chemotherapy regimens in an attempt to overcome drug resistance that may develop to a single combination. MOPP is most frequently alternated with *ABVD*: doxorubicin, bleomycin, vincristine, and dacarbazine, a combination being used with increasing frequency.

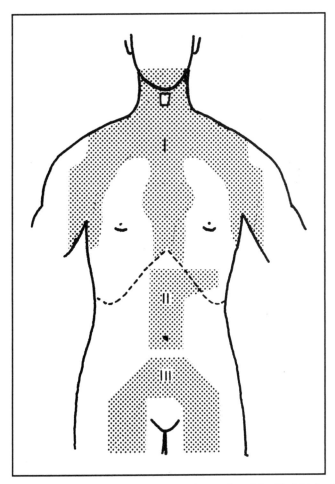

**Figure 1. Radiation fields (shaded) commonly employed in Hodgkin's disease.
I = Mantle. II = Para-aortic-splenic pedicle. III = Pelvic. I + II = Subtotal nodal
irradiation (STNI); I + III = Total nodal irradiation (TNI).**
Source: From *Clinical Oncology: A Multidisciplinary Approach (6th ed.)* (p. 352) by P. Rubin (Ed.),
1983, Atlanta: American Cancer Society. Reprinted with permission of publisher.

The most frequently observed acute side effects of chemotherapy
include nausea and vomiting, bone marrow suppression, alopecia,
and the mood changes associated with steroid therapy. Vinca
neurotoxicity is also prevalent.

Bone Marrow Transplant: The use of autologous bone marrow
transplant with high-dose chemotherapy is an investigational treatment option for refractory and relapsed stage III and IV Hodgkin's
disease.

Treatment Concerns

Treatment approaches for Hodgkin's disease are frequently complex. Nurses may need to help patients and families to understand the therapy and its impact. Nurses also play a crucial role in the management of chemotherapy and radiation side effects, and in explaining the importance of long-term surveillance.

Because a large proportion of patients with Hodgkin's disease are young adults, issues related to long-term effects of radiation and chemotherapy arise. Two major concerns are the effects on reproductive ability and the risk of a second malignancy.

Forty to fifty percent of female patients, usually women over age 35, experience ovarian dysfunction following MOPP therapy. Although younger women may not initially experience this difficulty, they may be at risk for premature menopause from ovarian failure. If the abdomen will be irradiated during treatment, the ovaries can be shielded or surgically displaced to maintain fertility. Since fertility cannot be assured following treatment, patients should be encouraged to discuss their concerns before therapy starts.

Males who receive MOPP have a greater than 80% chance of irreversible sterility. These patients may wish to consider storing sperm through a banking program before starting treatment.

All sexually active patients undergoing treatment should be advised to use contraceptives during treatment and for at least 6 months following therapy. Patients may still be able to conceive during therapy, and the effects of treatment on eggs and sperm are not known.

An increased incidence of second malignancies has been observed in Hodgkin's disease patients who receive intensive radiation and/or chemotherapy. Although patients should be informed of this risk, the need to balance the long-term risks of therapy with the benefits of treating a life-threatening disease should be emphasized. The incidence of second malignancies following chemotherapy treatment is approximately 6%; following both radiation therapy and chemotherapy, second malignancy incidence is about 12%.

NON-HODGKIN'S LYMPHOMAS

Incidence

Approximately 30,000 new cases of non-Hodgkin's lymphoma are diagnosed each year. The average age at diagnosis is 42 and the incidence increases with age; non-Hodgkin's lymphomas are also more common in men. Individuals with congenital or acquired immunodeficiencies, including people with AIDS, those undergoing organ transplantation, and those with autoimmune diseases such as rheumatoid arthritis, are at increased risk for developing non-Hodgkin's lymphomas.

Pathology

Non-Hodgkin's lymphoma is a malignancy of the B- and T-lymphocyte cell systems. The classification terminology for lymphomas can be confusing, as several different methods have been suggested (Table 2). Nevertheless, most patients with non-Hodgkin's lymphoma fall into two broad categories related to their clinical behavior: the nodular, indolent type and the diffuse, aggressive lymphomas. For treatment purposes, they may also be classified as low, intermediate, or high-grade lymphomas.

Non-Hodgkin's lymphoma is frequently disseminated at the time of diagnosis, and the pattern of spread is less predictable than with Hodgkin's disease. Early involvement of oropharyngeal lymphoid tissue or the gastrointestinal tract and infiltration of bone marrow are more common in non-Hodgkin's lymphoma than in Hodgkin's disease.

Clinical Manifestations

Presenting symptoms of this lymphoma are similar to those of Hodgkin's disease. Patients may have localized or generalized lymphadenopathy. In addition, if the gastrointestinal tract is involved, patients may present with an abdominal mass or pain, as well as nausea, vomiting, or signs of bowel obstruction. If the bone marrow is infiltrated, anemia, granulocytopenia, and thrombocytopenia may be present. The central nervous system may also be involved.

Diagnosis

The studies used to confirm the diagnosis of non-Hodgkin's lymphoma are the same as those for Hodgkin's disease. Bone marrow biopsies are routinely done because of the likelihood of bone marrow involvement. The Ann Arbor Staging System (Table 1) is also used for staging cases of non-Hodgkin's lymphoma; however, it is of less value because it does not account for the *histology*, or type, of tumor, which is more important to prognosis than the extent of disease.

Treatment

Therapy for low-grade lymphomas is controversial, because this type of disease is rarely cured regardless of treatment. The overall goal is control of disease for as many years as possible. Treatment may be deferred in selected asymptomatic patients while they are followed closely for changes in the clinical status. In symptomatic

Table 2. Pathologic Classifications of Non-Hodgkin's Lymphomas

Rappaport Classification	Working Formulation of the Non-Hodgkin's Lymphomas for Clinical Usage	Lukes and Collins
	Low Grade	
Diffuse lymphocytic, well differentiated	ML,* small lymphocytic	Small lymphocytic and plasmacytoid lymphocytic
Nodular, poorly differentiated lymphocytic	ML, follicular, predominantly small cleaved cell	Small cleaved FCC,** follicular only or follicular and diffuse
Nodular, mixed lymphocytic-histiocytic	ML, follicular, mixed small cleaved and large cell	Small cleaved FCC, follicular; large cleaved FCC, follicular
	Intermediate Grade	
Nodular histiocytic	ML, follicular, predominantly large cell	Large cleaved and/or non-cleaved FCC, follicular
Diffuse lymphocytic, poorly differentiated	ML, diffuse small cleaved cell	Small cleaved FCC, diffuse
Diffuse mixed lymphocytic-histiocytic	ML, diffuse, mixed small and large cell	Small cleaved, large cleaved or large noncleaved FCC, diffuse
Diffuse histiocytic	ML, diffuse large cell	Large cleaved or noncleaved FCC, diffuse
	High Grade	
Diffuse histiocytic	ML, large cell immunoblastic	Immunoblastic sarcoma, T-cell or B-cell type
Lymphoblastic convoluted/nonconvoluted	ML, lymphoblastic	Convoluted T-cell
Undifferentiated, Burkitt's and non-Burkitt's	ML, small noncleaved cell	Small noncleaved FCC
	Miscellaneous Composite Mycosis fungoides Histiocytic Extramedullary plasmacytoma Unclassifiable	

Note. ML = malignant lymphoma; FCC = follicular center cell.
Source: From "The Non-Hodgkins Lymphomas" by J. E. Ullman and R. H. Jacobs, 1985, *CA—A Cancer Journal for Clinicians, 35*(2), p. 67. Reprinted with permission of The American Cancer Society.

patients, comparable response rates can be achieved with either single-agent or combination chemotherapy, whole-body irradiation, or a combination of chemotherapy and radiation therapy.

Patients with intermediate and high-grade, aggressive lymphomas are routinely treated with combination chemotherapy with or without radiation therapy. One type of lymphoma, *diffuse histiocytic lymphoma*, is potentially curable. Although radiation therapy may be used alone in stage I diffuse histiocytic lymphoma, most patients will be treated with intensive combination chemotherapy regimens. The patient's age and clinical condition, as well as the histology of the tumor, may affect the choice of treatment.

Research is in progress into the roles of interferon, monoclonal antibodies, or autologous bone marrow transplants in the management of non-Hodgkin's lymphoma. (Chapters 4 and 5 of Unit III describe these therapies).

Because adults with non-Hodgkin's lymphoma frequently exhibit central nervous system involvement, the treatment regimen for certain patients will be augmented with intrathecal chemotherapy (administered via lumbar puncture or Ommaya-type reservoir into the cerebrospinal fluid) and/or cranial irradiation in addition to systemic chemotherapy.

The nurse can help the patient and family to understand various treatment approaches and the possible treatment side effects. Side-effect management is also an important nursing function in this patient population. Many patients receiving chemotherapy remain neutropenic throughout their treatment so it is important that nurses monitor them and educate them about this condition.

In addition, bulky tumor in these patients often causes obstruction and pressure, resulting in complications such as spinal cord compression, superior vena cava syndrome, ascites, gastrointestinal obstruction, or ureteral obstruction. The nurse should alert patients and families to the signs and symptoms of these complications and to the need for prompt intervention. These oncologic complications are discussed in Unit IV, Chapter 4.

MULTIPLE MYELOMA

Incidence

Multiple myeloma accounts for approximately 1.1% of all malignancies in whites and 2.1% in blacks. It is seen primarily in older individuals, with less than 2% of patients younger than 40 at diagnosis.

Pathology

Multiple myeloma is a malignant disorder resulting from the proliferation of immunoglobulin-secreting plasma cells, which are the mature form of B lymphocytes. This disease originates in the bone marrow. As the malignant plasma cells proliferate, they crowd out the normal hematopoietic cells produced by the bone marrow.

Clinical Manifestations

The clinical complications observed in patients with multiple myeloma are due to bone marrow involvement and the systemic effects of the substances secreted by the malignant plasma cells.

Bone pain is the most frequent presenting symptom, and pathologic fractures secondary to bone involvement are common. Large amounts of calcium are released as bone is destroyed, so approximately 33% of patients have hypercalcemia at diagnosis and another 33% develop this complication during therapy. Renal failure, often precipitated by hypercalcemia and protein deposits in the kidney, occurs in about 50% of multiple myeloma patients. Patients may be anemic, resulting in general fatigue and weakness. Platelets and white blood cells (particularly lymphocytes) are also affected. Even though platelets may be present in normal numbers, abnormalities of platelet function may lead to excessive bleeding and bruising. Impaired immune responses increase the risk of infection. In fact, infection is the primary cause of morbidity and mortality with this disorder.

Diagnosis

The disease is diagnosed by bone marrow examination and analysis of the serum and urine for *Bence-Jones proteins*, which are indicative of this disease. Immunoelectrophoresis is performed to identify the type of immunoglobulin produced by the plasma cells. X-ray examination will also reveal characteristic coin-shaped areas of bone destruction.

Treatment

Although major strides have been made in the treatment of multiple myeloma, the median survival for patients receiving standard therapy is only about 30 to 40 months. During the initial phase of the disease, which generally lasts for 2 to 3 years, patients respond well to systemic chemotherapy. This is followed by a "plateau phase," in which the disease does not respond to chemotherapy but remains stable. During the final phase of multiple myeloma, patients usually exhibit a resistance to the antitumor effects of chemotherapy and progression of disease. At that point, the focus of care shifts to palliation of the complications of myeloma.

The chemotherapeutic agents most often used include melphalan, cyclophosphamide, chlorambucil, and carmustine. Concurrent steroid therapy may be administered to treat hypercalcemia and improve tumor response. Long-term treatment with alkylating agents is associated with an increased risk of secondary leukemias. The nurse can assist the patient and family in understanding this risk and balancing it with the need for immediate treatment.

Radiation therapy is used primarily to palliate painful bony lesions and to prevent pathologic fractures of diseased bones.

Supportive Care

Myeloma patients may require frequent transfusions of platelets and red blood cells to prevent the clinical complications associated with anemia and thrombocytopenia. In addition, patients should be monitored closely for signs of infection, since this complication can be life-threatening. The risk of infection is further compounded in patients who are immunosuppressed from the effects of chemotherapy. The nurse should teach the patient and family members ways to reduce exposure to infectious agents and how to recognize early symptoms of infection.

Pain medication should be administered to minimize bone pain and facilitate ambulation, because weight bearing helps avoid further demineralization and weakening of the bones. The nurse can evaluate the patient's pain and assist with dose determinations and schedules for pain medication administration.

Because of the risk of renal failure, patients should be encouraged to maintain a fluid intake of 2000-3000 ml per day. Hydration is also helpful in the management of hypercalcemia. The nurse should explain the need for hydration to the patient and family.

Nurses can also provide valuable assistance to patients and family members by focusing on ways to maximize the patient's quality of life. In particular, the nurse can identify areas of daily activity in which the patient can retain independence and control.

Bibliography

Cook, M. B. (1989). Multiple myeloma. In. S. Groenwald, M. H. Frogge, M. Goodman, & C. H. Yarbro (Eds.), *Cancer nursing: Principles and practice* (pp. 990-998). Boston: Jones and Bartlett Publishers, Inc.

Cooley, M. & Copley, S. (1986). Sexual and reproductive issues for women with Hodgkin's disease: 1. Overview of issues. *Cancer Nursing, 9*(4), 188-193.

Hellman, S., Jaffe, E. S., & DeVita, V. T. (1989). Hodgkin's disease. In V. DeVita, S. Hellman, & S. Rosenberg, (Eds.), *Cancer: Principles & practice of oncology* (3rd ed.). (pp. 1696-1740). Philadelphia: J. B. Lippincott Company.

Lacher, M. (1985). Hodgkin's disease: Historical perspective, current status, and future directions. *CA—A Cancer Journal for Clinicians, 35*(2), 88-94.

Schnipper, L., Wagner, H., & McCaffrey, R. (1986). Multiple myeloma and plasma cell dyscrasias. In B. Cady (Ed.), *Cancer manual* (pp. 309-317). Massachusetts: American Cancer Society.

Sporn, J., & McIntyre, O. (1986). Chemotherapy of previously untreated multiple myeloma patients: An analysis of recent treatment results. *Seminars in Oncology, 13*(3), 318-325.

Yarbro, C. H., & Perry, M. C. (1985). The effect of cancer therapy on gonadal function. *Seminars in Oncology Nursing, 1*(1), 3-8.

Yarbro, C. H. (1989). Lymphomas. In. S. Groenwald, M. H. Frogge, M. Goodman, & C. H. Yarbro (Eds.), *Cancer nursing: Principles and practice* (pp. 974-989). Boston: Jones and Bartlett Publishers, Inc.

15 CHILDHOOD CANCER

Teresa Ely, Denise Giesler, and Ki Moore

Each year approximately 7,600 children in the United States are diagnosed with cancer. Because of significant advances in multimodal therapy, 65% of these children will survive 5 years or more, an increase of almost 40% since the early 1960s. Advances in clinical supportive care that maximize the benefits and minimize the side effects of cancer therapy, such as indwelling venous access lines, enteral and parenteral nutrition, blood products, and antibiotic therapy, have greatly reduced the number of treatment-related deaths. Despite the impressive strides in treatment and supportive care, cancer is still the leading cause of death from disease in children, second only to accidents in most age groups.

The types of cancers that occur in children vary greatly from those seen in adults. Leukemias, brain tumors, embryonal tumors, and sarcomas are the most common pediatric malignancies, while adenocarcinomas (i.e., lung, breast, colorectal cancer) are more common in adults. The stage of growth and development is another important difference between adults and children; the immaturity of children's organ systems often has important treatment implications. Similarly, the stage of psychosocial and cognitive development will greatly influence the child's emotional response to the illness.

ACUTE LYMPHOBLASTIC LEUKEMIA

Acute lymphoblastic leukemia (ALL), the most common childhood malignancy, accounts for almost one third of all pediatric cancers. The incidence of ALL is 1 per 23,000 children; approximately 2,000 new cases are diagnosed annually in the United States. The incidence of ALL is higher in white than in nonwhite children, and higher in males than in females. The exact cause of ALL is unknown; however, radiation, chromosomal abnormalities, viruses, and congenital immunodeficiencies have all been associated with an increased incidence of leukemia.

The pathophysiology of ALL involves unregulated proliferation and incomplete maturation of lymphocytes. Replacement of normal hematopoietic cells in the bone marrow by lymphoblasts accounts for the signs and symptoms usually present at diagnosis: thrombocytopenia with numerous bruises and petechiae; recurrent infections and fever; anemia with irritability and fatigue; and bone pain. The white blood cell (WBC) count may be low (less than 10,000) or high (greater than 100,000). Invasion of the liver, spleen, testes, and lymph nodes by circulating lymphoblasts is manifested as organomegaly and lymphadenopathy. The disease can also involve the central nervous system (CNS): approximately 10% of children have lymphoblasts in the cerebral spinal fluid at diagnosis. The presence of lymphoblasts in the peripheral blood may indicate ALL and the diagnosis is confirmed by an increased percentage of lymphoblasts in the bone marrow.

Large, multi-institutional clinical studies have identified factors that suggest outcome and determine the intensity of ALL therapy. *French-American-British (FAB) morphology*, initial WBC counts, and age at diagnosis are the most important prognostic factors. The lower the WBC count (less than 10,000) the better the prognosis; an initial WBC count greater than 50,000 is associated with a poor prognosis. Cell morphology is also an important factor. Predominantly small lymphoblasts with a scant amount of cytoplasm and regular nuclear shapes with occasional clefting (FAB L_1 morphology) warrant the best prognosis. Cells that are large, have prominent nucleoli and cytoplasmic vacuoles, and moderately abundant cytoplasm (L_3 morphology) warrant the poorest prognosis. Children who are diagnosed between the ages 2 and 10 have a more favorable prognosis than adolescents or children less than age 1. The presence of CNS leukemia, Down's syndrome, hepatosplenomegaly, or mediastinal lymphadenopathy at diagnosis and lack of a prompt disease response to induction therapy are other important predictors of poor survival.

ALL treatment involves several phases. The goal of *remission induction* is to rapidly decrease the leukemic cell burden with combination chemotherapy. *Central nervous system prophylaxis* with whole brain radiation and/or intrathecal chemotherapy is essential to preventing leukemic involvement of the brain and meninges. An *intensification or consolidation phase* is commonly included in the treatment of children at high risk for relapse. The purpose of intensification is to eradicate any residual tumor cells. Finally, 1½ to 3 years of *maintenance therapy* are required to sustain a complete remission. Drug regimens used in the treatment of ALL vary, depending upon patient factors and institutional preference. Common regimens are outlined in Table 1.

With current ALL therapy, 95% of children achieve a complete remission, and 70% will remain in remission for 5 years or longer. The bone marrow is the most common site of initial relapse, but relapses in the central nervous system or testes can also occur alone or along with marrow relapse. Some children have had a

**Table 1. Therapy for Childhood Acute Lymphoblastic Leukemia:
Commonly Used Chemotherapeutic Agents**

Treatment Phase	Chemotherapy
Remission induction	vincristine prednisone L-asparaginase*
Central nervous system	intrathecal methotrexate triple intrathecal therapy with methotrexate, arabinoside cytosine and hydrocortisone intermediate or high dose methotrexate in conjunction with intrathecal therapy cranial or craniospinal radiation**
Consolidation/ intensification	L-asparaginase vincristine prednisone methotrexate arabinoside cytosine* cyclophosphamide* VM-26*
Maintenance	6-mercaptopurine methotrexate vincristine prednisone

*Used to improve duration of remission especially for patients with poor prognostic features.
**Used in conjunction with intrathecal chemotherapy for patients with CNS disease or in some patients with poor prognostic features.

relapse in the bone marrow while on therapy. In these cases, a second remission can usually be induced, but is of short duration, especially in children who relapse within 1½ years of diagnosis.

Relapses in other tissues or organs are treated vigorously, and the bone marrow assessed regularly for signs of involvement. Those who relapse more than 6 to 12 months after initial treatment may do very well for long periods. The number of patients who attain 5-year disease-free survival following relapse has been significantly increased by the application of allogeneic bone marrow transplantation.

WILMS' TUMOR

Wilms' tumor is a renal malignancy that may involve one or both kidneys. The incidence of Wilms' tumor is 7.8 per one million children under the age of 14 and is slightly higher in females than males. The disease represents 5-6% of all childhood cancers in the United States, with 350 new cases per year; it is most frequently found in children between 2 and 3 years old.

Wilms' tumor is associated with certain congenital anomalies, including genitourinary malformations, hemihypertrophy of an organ or body part, and aniridia. Epidemiologic research suggests an increased incidence in children of men exposed to lead or hydrocarbons. Recently, an association between Wilms' tumor and chromosomal abnormalities has been established: deletion of a suppressor gene located on the short arm of chromosome 11 has been detected in Wilms' tumor cell lines.

When present, chromosomal anomaly associated with Wilms' tumor is transmitted as an autosomal dominant trait, therefore other family members need to be checked for it as well. It is unclear how many cases involve this mode of transmission, but it is frequent enough that Wilms' tumor in more than one child in a family is not unusual.

Wilms' tumor is often discovered by a parent who notices an increase in the child's abdominal size, or by a physician during a routine physical examination. Approximately half of affected children have additional signs or symptoms, such as abdominal pain, vomiting, fever, and gross or microscopic hematuria. Hypertension is present at diagnosis in 30–60% of children. Radiologic studies, abdominal ultrasound, abdominal computerized tomography (CT), and magnetic resonance imaging (MRI) are used for optimal imaging and to determine the location, extent, and stage of the primary tumor.

The most common metastatic site for Wilms' tumor is the lung; the disease may also spread to regional lymph nodes and the liver. The extent of disease is known to be an important prognostic criterion and is used to determine tumor group (Table 2). Tumor histology is also of prognostic significance. Well-differentiated

Table 2. National Wilms' Tumor Study Grouping Criteria

Group	Features
I	Tumor limited to kidney and completely excised. Surface of renal capsule is intact. Tumor was not ruptured before or during removal. No residual tumor apparent beyond margins of resection.
II	Tumor extended beyond kidney but is completely excised. Local extension into perirenal soft tissues, or periaortic lymph node involvement. No residual tumor apparent beyond margins of resection.
III	Residual nonhematogenous tumor confined to abdomen. Any of the following may occur: a) tumor rupture before or during surgery; b) implants on peritoneal surfaces; c) lymph node involvement beyond abdominal periaortic chains; d) incomplete tumor resection because of local infiltration into vital structures.
IV	Hematogenous metastases. Deposits are beyond Group III, affecting lung, liver, bone, and brain.
V	Bilateral renal involvement either initially or subsequently.

tumors are the most common and are associated with an excellent prognosis. Tumors of unfavorable histology, and accompanying poor prognosis, include those with anaplastic cytology and clear-cell sarcoma and rhabdoid tumors of the kidney.

Nephrectomy is required for all patients with unilateral disease. Surgical treatment of those with extensive bilateral disease involves excision of tumor with preservation of normal renal tissue if possible. Preoperative radiotherapy or chemotherapy is used only when surgical risk is high. Clinical trials conducted by the National Wilms' Tumor Study Group have led to significant strides in treatment. Adjuvant combination chemotherapy is recommended for group I and II patients; radiation to the tumor bed, in addition to chemotherapy, is recommended for children with more advanced disease and for the majority of patients with unfavorable histology.

With current therapy, the outlook for children with Wilms' tumor is excellent. Ninety-five percent of children with group I or II disease will achieve long-term, disease-free survival. Even children with advanced or bilateral disease at diagnosis are curable, with long-term survival rates exceeding 50%.

NEUROBLASTOMA

Neuroblastoma is the most common extracranial solid tumor in children and the most commonly diagnosed neoplasm during the first year of life. Approximately 500 new cases are diagnosed annually in the United States; the incidence is higher among whites than nonwhites.

Neuroblastoma originates from neural crest cells that are normally the progenitors of the sympathetic nervous system. The precise cause(s) of the disease is unknown; however, chromosomal abnormalities and an increased number of copies of the *N-myc* oncogene have been found in some neuroblastoma cells. About 20% of cases are familial—again because of autosomal dominant gene transmission—with an increased incidence among siblings and identical twins.

Neuroblastoma can originate anywhere along the sympathetic nervous system. More than half the tumors occur in the retroperitoneal area and present as an abdominal mass. Other common sites include the posterior mediastinum, pelvis, and neck. Nutritional problems, including weight loss, anorexia, cachexia, and diarrhea may be present at diagnosis. Urinary catecholamines are elevated in 80% of children; symptoms related to increased catecholamines that may also be present include hypertension, flushing, periods of excessive sweating, and irritability. If the bone marrow is involved, the child may also experience bone pain and exhibit anemia, thrombocytopenia, and leukopenia. Spread to the orbits can cause ecchymosis and sometimes proptosis. Bluish movable cutaneous or subcutaneous nodules are seen almost exclusively in infants.

Age at diagnosis, site of origin, and clinical stage of the disease (Table 3) affect survival. Age is the most important factor. Children under age 1 have a 75% survival rate. Spontaneous remission without treatment can occur in infants with stage IV-S (stage IV-S means that patients have local stage I or II disease but also have remote disease confined to one or more of the following: liver, skin, or bone marrow). The survival rate for children diagnosed at age 2 or older drops to 12%.

Table 3. Staging Criteria for Neuroblastoma

Stage	Criteria
I	Tumor limited to organ of origin.
II	Regional spread that does not cross the midline.
III	Tumor spread over the midline.
IV	Metastases to lymph nodes, bone, brain, or lung.
IV-S	Small primary tumor with metastases limited to liver, skin, and/or bone marrow without radiologic evidence of bony metastases.

Children with an abdominal primary mass have a poorer survival record than those with a chest, neck, or pelvic primary tumor. Sites of metastatic spread include the lymph nodes, bone, bone marrow, liver, and subcutaneous tissue. Unfortunately, 50% of infants and 66% of older children have widespread metastatic disease (stage IV) at diagnosis. Children with stage IV disease have the best prognosis if younger than 1 or older than 6 years of age, but the average age at diagnosis is 2 years. In addition, tumors often progress rapidly in patients with multiple copies of the *N-myc* oncogene in the neuroblastoma cells.

Treatment for neuroblastoma involves surgery for staging and tumor removal and aggressive combination chemotherapy. The rate of 2-year, relapse-free survival achieved in patients in stages I and II combined is 91%; in stage III, 58%. The 3-year survival rate for stage IV patients is about 20%; however, improved survival has recently been demonstrated in children treated with aggressive short-term chemotherapy followed by bone marrow transplant.

RETINOBLASTOMA

Retinoblastoma is a cancer of the eye. Although relatively rare, it accounts for 5% of childhood blindness. Approximately 70% of children present with a unilateral tumor, while 30% have bilateral disease. Retinoblastoma can be hereditary or nonhereditary. The hereditary type is autosomal dominant, with an 88-100% transmission rate; it accounts for 40% of all cases and is usually bilateral. A deletion on the short arm of chromosome 12 has been identified in patients with the inherited form of the tumor. Hereditary retinoblastoma also carries an increased risk for other malignancies. Approximately 60% of affected children have the nonhereditary form of the disease. The tumor is usually unilateral and not associated with an increased risk of other tumors.

Retinoblastoma is usually confined to the globe of the eye. If so confined, the child has an excellent prognosis, with a current survivial rate of 85-100%. Two types of growth patterns have been identified in retinoblastoma. Endophytic tumors grow mainly in the inner layers of the retina and fill the vitreous body. Exophytic tumors grow along the outer retinal layer and can spread to the subretinal space, causing retinal detachment. This commonly occurs with very large tumors, but can be corrected after starting treatment. Most cases of retinoblastoma are a combination of both growth patterns.

Extraocular tumor growth usually occurs along the optic nerve. Invasion of the optic nerve with 10-15 millimeters of tumor growth can cause subarachnoid and intracranial spread. Optic nerve involvement carries a poor prognosis.

The tumor is usually painless; symptoms include strabismus and leukokoria (white spots in the pupil of the eye). Leukokoria is the most common presenting symptom. Loss of vision also occurs, but is difficult for small children to identify.

Early tumor detection is critical. The extent to which vision is preserved is directly related to the size of the tumor at the start of therapy. If the tumor is detected early, cure is possible with radiation therapy alone, and the vision is preserved. Most cases of unilateral retinoblastoma are so far advanced that there is little or no hope of preserving vision. Enucleation is the treatment of choice.

Bilateral disease treatment includes radiation and possible enucleation of one or both eyes if no vision can be saved. Chemotherapy is also used for extraocular disease or distant tumor spread. Finally, genetic counseling is recommended if a family history of retinoblastoma is identified. Nurses can emphasize to families the importance of monitoring siblings of affected children and also of monitoring a child with a history of retinoblastoma.

RHABDOMYOSARCOMA

Rhabdomyosarcoma is the most common soft tissue sarcoma and the seventh leading cause of cancer in children. The tumor, which is more prevalent in males than females, originates from the same embryonic cells that give rise to striated muscle. The peak incidence is between the age of 2 and 5; a second peak occurs between the ages of 15 and 19.

The most common tumor sites are the head and neck, including the orbit (38%); the genitourinary tract (21%); and the extremities (18%). A painless mass is the major symptom at diagnosis. Orbital tumors can cause pain, nose bleeds, and difficulty with breathing, swallowing, and speech. One third of patients with lesions in the nasopharynx, nasal cavity, paranasal sinuses, or middle ear have CNS involvement. This can lead to cranial nerve palsies, meningeal symptoms, and respiratory paralysis. Ninety percent of children with lesions extending into the CNS eventually die. Involvement in the genitourinary area can cause hematuria, urinary obstruction, and vaginal bleeding.

Rhabdomyosarcoma is staged similarly to neuroblastoma. Stage I is localized and completely resectable. Disease with distant metastasis is categorized as stage IV. Those patients without metastases at diagnosis have a much better prognosis. Treatment for rhabdomyosarcoma includes surgical removal (if possible), radiation, and chemotherapy. Chemotherapy can be administered before surgery to reduce the tumor size. With tumor shrinkage, less radical surgery is possible, resulting in less damage to adjacent tissues. Chemotherapy and radiation are used after surgery to eradicate any residual tumor cells. Chemotherapy is continued for 1 to 2 years because the majority of patients relapse during this period. Patients who recieve radiation for head, neck, and bladder tumors are at increased risk for late effects such as short stature (growth hormone impairment) and impaired secondary sexual development.

OTHER CHILDHOOD CANCERS

Other common cancers seen in children are bone cancers—both osteogenic and Ewing's sarcomas (see Unit V, Chapter 12)—lymphoma (see Unit V, Chapter 14), and brain tumors (see Unit V, Chapter 10). Further discussion of leukemia is found in Unit V, Chapter 13.

PSYCHOSOCIAL IMPACT

Childhood cancer affects the entire family. An honest and open discussion of treatment, side effects of therapy, and psychosocial issues is an important first step in family-centered care. It is important that the ill child and healthy siblings be given honest and developmentally appropriate information about the disease. Parents and other family members may need encouragement to ask questions about the child's cancer; parents may find it helpful to make a list of questions as they arise. Research has demonstrated that the first 6 months after diagnosis is the most critical time for providing education and emotional support.

A comprehensive assessment of the family by the multidisciplinary team is recommended. Important areas for assessment include: the family's developmental level, coping strategies, social support, current sources of stress, and the parents' marital status. Assessment of financial resources is also important, as the direct medical costs and out-of-pocket expenses for food, lodging, and sibling care during hospitalizations can cause considerable financial strain.

Health care professionals can help parents by continually providing new information about the child's disease and therapy. Educational materials for the family, child, and school teachers are available from the American Cancer Society and the National Cancer Institute. Support groups such as Candlelighters and family and sibling camps are also important resources for families.

Healthy siblings, in particular, experience a great deal of disruption as a result of their brother's or sister's illness. Siblings may feel isolated and abandoned, have a fear of catching the disease, or resent the special attention given to the ill child. They may also feel guilty because of thoughts they once had about their ill brother or sister, or convince themselves that they are responsible for the illness. An age-appropriate discussion about the ill child's disease, treatment, and prognosis is recommended. Parents also need to prepare the healthy siblings for the physical changes that the ill child may experience as a result of therapy. Finally, parents are encouraged to spend special time or make frequent phone contact with the healthy children and involve them in the care of their sick brother or sister.

The ill child's developmental level will influence his or her emotional response to the illness. The young child may experience separation anxiety from parents and fear of the hospital and medical procedures. Parents need to reassure their child that they will not be abandoned, and that the medical procedures are not punishment for bad behavior. It is especially helpful to younger children if parents assume an active role in the child's care.

Older children also experience separation anxiety and threats to body integrity, as well as concerns about their independence, appearance, peer acceptance, sexuality, and future plans. Age-appropriate information about treatment and side effects, preparation for painful procedures, and emotional support during those procedures is essential for all children, regardless of age. The older child's need for privacy should also be respected. In addition, the patient should be given ample opportunity to ask questions and participate in medical decisions, including the discussion of therapy options.

Prompt return to school and to extracurricular activities is crucial to the child's growth and development. Teachers need to be informed of the child's disease and treatment, as well as of any special needs the child may have during school. Preparing peers for the child's return to school by discussing the disease, treatment, and physical changes such as hair loss will minimize isolation, teasing, and embarrassment. Finally, parents and teachers must continue to expect developmentally appropriate behavior and to maintain discipline. It may be helpful to role-play with parents, because they may not be confident discussing emotionally distressing information.

Dealing with a Life-Threatening Illness and Bereavement

Religion, cultural background, previous experience with death and loss, communication and coping patterns within the family, and environmental factors can all influence the child's and family's response to life-threatening illness and death. Preparing the child for death is important because it can help the child to die more peacefully and help the family cope with the loss. The child should feel free to ask questions and express feelings of pain, fear, separation, and confusion, but not all children will choose to use the opportunities.

Children develop an understanding of death at different ages. Spinetta (1981) found that children with a life-threatening illness understand death at an earlier age than do healthy children. Such a child is experiencing day-to-day physical changes that have a dramatic impact on his or her awareness of the seriousness of the situation. Children between the ages of 6 and 10 sense that their illness is not ordinary and that they may not get well. Fears of separation and abandonment are compounded by fears of mutilation and bodily harm. As the child's physical condition deteriorates, awareness of death increases.

Parents often need assistance preparing the child and other family members for death. Families sometimes tend to avoid discussing death because it can arouse intense emotions and feelings of discomfort. This may be especially problematic when the child is in the terminal stages of the disease. Nurses can assist parents to find other ways to deal with the issues. It may be helpful to role play with the parents if they are uncomfortable discussing death. Pertinent books are also helpful for children and adults. *About Dying* (Stein, 1974) has simple explanations and pictures for children on one side of the page and an explanation for parents on the other side.

Families experience intense feelings of grief and loss after a child's death. A bereavement follow-up by a health care professional who has already established a relationship with the family is recommended. Family members may also benefit from Candlelighters or other support groups, especially if they were involved with the group before the child's death.

LATE EFFECTS

Survival of patients with childhood cancers continues to improve. It has been estimated that by the year 2000, 1 in 1,000 individuals between the ages of 20 and 29 will be survivors of childhood cancer. With increasing survival rates, the recognition of and concern about the late effects of disease and treatment have grown. The term "late effects" refers to the damaging effects of surgery, radiation, and chemotherapy on nonmalignant tissues, and to the social, emotional, and economic consequences of survival. These effects appear months to years after treatment and can range in severity from subclinical to clinical to life-threatening. Not all children experience such effects, but they are common enough to warrant study.

Late effects have been identified in almost every organ system. Treatments involving the central nervous system (CNS) can cause deficits in intelligence, hearing, and vision. Treatment involving the CNS, head and neck, or gonads can cause endocrine abnormalities such as short stature, hypothyroidism, or delayed secondary sexual development. Cardiomyopathy following anthracyclines can result in congestive heart failure. Surgery and radiation involving the musculoskeletal system have been associated with defects such as kyphosis, scoliosis, and spinal shortening. Finally, although the incidence of multiple malignancies is low, the child who has received radiation and/or alkylating chemotherapy drugs for a first cancer has a 10 times greater risk of a second malignancy than children who have never had cancer.

Nurses should stress the importance of regular health surveillance and prompt investigation of changes for former pediatric oncology patients. As these children reach adulthood, nurses in a variety of health care settings will have opportunities to assist with other concerns. For example, the college health or Ob/Gyn nurse may assist with fertility and family planning concerns and can assure patients that most survivors can have healthy babies.

Long-term surveillance is important because late effects can occur many years after treatment. The effects of childhood cancer treatment on aging organs is still unknown. The child who was treated at an early age may have little understanding of the disease, its treatment, and implications for health maintenance. These are all important topics for discussion during off-therapy evaluations.

Long-term emotional problems—such as the inability to plan for the future or develop relationships—can interfere with the child's normal growth and development. The child who has residual physical effects may be at increased risk for emotional problems. The family may also experience emotional and economic consequences. Fears about disease recurrence and about the child's health in general may make it difficult for parents to permit age-appropriate independence. Difficulties obtaining health and life insurance for the cancer survivor are among the economic problems faced by the child and family.

Although the late effects discussed here are obviously distressing, it is important to remember that patients do not necessarily experience these effects and that positive long-term effects occur as well. In *The Damocles Syndrome*, the authors note positive effects these children and their family experience: maturity, resilience, and pride.

CONCLUSION

Advances in pediatric cancer have outpaced other areas of oncology. As Hammond notes, dramatically improved childhood survival rates are directly correlated with improved treatment, development of physical and psychosocial supportive modalities, and the pioneering utilization of the multidisciplinary team. Nurses in all settings are likely to be involved with bereaved parents and siblings or with former patients as they mature, enter the work force, and begin their adult lives. Nurse-to-nurse consultation, especially between the generalist and the oncology specialist, can assist in promoting optimal outcomes for the children and their families.

Bibliography

American Cancer Society: *Cancer facts and figures.* (1990). Atlanta, GA: American Cancer Society.

Diamond, C. A., & Matthay, K. K. (1988). Childhood acute lymphoblastic leukemia. *Pediatric Annals, 17*(3), 156–170.

Donaldson, S. S., & Smith, L. M. (1989). Retinoblastoma: Biology, presentation and current management. *Oncology, 3*(4), 45–52.

Hammond, G. D. (1986). The cure of childhood cancers. *Cancer, 58*(2) (Supplement), 407–413.

Koocher, G. P., & O'Malley, J. E. (1981). *The Damocles syndrome: Psychosocial consequences of surviving childhood cancer.* New York: McGraw Hill Publishing Company.

Lopez-Ibor, B., & Schwartz, A. D. (1985). Neuroblastoma. *Pediatric Clinics of North America, 32*(3), 755–771.

Malogolowkin, M. H., & Schwartz, A. D. (1988). Rhabdomyosarcoma of childhood. *Pediatric Annals, 170*(4), 251–268.

Moore, I. M., & Klopovich, P. (Guest Eds.). (1989). Late effects of cancer treatment in children and adults. *Seminars in Oncology Nursing, 5*(1). Entire issue.

Pizzo, P. A., & Poplack, D. G. (Eds.). (1989). *Principles and practice of pediatric oncology.* Philadelphia: J. B. Lippincott Company.

UNIT 6

Resources in Cancer Care

Nurses are a vital part of the health care team at all levels of cancer care. They function as health educators and locators of resources in a variety of situations where they may be the first health care professional to interact with patients. The nurse's role in detection, treatment, and continuing care is multifaceted, requiring numerous technical skills, facility in interpersonal communications, knowledge of the disease, supportive care techniques, and awareness of care trends.

Agencies and resources do exist to assist the nurse, the patient, and the family. The variety of resources is enormous. This unit contains information on resources that cancer nurses have found valuable. At a time when patients and families have tremendous needs for assistance, they may not be able to readily identify sources of help. The nurse can then be of great assistance in identifying and explaining resources to patients and families.

RESOURCES IN CANCER CARE

Marilyn Frank-Stromborg and Rhonda Niles

The initial diagnosis of cancer is often emotionally, financially, and socially devastating to patients and their families. Although there are multiple community-based resources available to assist the patient and family with treatment, rehabilitation, and financing, the patient and family are frequently unaware of the services that are offered. Thus, one of the primary responsibilities of the health care provider is either to supply the patient with information about cancer-related resources or to refer the patient to a structured agency that could supply this information (i.e., the hospital's social service department, local American Cancer Society, local public health agency). As part of a national health care trend, cancer patients are spending less and less time in acute care settings. This means that their familiarity with community-based resources that can help with all aspects of the disease is more crucial than ever before.

ORGANIZATIONS SPONSORING SELF-HELP GROUPS AND RELATED SERVICES FOR CANCER PATIENTS AND THEIR FAMILIES

Encore
National Board, YWCA
726 Broadway
New York, NY 10003 (212)614-2827
Encore is a national program offered by the YWCA and sponsored by local YWCAs. It provides floor and pool exercises as well as discussion and support groups for women recovering from breast cancer surgery. Contact your local YWCA for a program near you.

Make-a-Wish Foundation of America
2600 North Central Avenue/Suite 936
Phoenix, AZ 85004 1-800-722-9474 (602)240-6600
This foundation grants wishes for people under age 18 who are suffering from life-threatening illnesses. The wish includes the immediate family and expenses. There are 68 chapters serving 44 states and 5 international affiliates. Contact the national office for a chapter near you.

Make Today Count
101½ South Union Street
Alexandria, VA 22314   (703)548-9674
Make Today Count is a mutual support group for persons with life-threatening illnesses. The purpose is to allow these people to discuss their personal concerns so that they may deal with them in a positive way. There are over 200 chapters in the United States, Canada, and Europe. Contact the national headquarters for the chapter near you.

TOUCH
513 Tinsley Harrison Tower
University Station
Birmingham, AL 35294   (205)934-3814
TOUCH stands for "Today Our Understanding of Cancer is Hope" and is cosponsored by the American Cancer Society Alabama Division, Inc. and the Comprehensive Cancer Center, Birmingham, AL. There are several hundred members in a number of different cities in Alabama. The program offers emotional and psychological support to cancer patients who are undergoing or have completed cancer treatment and their significant others.

Y-ME National Organization for Breast Cancer Information and Support.
18220 Hardwood Ave.
Homewood, IL 60430 (312)799-8228 Open 24 hours; (800) 221-2141 weekdays 9 to 5.
Y-ME has become the largest breast cancer support program in the USA. It provides hotlines staffed by volunteers who have personally experienced breast cancer. Y-ME offers preoperative counseling, open-door meetings, early detection workshops, a speakers bureau, a resource library, a wigs and prosthesis bank, and inservice workshops for health professionals.

NATIONAL ORGANIZATIONS PROVIDING INFORMATION AND OTHER SERVICES TO CANCER PATIENTS AND THEIR FAMILIES

American Cancer Society
1-800-ACS-2345 for information about cancer.
National Offices: 1599 Clifton Road, NE
          Atlanta, GA 30329   (404)320-3333
The American Cancer Society offers programs of cancer research, education, and patient service and rehabilitation. The ACS is organized into the national office, state or division offices, and local units. Many American Cancer Society Units provide equipment and

supplies to make home care as comfortable as possible. Both large items, such as beds and wheelchairs, and smaller items like walkers are available in many areas. Transportation to and from cancer treatments is also supplied by many local units. Local staff and volunteers can answer questions about cancer and assist patients with getting the help they need from organizations in their community. The ACS has extensive free professional and patient education materials including films, videotapes, booklets, pamphlets, books, national conference proceedings and posters. The ACS also sponsors many valuable patient and family support and educational groups.

CanSurmount: The CanSurmount Program is a "therapeutic community" composed of the patient, the family member, the CanSurmount volunteer, who is also a cancer patient, and the health professional. On physician referral, a trained CanSurmount volunteer meets with a patient and/or family members in the hospital and home and provides them with information and emotional support.

I Can Cope: I Can Cope is a formal educational program that addresses the educational and psychological needs of people with cancer. The course consists of eight classes taught by health professionals from the hospital and community that are usually offered through the local hospital.

International Association of Laryngectomees is a voluntary organization sponsored by the American Cancer Society, that promotes and supports the total rehabilitation of people with laryngectomies. At the invitation of the physician, members who are themselves laryngectomees call on hospitalized patients to offer moral support and encouragement. There are 257 domestic and 14 foreign clubs whose members are laryngectomees. For the location of the "Lost Chord," "New Voice," or "Anamile" club nearest a patient, contact the local Unit of the American Cancer Society. The goals of the Lost Chord clubs are to help new patients make early adjustments to the loss of voice and to overcome psychosocial problems.

Reach to Recovery is one of the best known self-help groups. Reach to Recovery provides rehabilitation support for women who have had breast cancer. Designed to meet physical, psychological, and cosmetic needs, the program works through volunteer visitors who have adjusted successfully to their surgery. With referral from the patient's physician, the volunteers make hospital visits after surgery, bringing information about rehabilitative exercises and a temporary breast form. They also demonstrate the exercises and provide literature for the patient's family. In addition, Reach to Recovery distributes educational materials and provides lectures and demonstrations for health professionals.

Consult your telephone directory for the number of your local Unit for complete information about all programs. A listing of Division offices follows this chapter.

Association of Brain Tumor Research
3735 North Talman Avenue
Chicago, IL 60618   (312)286-5571
This organization raises funds for brain tumor research and patient education materials. They furnish on request a list of experimental treatment centers and brain tumor study groups. Twelve publications, in lay language, are available free of charge to patient and family members.

Cancer Care
1180 Avenue of the Americas
New York, NY 10036   (212)221-3300
The service arm of the National Cancer Foundation, Cancer Care is a nonprofit social service agency dedicated to helping patients and families cope with the emotional, psychological, and financial consequences of cancer. Although the organization primarily serves New York City and its tri-state, metropolitan region, it also responds to letters and phone calls from all over the United States, providing information and referrals whenever possible.

Cancer Information Service
1-800-4-CANCER
HAWAII: OAHU 524-1234 (Call collect from neighbor islands)
Alaska: 1-800-638-6070
National Office: 1-800-638-6694
The Cancer Information Service, a program of the National Cancer Institute, is a network of regional offices with trained staff and volunteers who provide accurate and confidential telephone information to questions concerning cancer rehabilitation, research, causes, prevention and detection, diagnosis, treatment, support services, etc.

Candlelighters
1901 Pennsylvania Avenue/Suite 1011
Washington, D.C. 20006   (202)659-5136
Candlelighters has two primary goals: to obtain consistent and adequate federal support for cancer research and to help parents and other family members who share the particularly difficult experience of living with a child with cancer. Candlelighters main-

tains communications between parents and professionals through quarterly newsletters and between groups through bimonthly news-letters. It also publishes a resource list of childhood cancer education materials. There are 250 chapters in the United States; contact the national office for the chapter nearest you.

Concern for the Dying
250 West 57th Street
New York, NY 10107   (212)246-6962
Concern for the Dying is a nonprofit educational council that advocates an individual's right to participate in decisions regarding her/his treatment, particularly those decisions when a person is near death. Services provided include: information regarding the living will and up-to-date information on the current laws of each state concerning euthanasia, death, and dying; psychological and legal counseling; and referral to local organizations for other types of assistance.

Corporate Angel Network, Inc.
Westchester County Airport
Building One
White Plains, NY 10604   (914)328-1313
This is a nonprofit organization that arranges free air transportation for cancer patients going to or from health care centers for recognized treatments, consultations, or check-ups. The program utilizes available seats on corporate aircraft and is free of charge for both the ambulatory cancer patient and one attendant or family member.

Leukemia Society of America, Inc.
733 Third Avenue
New York, NY 10017   (212)573-8484
The Leukemia Society of America offers financial assistance and consultations for referrals to cancer patients with leukemia and related disorders. Financial coverage is reserved for outpatient care. The program includes payment for drugs used in the cure, treat-ment, and/or control of leukemia; laboratory costs associated with blood transfusion; transportation; radiotherapy in the first stages of Hodgkin's disease, and prophylactic radiation for children with acute leukemia. Fifty-six chapters operate in 31 states and the District of Columbia.

National Coalition for Cancer Survivorship
323 Eighth Street, S.W.
Albuquerque, NM 87102 (505)764-9956
The National Coalition for Cancer Survivorship is a fairly new organization comprised of independent groups and individuals interested in issues of cancer survivorship and support of cancer survivors and their significant others. It provides a national communication network between people and organizations involved with survivorship; advocates for the issues, research, and interests of cancer survivors; and collects and distributes information.

National Hospice Organization
1901 North Moore Street/Suite 901
Arlington, VA 22209 (703)243-5900
National Hospice Organization (NHO) is a nonprofit organization promoting quality care to the terminally ill and their significant others. The number of hospices has increased in the United States from one in 1974 to over 1,725 today. There are several different membership categories to meet the diverse needs of people working with hospice. Members receive *The Hospice Journal* among numerous other publications and workshops.

Ronald McDonald Houses
500 North Michigan Avenue
Chicago, IL 60611 (312)836-7100
The purpose of the house is to provide temporary lodging for families of children who are undergoing treatment at a nearby hospital for cancer, leukemia, or other serious illnesses. One hundred Ronald McDonald Houses currently operate in the United States and in some foreign countries.

Society for the Right to Die
250 West 57th Street
New York, NY 10107 (212)246-6973
The Society for the Right to Die is a national nonprofit organization in the United States that pursues a program on several fronts: legal services, legislation, and promotion for citizens' rights. A copy of a living will for each of 40 states will be sent free of charge upon request. A declaration in general language is provided for those states that still lack living will legislation.

United Ostomy Association
36 Executive Park/Suite 120
Irving, CA 92714 (714)660-8624
Local chapters of the United Ostomy Association are composed of ostomates who provide mutual aid, moral support, and education

to those who have a colostomy, ileostomy, or urostomy surgery. All local chapters (there are more than 500) are volunteer organizations; a list of them is available from the UOA. The organization publishes a magazine, *Ostomy Quarterly*, and has publications and slide programs that cover every aspect of ostomies.

NATIONAL CANCER NURSING ORGANIZATIONS AND RELATED ORGANIZATIONS

American Association for Cancer Education
Samuel Brown, Ed.D., Secretary, AACE
Educational Research and Development
University of Alabama at Birmingham
401 CHSD University Street
Birmingham, AL 35294
This is a multidisciplinary organization that holds an annual fall meeting. Members receive the *Journal of Cancer Education* and other publications on cancer education.

Association of Pediatric Oncology Nurses
11508 Allecingie Parkway, Suite C
Richmond, VA 23235   (804)379-9150
Membership is open to all registered nurses who are either interested in or engaged in pediatrics or pediatric oncology. Members receive a copy of the quarterly journal, *JAPON*, the APON *Newsletter*, and other pertinent publications; members can also attend all business meetings and programs at a reduced rate.

International Society of Nurses in Cancer Care
Carol Reed Ash, Ed.D., R.N., F.A.A.N.
Secretary/Treasurer
Adelphi University School of Nursing/Box 516
Garden City, NY 11530   (516)663-1001
This society's goal is to enable cancer nurses to share their knowledge and concerns on a worldwide basis. Members receive the bimonthly journal, *Cancer Nursing: An International Journal for Cancer Care*, and can attend the biannual international meetings.

International Union Against Cancer (UICC)
Rue de Consil-General 3
1205 Geneva, Switzerland   Tel: (41-22)20 18-11
UICC is composed of multidisciplinary cancer organizations. Its purpose is to encourage the fight against cancer worldwide, promoting international communication in cancer research, treatment,

and prevention. Membership dues are based on an organization's ability to pay; congresses are held every four years.

Oncology Nursing Society
1016 Greentree Road
Pittsburgh, PA 15220-3125 (412)921-7373
Founded in 1975, the Oncology Nursing Society (ONS) presently has more than 17,000 members and 100 chapters across the country. Members get the society's refereed journal, *Oncology Nursing Forum*, and its newsletter, *ONS NEWS*, as well as reduced registration at the ONS Annual Congress. ONS has multiple publications related to cancer nursing, including standards of care. Information on certification is also available.

FEDERAL AGENCIES THAT RELATE TO ONCOLOGY

Food and Drug Administration
Office of Consumer Affairs
HFE-88
5600 Fishers Lane
Rockville, MD 20857 (301)443-3170

National Institute for Occupational Safety and Health
U.S. Department of Health and Human Services
Room 714B
200 Independence Avenue, SW
Washington, D.C. 20201 (202)472-7134 or (800) 35 NIOSH
(Clearinghouse)

APPENDIX I
Antineoplastic Agents

Class	Name	Route	Major Toxicities
Alkylating agents	Aziridinylbenzoquinone (AZQ)	IV	BMD, N/V, stomatitis, diarrhea.
	Busulfan	PO	Prolonged BMD, hyperpigmentation, pulmonary fibrosis, gynecomastia.
	Carboplatin	IV	BMD, N/V, mild neurotoxicity.
	Chlorambucil	PO	BMD, occasional dermatitis.
	Cisplatin	IV, IP, IA	Renal toxicity, N/V, anaphylaxis, ototoxicity peripheral neuropathy, Mg^{++} wasting.
	Cyclophosphamide	IV, PO	BMD, N/V, hemorrhagic cystitis/hematuria, alopecia.
	Decarbazine	IV, IA	Mild BMD, N/V, alopecia, hepatic necrosis, flu-like syndrome, local pain with infusion (irritant).
	Ifosfamide	IV	Mild BMD, bladder toxicity, (Mesna is routinely used to prevent hemorrhagic cystitis), alopecia, lethargy and confusion at higher doses.
	Melphalan	PO	Delayed BMD, N/V, pulmonary fibrosis.
	Nitrogen Mustard	IV, Topical	BMD, N/V, fever, diarrhea, alopecia, tissue necrosis.
	Thiotepa	IV, IM, IT, IC	BMD, dermatitis, paresthesia reported after IT administration.
Nitrosoureas	Carmustine (BCNU)	IV	Severe N/V, local pain and tissue necrosis, facial flushing, pulmonary, renal, and hepatotoxicity.
	Lomustine (CCNU)	PO	N/V, BMD, alopecia, stomatitis, pulmonary and renal toxicity.
	Semustine	PO	N/V, BMD, stomatitis, renal and pulmonary toxicity.
	Streptozotocin	IV	N/V, anorexia, BMD, hypoglycemia, tissue necrosis.
Antimetabolites	Cytarabine (AraC)	IV, SC, IT	N/V, BMD, stomatitis, cerebellar toxicity, conjunctivitis.
	Floxuridine (FUDR)	IA, IV	BMD, anorexia, N/V, hepatic toxicity, stomatitis.
	5-Fluorouracil	IV, IP, IA, Topical	BMD, stomatitis, diarrhea, N/V, ataxia, visual disturbances.
	Hydroxyurea	PO	BMD, N/V, rash, renal and neurotoxicity.
	6-Mercaptopurine	PO	N/V, BMD, cholestasis, hepatotoxicity.
	Methrotrexate (MTX)	IV, IM, IT, SC, PO, IA	BMD, N/V, GI ulceration, pulmonary and hepatotoxicity. (High-dose MTX $>$ 1 gm/m^2 must be followed by leucovorin rescue.)
	6-Thioguanine	PO, IV	BMD, stomatitis, diarrhea.
Antitumor antibiotics	Bleomycin	IV, IM, SC	N/V, chills/fever, anaphylaxis, alopecia, stomatitis, hyperpigmentation, erythema.
	Dactinomycin	IV	N/V, BMD, tissue necrosis, alopecia, mucositis.
	Daunorubicin	IV	N/V, tissue necrosis, BMD, alopecia, stomatitis, cardiotoxicity.

APPENDIX I (Continued)
Antineoplastic Agents

Class	Name	Route	Major Toxicities
	Doxorubicin	IV, IP, IC	N/V, tissue necrosis, BMD, alopecia, stomatitis, cardiotoxicity.
	Mitomycin C	IV	BMD, stomatitis, tissue necrosis, pulmonary toxicity, renal toxicity, N/V.
	Mitoxantrone	IV	BMD, cardiotoxicity, alopecia (rare), N/V, diarrhea, abdominal pain, hepatic dysfunction.
	Plicamycin	IV	N/V, BMD, coagulation abnormalities, tissue necrosis, CNS and renal toxicity.
Plant alkaloids	Etoposide (VP-16-213)	IV	BMD, mild N/V, hypotension, anaphylaxis, alopecia, headache, peripheral neuropathy, fever and chills.
	Teniposide (VM 26)	IV	BMD, tissue necrosis, fever, hypotension, anaphylaxis, alopecia.
	Vinblastine	IV	BMD, stomatitis, alopecia, neurotoxicity, tissue necrosis with infiltration.
	Vincristine	IV	N/V, BMD, tissue necrosis, peripheral neuropathy, constipation, paralytic ileus, SIADH.
	Vindesine	IV	BMD, neurotoxicity, tissue necrosis, stomatitis.
Miscellaneous agents	Hexamethamelamine (HMM)	PO	N/V, neurotoxicity, rash.
	L'asparaginase	IV	Anaphylaxis, N/V, malaise, hepatotoxicity, hyperglycemia, pancreatitis, coagulation abnormalities, CNS depression.
	Amsacrine (M-AMSA)	IV	BMD, tissue necrosis, N/V, stomatitis, mucositis, cardiac arrhythmias, renal toxicity.
	Mitotane (O,P'-DDD)	PO	N/V, anorexia, CNS toxicity, adrenal insufficiency, rash.
	Procarbazine	PO	N/V, flu-like syndrome, BMD, hypersensitivity reactions, disulfiram like reaction with alcohol. Drug interaction with MAO inhibitors, tricyclic antidepressants, and sympathomimetics causing hypertensive crisis. CNS and pulmonary toxicity.

BMD = bone marrow depression
IA = intra-arterially
IC = intracavitary
IM = intramuscular
IP = intraperitoneal
IT = intrathecal
N/V = nausea and/or vomiting
SC = subcutaneous

APPENDIX II
Cancer Treatment: Side Effects Associated with Hormone Therapy

	Edema	Weight Gain	Appetite	Salt/Water Retention	Nausea/Vomiting	Hot Flashes	Vaginal Bleeding	Menstrual Irregularity	Headache	Gynecomastia	Virilization	Lethargy	Altered Libido	Erectile Impotence	Tumor Flare	Cardiovascular Dis	Hypercalcemia	Skin Rash	Thrombocytopenia	Comments
Tamoxifen Citrate	+	+			+	++	+	+	+						+		+	+	+	Patients may take Tamoxifen Citrate for three to five years as adjuvant therapy. Monitor calcium level. Advise use of non-hormonal contraception during therapy. Avoid taking antacid within two hours of taking enteric coated tablets.
Estrogen	+			+	++		+	+	+	++			→	++	+	++	+			Estrogens may be poorly metabolized in patients with liver dysfunction. Vaginal candidiasis may occur. Gingivitis can occur—encourage oral hygiene. Thrombophlebitis can occur. Take with food to minimize nausea.
Fluoxymes-terone	+	+	←	+				+	+		+		←		+		+			Therapeutic effect is seen after one or two months. Voice changes may not improve after drug is discontinued. Skin acne may occur. Alopecia (virilism).
Megestrol Acetate		++	←			+	+								+					DVT have been reported. Alopecia may occur. Therapeutic effect is seen after two months. Relatively non-toxic.

Drug	Comments
Flutamide	Currently not FDA-approved. Obtained through Canada under the cooperation of specific oncologists in the U.S. Use with caution in people with renal impairment.
Aminoglutethimide	Hypotension may occur. Liver function tests may be elevated. Nausea improves over time. Suppresses adrenal function in three to five days. Lethargy more frequent in the elderly. Consider drug withdrawal if rash persists longer than five to eight days.
Leuprolide	Given by daily SQ injections. Constipation, dizziness, and breast tenderness have been reported.
Prednisone	Cushingoid symptoms may occur. GI upset is common. Anxiety, irritability, insomnia, and depression can be minimized by tapering dosage over three to four days.
Cyproterone Acetate	Mood changes. Gastrointestinal disturbances. Use with caution in person with liver dysfunction.

(+) Occurrence is common with mild intensity. (++) Occurrence is more frequent and usually more intense. (↑) Increased frequency or intensity. (↓) Decreased frequency or intensity.

Source: From "Concepts of hormonal manipulation in the treatment of cancer." by M. Goodman, 1988, Oncology Nursing Forum, 15(5), pp. 639–647. Reprinted with permission of The Oncology Nursing Press.

APPENDIX III
Chartered Divisions of the American Cancer Society, Inc.

Alabama Division, Inc.
402 Office Park Drive
Suite 300
Birmingham, Alabama 35223
(205) 879-2242

Alaska Division, Inc.
406 West Fireweed Lane
Suite 204
Anchorage, Alaska 99503
(907) 277-8696

Arizona Division, Inc.
2929 East Thomas Road
Phoenix, Arizona 85016
(602) 224-0524

Arkansas Division, Inc.
901 North University
Little Rock, Arkansas 72207
(501) 664-3480

California Division, Inc.
1710 Webster Street
P.O. Box 2061
Oakland, California 94612
(415) 893-7900

Colorado Division, Inc.
2255 South Oneida
P.O. Box 24669
Denver, Colorado 80224
(303) 758-2030

Connecticut Division, Inc.
Barnes Park South
14 Village Lane
Wallingford, Connecticut 06492
(203) 265-7161

Delaware Division, Inc.
92 Read's Way
New Castle, DE 19720
(302) 324-4227

District of Columbia Division, Inc.
1825 Connecticut Avenue, N.W.
Suite 315
Washington, D.C. 20009
(202) 483-2600

Florida Division, Inc.
1001 South MacDill Avenue
Tampa, Florida 33629
(813) 253-0541

Georgia Division, Inc.
46 Fifth Street, NE
Atlanta, Georgia 30308
(404) 892-0026

Hawaii/Pacific Division, Inc.
Community Services Center Bldg.
200 North Vineyard Boulevard
Honolulu, Hawaii 96817
(808) 531-1662

Idaho Division, Inc.
2676 Vista Avenue
P.O. Box 5386
Boise, Idaho 83705
(208) 343-4609

Illinois Division, Inc.
77 East Monroe
Chicago, Illinois 60603
(312) 641-6150

Indiana Division, Inc.
8730 Commerce Park Place
Indianapolis, Indiana 46268
(317) 872-4432

Iowa Division, Inc.
8364 Hickman Road, Suite D
Des Moines, Iowa 50322
(515) 253-0147

Kansas Division, Inc.
1315 SW Arrowhead Road
Topeka, Kansas 66604
(913) 273-4114

Kentucky Division, Inc.
701 West Muhammad Ali Blvd.
P.O. Box 1807
Louisville, Kentucky 40201-1807
(502) 584-6782

Louisiana Division, Inc.
Fidelity Homestead Bldg.
837 Gravier Street
Suite 700
New Orleans, Louisiana 70112-1509
(504) 523-4188

Maine Division, Inc.
52 Federal Street
Brunswick, Maine 04011
(207) 729-3339

Maryland Division, Inc.
P.O. Box 82
White Marsh, Maryland 21162-0082
(301) 931-6868

Massachusetts Division, Inc.
247 Commonwealth Avenue
Boston, Massachusetts 02116
(617) 267-2650

Michigan Division, Inc.
1205 East Saginaw Street
Lansing, Michigan 48906
(517) 371-2920

Minnesota Division, Inc.
3316 West 66th Street
Minneapolis, Minnesota 55435
(612) 925-2772

Mississippi Division, Inc.
1380 Livingston Lane
Lakeover Office Park
Jackson, Mississippi 39213
(601) 362-8874

Missouri Division, Inc.
3322 American Avenue
Jefferson City, Missouri 65102
(314) 893-4800

Montana Division, Inc.
313 N. 32nd Street
Suite #1
Billings, Montana 59101
(406) 252-7111

Nebraska Division, Inc.
8502 West Center Road
Omaha, Nebraska 68124-5255
(402) 393-5800

Nevada Division, Inc.
1325 East Harmon
Las Vegas, Nevada 89119
(702) 798-6857

New Hampshire Division, Inc.
360 Route 101, Unit 501
Bedford, New Hampshire 03102-6800
(603) 472-8899

New Jersey Division, Inc.
2600 Route 1, CNN 2201
North Brunswick, New Jersey 08902
(201) 297-8000

New Mexico Division, Inc.
5800 Lomas Blvd., NE
Albuquerque, New Mexico 87110
(505) 260-2105

New York State Division, Inc.
6725 Lyons Street
P.O. Box 7
East Syracuse, New York 13057
(315) 437-7025

☐ Long Island Division, Inc.
145 Pidgeon Hill Road
Huntington Station, New York 11746
(516) 385-9100

☐ New York City Division, Inc.
19 West 56th Street
New York, New York 10019
(212) 586-8700

☐ Queens Division, Inc.
112-25 Queens Boulevard
Forest Hills, New York 11375
(718) 263-2224

☐ Westchester Division, Inc.
30 Glenn St.
White Plains, New York 10603
(914) 949-4800

North Carolina Division, Inc.
11 South Boylan Avenue
Suite 221
Raleigh, North Carolina 27603
(919) 834-8463

North Dakota Division, Inc.
123 Roberts Street
P.O. Box 426
Fargo, North Dakota 58107
(701) 232-1385

Ohio Division, Inc.
5555 Frantz Road
Dublin, Ohio 43017
(614) 889-9565

Oklahoma Division, Inc.
3000 United Founders Blvd.
Suite 136
Oklahoma City, Oklahoma 73112
(405) 843-9888

Oregon Division, Inc.
0330 SW Curry
Portland, Oregon 97201
(503) 295-6422

Pennsylvania Division, Inc.
P.O. Box 897
Route 422 & Sipe Avenue
Hershey, Pennsylvania 17033-0897
(717) 533-6144

☐ Philadelphia Division, Inc.
1422 Chestnut Street
Philadelphia, Pennsylvania 19102
(215) 665-2900

Puerto Rico Division, Inc.
Calle Alverio #577,
Esquina Sargento Medina,
Hato Rey, Puerto Rico 00918
(809) 764-2295

Rhode Island Division, Inc.
400 Main Street
Pawtucket, Rhode Island 02860
(401) 722-8480

South Carolina Division, Inc.
128 Stonemark Lane
Columbia, South Carolina 29210
(803) 750-1693

South Dakota Division, Inc.
4101 Carnegie Place
Sioux Falls, South Dakota 57106-2322
(605) 361-8277

Tennessee Division, Inc.
1315 Eighth Avenue, South
Nashville, Tennessee 37203
(615) 255-1ACS

Texas Division, Inc.
2433 Ridgepoint Drive
Austin, Texas 78754
(512) 928-2262

Utah Division, Inc.
610 East South Temple
Salt Lake City, Utah 84102
(801) 322-0431

Vermont Division, Inc.
13 Loomis Street, Drawer C
P.O. Box 1452
Montpelier, Vermont 05601-1452
(802) 223-2348

Virginia Division, Inc.
4240 Park Place Court
Glen Allen, Virginia 23060
(804) 270-0142/(800) ACS-2345

Washington Division, Inc.
2120 First Avenue North
Seattle, Washington 98109-1140
(206) 283-1152

West Virginia Division, Inc.
2428 Kanawha Boulevard East
Charleston, West Virginia 25311
(304) 344-3611

Wisconsin Division, Inc.
615 North Sherman Avenue
Madison, Wisconsin 53704
(608) 249-0487

Wyoming Division, Inc.
2222 House Avenue
Cheyenne, Wyoming 82001
(307) 638-3331

National Headquarters: American Cancer Society, Inc., 1599 Clifton Road N.E.,
Atlanta, GA 30329

GLOSSARY

Linda Yoder

ABVD: A chemotherapy regime that consists of a combination of doxorubicin + bleomycin + vinblastine + dacarbazine.

Abdominal-perineal resection: Surgical procedure used in the treatment of colorectal cancer that requires a combined approach through the abdomen and the perineum. Complications include ureteral injury, urinary dysfunction, urinary tract infections, sexual dysfunction, perineal and abdominal wound infections, and stomal complications.

Addiction: A combination of physical and psychological dependence on a drug; a behavioral pattern of compulsive drug use.

Adjuvant therapy: A therapy that aids another, such as chemotherapy after surgery.

Adrenocorticotropic hormone (ACTH): A hormone secreted by the anterior pituitary gland that has a stimulating effect on the adrenal cortex.

Allogeneic bone marrow transplantation: Transplanting bone marrow from one person to another person who is of the same tissue type.

Alopecia: Loss of hair resulting from the destruction of the hair follicle. Sometimes a side effect of chemotherapy or radiation therapy to the head. May be transient or permanent depending on course of treatment.

Alpha-fetoprotein (AFP): An antigen tumor marker associated with testicular germ cell tumors, liver cancers, and gastric malignancies.

Anorexia: Loss of appetite.

Antibody: Proteins produced by B lymphocytes in response to an antigen. Important components in humoral immunity. *Also called immunoglobulins.*

Antigen: A molecule that stimulates an immune response and is capable of reacting with antibodies or other sensitized cells of the immune system, such as T lymphocytes.

Anti-oncogenes: Genes having the ability to regulate growth and inhibit carcinogenesis.

Anxiolytics: Mild sedatives, such as Valium, used for the relief of anxiety; also referred to as minor tranquilizers.

Astrocytoma: A tumor composed of neuroglial cells of ectodermal origin, characterized by fibrous or protoplasmic processes. This tumor is classified in order of malignancy as grade I (consists of fibrillary or protoplasmic astrocytes), grade II (Astroblastoma), grades III or IV (glioblastoma multiforme).

Attributable risk: This is the arithmetic difference in the disease rates between the group exposed to the factor and unexposed groups. The attributable risk is used to calculate the magnitude of change of a disease rate outcome with the removal of the suspected antecedent factor.

Autologous bone marrow transplantation: Transplanting the patient's own bone marrow after ablative treatment.

B cells: Another term for a B lymphocyte (bursa-equivalent lymphocyte). These cells develop from the stem cell and are involved in humoral immunity, and the secretion of antibodies.

BCG: *Bacille Calmette Guérin* vaccine, a tuberculosis vaccine, containing living, avirulent, bovine-strain tubercle bacilli. It is administered by a special technique using a multiple puncture disk and is used in immunotherapy for the treatment of cancer, particularly malignant melanoma.

Bence-Jones Protein: A low molecular weight, heat sensitive protein found in patients with multiple myeloma. The presence of these proteins in the urine may lead to the formation of precipitates in the tubules, resulting in tubular obstruction, foreign body reaction, and tubular degeneration.

Benign: Not malignant; not recurrent; favorable for recovery.

Beta antagonists: Drugs that bind to beta receptors, blocking the neurotransmitter action, without producing any physiologic effect itself.

Bilroth I: Pylorectomy with end-to-end anastomosis of the upper portion of the stomach to the duodenum.

Bilroth II: Partial gastric resection, with closure of duodenal stump and gastrojejunostomy.

Biopsy: Removal and examination, usually microscopic, of tissue from the living body. Biopsies are done to determine whether a tumor is malignant or benign.
  A. Excisional: Entire lesion is removed by surgical cutting.
  B. Incisional: Biopsy of a selected portion of a lesion.
  C. Needle aspiration: Biopsy in which tissue is obtained by application of suction through a needle attached to a syringe.

Blast crisis: A sudden severe change in the course of chronic myelocytic leukemia, in which the clinical picture resembles that seen in acute myelogenous leukemia with an increase in the proportion of myloblasts.

Blocks: Devices used in radiotherapy to prevent radiation beams from striking areas of the body that do not require treatment or require shielding, such as the heart.

Brachytherapy: Radiation from a source placed within the body or a body cavity.

Breast self-exam: One early detection method that can aid in decreasing mortality provided that women have regular physical exams, undergo mammography as recommended, and seek advice as soon as an abnormality is detected. Consists of visual and manual examination of the breast which should be done after menstruation when the breasts are normally soft. A physician should be contacted if any lump in the breast can be felt.

Central nervous system prophylaxis: Administration of intrathecal chemotherapy and/or cranial irradiation, designed to eradicate leukemic cells that may sequester themselves behind the blood-brain barrier, thus out of reach of most chemotherapy.

Cachexia: A condition of severe malnutrition, emaciation, and debility.

Cancer: Encompasses a group of neoplastic diseases in which there is a transformation of normal body cells into malignant ones, with uncontrolled proliferation.

Carcinoembryonic antigen (CEA): A tumor marker associated with malignancies of the gastrointestinal tract.

Carcinogen: A substance that causes cancer.

Carcinogenesis: Production of cancer.

Carcinoma: A malignant growth consisting of epithelial cells tending to infiltrate surrounding tissues and give rise to metastases. Carcinomas comprise the majority of cases of cancers of the breast, uterus, intestinal tract, skin, and tongue.
  A. Basal cell carcinoma: An epithelial tumor of the skin that seldom metastasizes, but has the potential for local invasion and destruction.
  B. Carcinoma in situ: Neoplastic activity where the tumor cells have not yet invaded the basement membrane, but are still confined to the epithelium of origin; a lesion with all the histological characteristics of malignancies except invasion.
  C. Squamous cell carcinoma: Neoplastic cells arising from squamous epithelium and having cuboid cells.

Cell-mediated immunity: Type of immune response dependent upon T lymphocytes, which are primarily concerned with a type of delayed immune response. Examples of this type of immunity are transplant rejection or defense against a slowly developing bacterial disease that results from intracellular infection.

Cholecystojejunostomy: Surgical anastomosis of the gallbladder and jejunum.

Chondrosarcoma: A malignant tumor derived from cartilage cells or their precursors.

Choriocarcinoma: A malignant neoplasm of trophoblastic cells formed by the abnormal proliferation of the placental epithelium, without the production of chorionic villi.

Citrovorum factor: Folinic acid. Also called leucovorin. A metabolically active derivative of folic acid used to treat folic acid deficiency and as an antidote to folic acid antagonists, such as methotrexate.

Colony stimulating factor (CSF): Soluble protein factors that stimulate division and maturation of bone marrow stem cells. All CSFs are named as a function of the cell most responsive to the factor, e.g. granulocyte-stimulating factor.

Colposcopy: The process of examining the vagina and cervix by means of a speculum and a magnifying lens; procedure used for the early detection of malignant changes on the cervix/vaginal cuff.

Complement cascade: Series of steps or stages within the immune system that, once initiated, continues to the final steps of complement activation resulting in the formation of many biologically active complement fragments that act as anaphylatoxins, opsonins, or chemotactic factors. There are two classic pathways in the complement system; both play a vital role in immunity.

Computerized tomography: A radiologic imaging technique that produces images of "slices" 1 cm thick through a patient's body. Also referred to as computerized axial tomography, CAT scan, or CT scan.

Conditioning or preparative regimen: Doses of chemotherapy and/or total body irradiation lethal to bone marrow given in an effort to eradicate the population of tumor cells in the body. Commonly used in the treatment of leukemia.

Congenital melanocytic nevi: A mole present since birth, which is composed of melanocytes; usually pigmented.

Conization: The removal of a "cone" of tissue, as a partial excision of the cervix. This can be done with a scalpel or electrocautery; the scalpel technique preserves the histologic elements of the tissue better.

Consolidation chemotherapy: A phase of treatment in leukemia consisting of one to three intensive cycles of chemotherapy designed to bring together the gains made during remission-induction therapy. This therapy begins as soon as a complete remission is documented, to ensure that any remaining leukemic cells will be eradicated. Doses of chemotherapy drugs are given so as to give an anticipated marrow hypoplasia from which the patient will recover in 7–14 days.

Continent urinary reservoir (Continent ileal reservoir): Also called the "Kock pouch"; A surgical procedure which provides an intra-abdominal pouch that stores urine and has two nipple valves that maintain continence and prevent ureteral reflux.

Corynebacterium parvum (c. parvum): A gram-positive, nonviable, formalin-treated bacillus found to be a strong stimulator of the reticuloendothelial system; thought to be an immunopotentiating agent.

Craniotomy: Any surgical operation on the cranium.

Cystectomy: Excision of the urinary bladder or a part of it.

Cytokines: Cell products used as biologic response modifiers. These soluble proteins have a variety of activities that may alter the growth and metastasis of cancer cells by enhancing the immune responsiveness of non-cancerous cells. Most are still highly experimental and are undergoing clinical trials.

Cytotoxic: An agent capable of specific destructive action on certain cells; usually used in reference to antineoplastic drugs that selectively kill dividing cells.

Debulking: Surgery to reduce tumor burden to aggregates of 2 cm or less; improves the response to postoperative chemotherapy.

DIC (Disseminated Intravascular Coagulation): Widespread formation of clots (thromboses) in the microcirculation, mainly within the capillaries. This intravascular clotting ultimately produces hemorrhage because of the rapid consumption of fibrinogen, platelets, prothrombin, and clotting factors V, VIII, and X. It is a secondary complication of a diverse group of hemolytic and neoplastic disorders that in some way activate the intrinsic coagulation sequence.

Detection: To find or discover the existence of disease. In relation to cancer this can occur via screening methods or tests such as breast self-examination or mammography.

Diagnosis: A concise, technical description of the cause, nature, or manifestations of a condition, situation, or problem.

Diethylstilbestrol (DES): A synthetic nonsteroidal estrogen, used to relieve vasomotor symptoms associated with menopause; also used for female hypogonadism, atrophic vaginitis, primary ovarian failure, palliative treatment for female breast carcinoma, and to relieve the symptoms of prostatic cancer. It was widely used to prevent threatened abortion and premature labor in the 1950s/1960s and the female children who were exposed to the drug as fetuses tend to have a variety of cervical abnormalities that may progress to malignancy.

Differentiation: The act or process of having recognizable, specialized structures and functions; usually refers to a cellular process that causes an increase in morphological heterogeneity.

Diffuse histiocytic lymphoma: Characterized by the presence of large tumor cells that resemble histiocytes morphologically, but are considered to be of lymphoid origin. The neoplastic cells infiltrate the entire lymph node without any organized pattern.

Dumping syndrome: A symptom complex of uncomfortable epigastric fullness, nausea, weakness, sweating, palpitations, and diarrhea that occurs after meals in patients who have had gastric surgery that interferes with the function of the pylorus.

Dyspareunia: Painful intercourse experienced by women.

Dysphagia: Difficulty in swallowing.

Dysplastic nevi: Moles that have a greater tendency to be malignant; they differ from regular moles in that they are irregular in shape, variably pigmented, larger in size, and located in unusual places (scalp, buttocks, breasts).

Endoscopic retrograde cholangiopancreatogram (ERCP): A procedure consisting of a combination of retrograde cholangiography and transhepatic cholangiography used to visualize all portions of the biliary tree.

Endoscopic laser therapy: Laser therapy administered via visual examination of interior structures of the body using an endoscope.

Epidemiology: The science concerned with the study of factors determining and influencing the frequency and distribution of disease, injury, and other health-related events.

Esophagoscopy: Direct visual examination of the esophagus with an esophagoscope.

Extravasation: Escape from the blood vessel into the tissue; term used to describe chemotherapy escaping from a blood vessel into the tissue, resulting in tissue damage.

FAB morphology: The French-American-British morphologic classification system used to describe cellular morphology.

Fractions: Divisions of the total dose of radiation into small doses given at intervals.

Gestational trophoblastic disease: A neoplasm which occurs as the result of the excessive proliferation of chorionic epithelium during very early pregnancy.

Glioblastoma multiforme: Astrocytoma Grade III or IV; a rapidly growing tumor, usually of the cerebral hemispheres, composed of spongioblasts, astroblasts, and astrocytes.

Glioma: A tumor composed of neuroglia in any state of development; sometimes extended to include all intrinsic neoplasms of the brain and spinal cord, such as astrocytomas.

Gonadotropin releasing hormone (GnRH): A decapeptide hormone of the hypothalamus that stimulates the release of follicle-stimulating hormone and luteinizing hormone from the pituitary gland; used in the differential diagnosis of hypothalamic, pituitary, and gonadal dysfunction.

Graft versus host disease (GVHD): A frequent complication of bone marrow transplant. Immunocompetent T lymphocytes derived from the donor tissue recognize the recipient's tissue as "foreign" and react to it, producing clinical manifestations which include edema, erythema, ulceration, loss of hair, and heart and joint lesions similar to those occurring in connective tissue disorders.

Granulocytopenia: A decrease in white blood cells.

Gray: The SI (Systéme International d'Unités) unit of absorbed radiation dose, defined as the transfer of 1 joule of energy per Kg of absorbing material. 1 Gray = 100 rads.

Gynecomastia: Abnormally large mammary glands in the male; may secrete "milk."

Histology: Examination of tissue dealing with the minute structure, composition, and function of tissues as seen through a microscope.

Hodgkin's disease: A specific type of lymphoma, differing from all other lymphomas in its predictability of spread, microscopic characteristics, and occurrence of extranodal tumors. The Reed-Sternberg cell is essential to the diagnosis. The accepted histopathologic classification distinguishes four different disease patterns:

A. Nodular sclerosing—characterized by the lymph node being divided into nodules by sclerosing bands of collagen. The lymphocytes in the collagen-bound nodules may be of various types, from predominantly small lymphocytes to the large histiocytic forms.

B. Lymphocyte-predominant—characterized by sheets of mature-appearing small lymphocytes with few Reed-Sternberg cells; has a good prognosis.

C. Lymphocyte-depleted—characterized by a small quantity of the small lymphocytes, a large number of Reed-Sternberg cells, and a predominance of histiocytes; has a poor prognosis.

D. Mixed cellularity—characterized by a histology between lymphocyte predominant and lymphocyte-depleted.

Hormone receptor assay: A laboratory test used to determine the quantity of autoantibodies to the particular hormone receptor in question and to identify those tumors that are endocrine sensitive. Used commonly in breast cancer, this information is used for planning treatment. About two-thirds of patients have receptors present and about half of estrogen receptor-positive patients will respond to hormones.

Human chorionic gonadotropic (HCG): A glycopeptide hormone produced by the fetal placenta that is thought to maintain the function of the corpus luteum during the first few weeks of pregnancy. It is also present in certain neoplastic conditions; used as a tumor marker in choriocarcinoma and testicular cancer. It can be detected by immunoassay in the urine within days after fertilization and is therefore the basis of the most common pregnancy tests.

Human-leukocyte antigen (HLA): The human major histocompatibility complex located on the short arm of chromosome number 6. Transplants, platelet, and leukocyte transfusions are least likely to be rejected by the recipient when the donor and the recipient are HLA-identical.

Humoral immunity: A response that begins as soon as a substance enters the body and is interpreted as being foreign. Antibodies are released from plasma cells and enter the body fluids, where they can react with the specific antigens for which they were formed. This release of antibodies is stimulated by antigen-specific groups of B lymphocytes.

Hydatidiform mole: An abnormal pregnancy resulting from a pathologic ovum, with proliferation of the epithelial covering of the chorionic villi. It results in a mass of cysts resembling a bunch of grapes. Also called hydatid mole.

Hyperalimentation: Nutritional supplementation of calories, protein, lipids, and other nutritional elements.

Hypercalcemia: Excessive quantity of serum calcium; usually seen in breast cancer patients. Weakness, confusion, and possible ventricular dysrhythmias are classic symptoms and require immediate intervention.

Ileal conduit: A surgical procedure that uses a segment of the ileum for the diversion of urinary flow from the ureters.

Immunotherapy: Passive immunization of an individual by administration of preformed antibodies actively produced in another individual (serum or gamma globulins). The term has also come to include the use of immunopotentiators, replacement of immunocompetent tissue (bone marrow), and infusion of specially treated white blood cells.

Incidence: The rate at which a certain event occurs, such as the number of new cases of a specific disease occurring during a certain period.

Incidence rate epidemiology: The science concerned with the study of the factors determining and influencing the frequency and distribution of disease.

Induction chemotherapy: The **initial** chemotherapy regimen used in the treatment of leukemia, when the greatest number of leukemic cells are affected. The combination of drugs is designed to cause severe bone marrow depression, and the goal of treatment is remission of the disease.

In situ: Confined to the site of origin.

Intensification therapy (also called reintensification therapy): This therapy has been proposed to prevent the return of the leukemic cell population. After 1 year of sustained, complete remission, the person undergoes the same intensive induction therapy as in the initial treatment period. The objective is bone marrow depression. After recovery of the bone marrow depression the person continues on maintenance therapy for another year.

Interferons: Natural glycoproteins released by cells invaded by viruses or certain infectious agents; acts as a stimulant to noninfected cells, causing them to synthesize another protein with antiviral capabilities. Interferons are divided into three subsets, with each originating from a different cell and having distinctive chemical and biologic properties:
Alpha: Produced by leukocytes in response to a viral infection.
Beta: Produced by fibroblasts in response to a viral infection.
Gamma: Produced by lymphoid cells in culture that are stimulated by a mitogen.

Interleukin-2: A glycoprotein produced by helper T cells that is an essential factor in the growth of T cells and seems to induce the production of interferon. It is used as an anti-cancer drug in the treatment of a wide variety of solid tumors.

Intrathecal chemotherapy: Cytotoxic drugs injected into the cerebrospinal fluid (CSF), thus bypassing the blood-brain barrier.

Intravenous hyperalimentation: Nutritional supplementation by peripheral intravenous or central intravenous line infusion; also known as total parenteral nutrition (TPN).

Intravesical chemotherapy: Chemotherapy administered via a foley catheter for the treatment of bladder cancer. The foley is then usually clamped for a period of time and then emptied. This procedure delivers a high local concentration to the tumor area. Patients receiving this therapy require life-long cytoscopic surveillance for recurrent disease.

Invasive mole (chorioadenoma destruens): A form of hydatidiform mole in which molecular chorionic villi penetrate into the myometrium and may invade the parametrium. Hydropic villi may be transported to distant sites, most often the lungs, but they do not grow as metastases.

In vitro fertilization: Fertilization within an artificial environment such as a test tube.

Lactose Intolerance: Lacking the soluble enzyme lactase, which breaks down lactose to dextrose and galactose. This can occur as a result of damage to the intestinal villi due to infection or a disease such as gastric cancer. This condition may result after a subtotal gastrectomy, gastrojejunostomy, or radiation therapy to the GI tract. Symptoms include gastrointestinal cramps, distention, and diarrhea. Individuals with this problem should have all sources of milk excluded from their diet.

Latency period: A seemingly inactive period like that between the time of tissue stimulation and the beginning of a response.

Leukemia: A progressive disease of the blood-forming organs, marked by distorted proliferation and development of leukocytes and their precursors in the blood and the bone marrow. It is accompanied by a reduced number of red blood cells and platelets, resulting in anemia and increased susceptibility to infection and bleeding. Leukemia is classified on the basis of duration and character of the disease—acute or chronic; the cell type—myelocytic, lymphoid, or monocytic; and increase in or maintenance of the number of abnormal cells in the blood.

A. Acute lymphocytic leukemia (ALL)—Most common type of pediatric leukemia. Infiltration and accumulation of immature lymphoblasts occurs within the bone marrow, as well as the extramedullary lymphatic tissue, causing painful lymphadenopathy and hepatosplenomegaly. Combination chemotherapy is the treatment modality most commonly used, and if refractory to this treatment, bone marrow transplant is an option.

B. Acute nonlymphocytic leukemia (ANLL)—A broad term referring to all leukemias that are not lymphocytic. This leukemia that occurs most commonly after treatment with alkylating agents and is characterized by pancytopenia, megaloblastic bone marrow, nucleated red cells in the peripheral marrow, and refractoriness to treatment, with a short survival time. Most patients have chromosomal abnormalities in marrow cells.

C. Acute myelocytic leukemia (AML)—A subtype of ANLL. These types of childhood leukemias encompass various subtypes, with myloblastic leukemia being the most common type. This type of leukemia is rare.

D. Chronic myelocytic leukemia (CML)—May occur in older adults as well as in children. The onset is insidious and the leukocytosis consists of predominantly mature white blood cells. Patients with CML usually progress to a blast crisis, which is associated with a poor prognosis.

E. Hairy-cell leukemia (HCL)—An adult leukemia marked by splenomegaly and by an abundance of large mononuclear abnormal cells with numerous irregular cytoplasmic projections that give them a flagellated or hairy appearance in the bone marrow, spleen, liver, and peripheral blood.

F. T-cell chronic lymphocytic leukemia—An adult onset form of leukemia in which the leukemic cells have T-cell properties, with frequent dermal involvement, lymphadenopathy, hepatosplenomegaly, and a subacute or chronic course. It is associated with the human T-cell leukemia-lymphoma virus.

Leukophoresis: Removing white blood cells from the patient; usually used in leukemic patients when the white blood cell count gets too high. Can be accomplished by continuous-flow cell separators or filtration techniques.

Leukoplakia: The development of white, thickened patches on the mucous membranes of the cheeks, gums, or tongue. These patches have a tendency to fissure and become malignant. They tend to grow into larger patches, or they may take the form of ulcers. Those in the mouth may cause pain during swallowing, eating, or talking.

Leukostasis: Occurs as a result of leukemic blast cells accumulating and invading vessel walls, causing rupture and bleeding.

Limb perfusion: Used in the treatment of malignant melanoma, where certain chemotherapeutic drugs (usually L-phenylalanine and DTIC) are instilled into the affected extremity by arterial perfusion. A pump system counteracts the normal arterial pressure, permitting a steady state of infusion, allowing the drugs to have the greatest effect at the disease site. Usually performed after surgical removal of the bulk of the tumor mass.

Lymphadenectomy: Surgical excision of one or more lymph nodes.

Lymphangiogram: The film produced by lymphangiography, which is an x-ray of the lymphatic channels after introduction of a contrast medium.

Lymphocyte: Any of the mononuclear, nonphagocytic leukocytes found in the blood, lymph, and lymphoid tissue. Divided into two classes, B and T lymphocytes, which are responsible for humoral and cellular immunity, respectively.

Lymphokines: Cytokines produced by lymphocytes and capable of regulating the immune response. Examples are Interleukin 2 and interferon.

Lymphokine-activated killer cells (LAK cells). Cells that are produced in the laboratory by incubating human lymphocytes with interleukin 2. These cells selectively lyse tumor cells that are resistant to natural killer cells, without affecting normal cells. They are part of a class of anti-cancer agents known as biologic response modifiers.

Lymphoma: Any neoplastic disorder of the lymphoid tissue, including Hodgkin's disease. Classifications are based on predominant cell type and degree of differentiation. Various categories may be subdivided into nodular and diffuse types, depending on the predominant pattern of cell arrangement.

MOPP: A chemotherapy regimen consisting of a combination of mechlorethamine vincristine + procarbazine + prednisone. This treatment is used against Hodgkin's disease.

Macrophages: Any of the large, mononuclear, highly phagocytic cells derived from monocytes that occur in the walls of the blood vessels and in loose connective tissue. They are usually immobile, but become mobile when stimulated by inflammation. They have a vital role in the immune system.

Magnetic resonance imaging (MRI): A noninvasive nuclear procedure for imaging tissues of high fat and water content that cannot be seen with other radiologic techniques. Provides information that allows the distinction between normal tissues versus cancerous, atherosclerotic, or traumatized tissues.

Maintenance chemotherapy: This leukemia therapy begins when the marrow and peripheral blood have recovered, after either induction or consolidation therapy. Drug doses are chosen to cause significant, but not life threatening, cytopenias.

Malignant: Having the properties of anaplasia, invasiveness, and metastasis.

Malignant melanoma: Least common form of malignant skin cancer, usually developing from a nevus and consisting of black masses of cells with a marked tendency to metastasis.

Meningioma: A hard, usually vascular tumor occurring mainly along the meningeal vessels and superior longitudinal sinus, invading the dura and skull, which leads to the erosion and thinning of the skull.

Metastasis: Secondary malignant lesions originating from the primary tumor but located in anatomically distant places.

Micrometastases: Tumor cells escaping into the smaller sections of the lymphatic or vascular flow where they can travel to other parts of the body.

Mohs surgery: A technique for microscopically controlled serial excisions of fresh tissue used for microscopic analysis in the diagnosis and treatment of skin cancer.

Monoclonal antibodies: Antibodies formed through a special process of immunizing mice with a desired antigen, removing immunized lymphocytes from the mice, and fusing the lymphocytes with mouse myeloma cells to form a hybridoma, which is capable of unlimited cell division. Cells that produce the desired antibody are selected, and those are cloned to produce large amounts of uniform antibodies specific to the target antigen. These antibodies are still under testing in an attempt to find antibodies which are tumor-cell specific for various cancers.

Monokines: Cytokines produced by macrophages and other cells that are capable of regulating the immune response.

Mucosal erythroplasia: A condition of the mucous membranes characterized by erythematous papular lesions.

Myelosuppression: A reduction in bone marrow function, resulting in a reduced release of erythrocytes, leukocytes, and platelets into the peripheral circulation and/or the release of immature cells into the circulating blood.

Nadir: The period of time when an antineoplastic drug has its most profound effects on the bone marrow.

Natural killer cells: A group of large, granular lymphocytes that have the intrinsic ability to recognize and destroy some virally infected cells and some tumor cells.

Non-seminomatous tumors: A histologic type of testicular cancer consisting of the embryonal (including yolk sac), teratocarcinoma, teratoma, and choriocarcinoma tumors, which can produce human chorionic gonadotropins, causing gynecomastia. Alpha-fetoprotein levels are also elevated in the presence of this type of tumor.

Non-small cell carcinoma of the lung: A broad term referring to all bronchogenic cancers that are not small cell; includes large cell, adenocarcinoma, and epidermoid lung cancers.

Odynophagia: Painful swallowing of food.

Ommaya™ Reservoir: This device is a subcutaneous cerebrospinal fluid (CSF) reservoir that is implanted surgically under the scalp and provides access to the CSF through a burr hole in the scalp. Drugs are injected into the reservoir with a syringe, and the domed reservoir is then depressed manually to mix the drug within the CSF. This device eliminates the need for multiple lumbar punctures in the repeated administration of intrathecal chemotherapy.

Oncogenes: Genes whose protein products may be involved in the processes of transformation of a normal cell to a malignant state. Classically, it is a normal cellular gene that has been incorporated into a RNA virus and causes the transformation when the virus infects the cell.

Orchiectomy: Surgical removal of one or both testes.

Osteoblast cells: A cell arising from a fibroblast, which, as it matures, is associated with bone production.

Osteoradionecrosis: Necrosis of bone as a result of excessive exposure to radiation.

Pancreaticoduodenectomy: Surgical excision of the head of the pancreas and the adjacent portion of the duodenum.

Papanicolaou Smear: A technique that uses exfoliated cells and subjects them to cytologic staining for the purpose of detecting abnormal cells. Most commonly used to detect cancer of the cervix and uterus, but may also be used in the diagnosis of lung, stomach, and bladder cancers.

Paraneoplastic syndrome: A collective term for disorders arising from metabolic effects of cancer on tissues remote from the tumor. These disorders may appear as primary endocrine, hematologic, or neuromuscular problems.

Pelvic exenteration: Total pelvic exenteration includes a radical hysterectomy, pelvic lymph node dissection, and removal of the bladder and rectosigmoid. Occasionally a posterior exenteration, which preserves the bladder, or an anterior exenteration, which preserves the rectum, can be performed. Used as a treatment for recurrent or persistent cervical cancer.

Pheochromocytoma: A usually benign tumor of the sympatho-adrenal system that produces catecholamines; produces a hypertension that may be sudden in nature.

Philadelphia Chromosome: An abnormality of chromosome 22, characterized by shortening of its long arms. This chromosome is seen in the marrow cells of most patients with chronic myelogenous leukemia.

Plasma cells: Descendants of B cells that are capable of producing antibodies.

Pluripotent stem cell: This is the cell that can generate all cell lineages in the bone marrow, such as red blood cells, white blood cells, and platelets.

Prevalence: The number of existing cases of a disease in a given population at a specific time.

Prostate-specific antigen: A tumor marker that has been used to monitor tumor activity of prostate carcinomas. An elevation of this enzyme is thought to indicate advanced disease regardless of whether the metastatic sites are obvious.

Proto-oncogenes: Genes in normal cells similar to viral transforming genes. Some proto-oncogenes encode proteins that influence the control of cellular proliferation and differentiation. Mutations, amplifications, and rearrangements of proto-oncogenes allow them to function as oncogenes.

Purged bone marrow: Bone marrow that has had tumor cells removed by a chemical treatment (purge) or by a mechanical removal (usually using a magnet which pulls off tumor cells that have attached to monoclonal antibodies), or a combination of both methods. Bone marrow is purged in children with neuroblastoma who receive autologous bone marrow transplants.

Radionuclide: A species of atom that is radioactive and disintegrates with the emission of corpuscular or electromagnetic radiations; used in nuclear medicine scanning for diagnostic and evaluative purposes.

Relative risk: A ratio comparing the rate of the disease among exposed individuals with the rate of disease among unexposed individuals. This risk *does not* reveal probability of disease occurrence; it measures the strength of the association between a factor and the outcome. The higher the relative risk, the greater the evidence for causation.

Sarcoma: A tumor that is often highly malignant, composed of cells derived from connective tissue such as bone and cartilage, muscle, blood vessel, or lymphoid tissue. These tumors usually develop rapidly and metastasize through the lymph channels. The different types of sarcomas are named for the different types of tissues they affect:
  A. Ewing's sarcoma—A malignant tumor of bone that arises in medullary tissue, occurring more often in cylindrical bones, with pain, fever, and leukocytosis as prominent symptoms.
  B. Fibrosarcoma—A sarcoma arising from collagen-producing fibroblasts.
  C. Kaposi's sarcoma—Malignant neoplastic vascular proliferation characterized by the development of bluish red cutaneous nodules, usually on the lower extremities, which spread slowly, increase in size and number, and spread to more proximal sites. The tumors often remain confined to the skin and subcutaneous tissue, but widespread visceral involvement may occur. Often seen in patients with acquired immunodeficiency syndrome (AIDS) and in transplant recipients.
  D. Osteogenic sarcoma—Malignant primary tumor of the bone composed of a malignant connective tissue stroma with evidence of osteoid, bone, and/or cartilage formation.

Schwannomas: A neoplasm originating from Schwann cells (of the myelin sheath) of neurons. These neoplasms include neurofibromas and neurilemomas.

Screening: Tests that are systematically applied to defined populations for the detection of early and asymptomatic disease.

Seminoma: A malignant tumor of the testes thought to arise from the primordial germ cells of the sexually undifferentiated embryonic gonad.

Seroma: A collection of serum in the body, producing a tumor-like mass.

Sigmoidoscopy: Direct examination of the interior of the sigmoid colon.

Small-cell carcinoma of the lung: A radiosensitive tumor composed of small, undifferentiated cells. Also called oat-cell carcinoma.

Spinal cord compression: A medical emergency that can lead to paraplegia, quadraplegia, loss of bowel and bladder function, and possibly death. Usually seen in cancers that have a tendency toward bony metastasis, such as breast cancer.

Staging: The classification of the severity of disease in distinct stages on the basis of established criteria.

Stereotactic surgery: A surgical technique used in neurology in which precise localization of the target tissue is possible through use of three-dimensional coordinates. Also known as stereotaxic surgery.

Subtotal esophagogastrectomy: Subtotal surgical excision of the stomach and the esophagus.

Superior vena cava syndrome: An oncologic emergency that occurs when tumors of the superior mediastinum on the right obstruct the return of blood to the heart by the superior vena cava. This produces a characteristic syndrome of edema of the upper half of the body associated with prominent collateral circulation. This condition necessitates prompt therapy aimed at relieving the pressure on the superior vena cava.

Support: Usually used in the term "social support," defined as that situation in which ill persons believe that they are loved, that they are an important part of a network of communication, that they are esteemed and valued, and that a network of mutual obligations exists exclusive of tangible or material aid.

Survivorship: The state of living with cancer in remission or having obtained a prognosis of "cured."

Syndrome of inappropriate ADH (SIADH): A disorder in which antidiuretic hormone is continually released despite a plasma osmolality below normal, leading to weakness, confusion, nausea and vomiting. Treatment aims to remove the underlying cause (the tumor), restrict fluid intake/output, and protect patients from injury.

Syngeneic bone marrow transplantation: Transplanting bone marrow from an identical twin.

T cells: Thymus-dependent lymphocytes, also called T-lymphocytes, which originate from stem cells and undergo differentiation in the thymus when triggered by thymin and thymopoietin. A type of white blood cells that produces lymphokines and is involved in cell mediated immunity. Differentiated T-cells play important roles in the immune system:
  A. Cytotoxic T cells—A subset of T cells capable of direct destruction of foreign cells.
  B. Helper T cells—A subset of T cells that stimulates other T cells and B cells.

TNM staging classification: A system of cancer staging where T stands for the primary tumor growth, N stands for spread to primary lymph nodes and M stands for metastasis. This is the staging system recommended by the American Joint Committee on Cancer.

Thermography: A technique wherein an infrared camera photographically portrays the body's surface temperature, based on self-emanating infrared radiations; used as a diagnostic aid in the detection of breast tumors.

Therapy: A procedure designed to treat disease, illness, or disability.

Thrombocytopenia: An abnormally low quantity of platelets in the circulating blood.

Thyroid cancer: Because the thyroid contains a variety of cells, malignant tumors may arise within the thyroid from any of these cells:
  A. Anaplastic thyroid carcinoma—Resembles a variety of other tumors such as sarcoma. Highly malignant and locally invasive. Invasion beyond the thyroid usually present at the time of diagnosis. Often presents with compression of the esophagus and trachea.
  B. Follicular thyroid carcinoma—Usually solitary and encapsulated. May be well circumscribed and well differentiated. Uncommon as pure follicular.
  C. Medullary thyroid carcinoma—Tends to be unencapsulated. Cells vary in morphology, but do not contain papillary or follicular cells.
  D. Papillary thyroid carcinoma—Usually multifocal and unencapsulated. Pure papillary is uncommon; usually mixed with follicular.

Tolerance: A reduced responsiveness to any effect of any drug as a consequence of prior administration of that drug, necessitating larger doses of the drug to produce an equivalent effect to that of the initial dose.

Total abdominal hysterectomy with bilateral salpingectomy and oophorectomy: Total removal of the uterus and the cervix performed through the abdominal wall rather than the vaginal route; in addition, the fallopian tubes and the ovaries are removed bilaterally.

Total parenteral nutrition (TPN): Nutritional supplementation by peripheral intravenous or central intravenous line infusion; also known as intravenous hyperalimentation.

Transurethral resection of prostate (TURP): Removal of a portion of the prostate gland by means of an instrument passed through the urethra. This procedure removes only enlarged prostatic tissue, as in benign prostatic hypertrophy. Normal prostatic tissue and the outer capsule are left intact.

Tumor: Neoplasm; a new growth of tissue in which cell growth is uncontrolled and progressive.

Tumor Lysis Syndrome: Severe hyperphosphatemia, hyperkalemia, hyperuricemia, and hypocalcemia occurring after effective induction therapy of rapidly growing malignant tumors; thought to be due to release of intracellular products after cell lysis.

Tumor necrosis factor (TNF): Produced primarily by activated macrophages, TNF is cytotoxic for some neoplastic cells. This factor induces hemorrhagic necrosis in some tumors and is similar to interleukin-1 in the inducement of acute phase reaction. This factor is also known as "cachectin."

Tumorocidal: Destructive to cancer cells.

Ultrasound: Radiologic technique in which deep structures of the body are visualized by recording the reflections of ultrasonic waves into the tissues; uterine tumors and other pelvic masses can be detected using this technique.

Ultraviolet (UV) light: The type of light that consists of electromagnetic radiation of wavelength shorter than that of the violet end of the spectrum, having wavelengths of 4–400 nanometers. It is used in the treatment of various diseases, particularly those affecting the skin; but is also thought to be a causative agent in some types of skin cancer.

Undifferentiated or anaplastic: A loss of differentiation of cells, an irreversible alteration in adult cells toward more primitive cell types; a characteristic of tumor cells.

Ureterosigmoidostomy: A surgically created anastomosis of one or both ureters to the sigmoid colon. In this form of diversion of urinary flow there is no need for an appliance because the urine flows into the colon, which acts as a kind of reservoir. The urine liquefies the stool and can create difficulties in patients who are unable to regulate themselves successfully. A disadvantage of this procedure is the constant danger of urinary infection by organisms from the bowel.

Veno-occlusive disease: An acute or chronic disease of the liver where there is partial or complete occlusion of the branches of the hepatic veins by endophlebitis and thrombosis, leading to centrilobular necrosis, fibrosis, and ascites. Seen in bone marrow transplant patients.

Vulvectomy: Excision of the vulva; en bloc dissection may be used for more advanced cancer, whereas more conservative surgical interventions are used for early diagnosis.

Xeroderma pigmentosa: A rare and frequently fatal pigmentary and atrophic disease in which the skin and eyes are extremely sensitive to light. It begins in childhood and progresses to early development of excessive freckling, keratosis, papillomas, carcinoma, and melanoma.

Xerostomia: Dryness of the mouth from salivary gland dysfunction. This is often seen in head and neck cancer patients.

INDEX

ABVD 288, *325*
Abdominal-perineal resection 146, *325*
Addiction 117, *325*
Adjuvant therapy 77–78, *325*
  in Breast cancer 221
Adrenal gland cancer 205–206
  Incidence 205
  Diagnosis 205
  Adrenocortical 206
  Adrenal Medula 206
Adrenocorticotropic hormone (ACTH) 51, *325*
  and Adrenal gland cancer 206
AIDS 36
Airway
  Alt in Lung cancer 181
  Alt in Head and Neck cancer 171
Allogeneic bone marrow transplantation 91, 94f, 94, *325*
Alopecia 77t, 81, 105–108, *325*
  re to body image 147
Ambulatory care 3
American Association for Cancer Education 316
American Cancer Society 4, 5, 6, 31, 34–35, 36, 41, 42t, 53, 61, 127
  and Breast self-examination 216
  and cervical screening recommendations 231
  and Colorectal screening recommendations 192
  and Endometrial cancer screening recommendations 228
  and Head and Neck cancer 174
  and Ostomy visitor program 197
  and Reach to Recovery 226–227
  and Rehabilitation 164
  and Smoking cessation 175
  and Testicular self-examination 247–248
  Programs 311–313
American Lung Association
  and Smoking cessation 175
Anemia 101, 103t
Anorexia 70, 121, 128t, *325*
Antibiotics 56

Antibody *325*
Antiemetics 101, 103, 104t
Antigens 83, *325*
Anti-oncogenes 25, *325*
Anxiolytics *325*
  in Lung cancer 181
Arteriography 51
Association of Brain Tumor Research 313
Association of Pediatric Oncology Nurses 316
Astrocytoma 27–28, 252, *325*
Attributable risk 33–34, *325*
Autologous bone marrow transplantation 91, 94, *326*
B-cells 84, 85f, 86t, 87, 277, *326*
  antigens 279
BCG 83, 212, *326*
Bence-Jones Proteins 294, *326*
Benign 23, 23t, 28t, *326*
Beta antagonists 182, *326*
Bile duct, cancer of
  Screening and detection 45t
Bilroth I 189, *326*
Bilroth II 189, *326*
Biologic response modifiers 56, 83–90, 258
Biopsy 52, 57, 58t
  Excisional 52, 57, 58t, *326*
  Incisional 52, 57, 58t, *326*
  Needle Aspiration 52, 57, 58t, *326*
Bladder cancer 65, 67, 68t, 208–213
  and Rehabilitation 163t
  and Sexual functioning 145
  Clinical Presentation and Diagnosis 208–209
  Incidence and Risk factors 208
  Pathology 208
  Penile implants 212
  Screening and detection 44t
  Staging 208, 209f
  Treatment 209
Blast Crisis 276, 283, *326*
Bleeding
  In bone marrow transplants 97
Blocks 67, *326*

Body image 147–148
 and breast cancer 226
 and Head and Neck Cancer 169–170
 and ostomies 147
Bone cancers 270–275
 Chondrosarcoma 272
 Clinical manifestations 270–271
 Diagnosis 271
 Ewing's sarcoma 272–273
 Fibrosarcoma 273
 Incidence 270
 Limb salvage procedures 274
 Metastatic bone cancer 273
 Nursing care 273–274
 Osteosarcoma 271–272
 Rehabilitation 163t
 Risk 270
Bone marrow
 Dysfunction 100–101, 102t–103t
 Response to radiation 68t, 69t, 77t
Bone marrow transplantation 91–98
 Conditioning or preparative regimen 93
 Harvest 94, 95f, 96
 in Hodgkin's disease 289
 Purged bone marrow 94, 335
Bowel dysfunction 103–105
 Constipation 129t
 Diarrhea 128t, 285
Brachytherapy 67, 70, 237, *326*
Breast cancer 56, 59, 65, 67, 92t, 216–227
 Arm and hand exercises after surgery 224f
 Diagnosis 218–219
 Incidence 216
 Rehabilitation 163t
 Risk factors 218
 Screening and detection 44t, 216
 Staging 219, 220f
 Treatment 220–226, 223t
Breast self examination 216, 217f, *326*
Cachexia 121, 122f, *326*
Cancer 10, 23, *326*
 Causes 31, 35–38
Cancer Care 313
Cancer Information Service (CIS) 313
Candlelighters 313
CanSurmount 227, 312
Carcinogens 23, *326*
 and Pancreatic cancer 200
Carcinogenesis 23–24, 24f, 25t, 35–38, *327*
Carcinoid syndrome 177
Carcinoma 27, *327*

Basal cell 259, 260t, *327*
 in situ *327, 331*
 in situ, breast 219
 in situ, cervical 231
 Squamous cell carcinoma 259, 260t, *327*
Cardiac tamponade 136–137
Cardiovascular system 69t
Causes of cancer 31, 35–38
 Alcohol 35–36, 184
 Diet 37–38, 187, 191
 Hormones 36
 Ionizing radiation 63
 Occupational exposure 36, 37t
 Radiological examination 43
 Tobacco 16, 35
 Ultraviolet rays 36, 259, *337*
 Viral 36
 X-rys 36, 43
Cell mediated immunity 84, 85t, *327*
Central nervous system tumors 65, 67, 69t, 88, 92t, 252–258
 Classification 252–253, 253t
 Clinical presentation 253–254, 254t
 Diagnosis 255
 Etiology 253
 Incidence 252
 Metastatic tumors 257
 Neuroblastoma 300–301, 301t
 Prophylaxis *326*
 Rehabilitation 163t
 Screening and detection 44t
 Treatment 255–257
Certification 5
Cervical cancer 65, 67, 230–234
 Classification 231t
 Clinical manifestations 233
 Diagnosis 233
 Incidence and etiology 230–231
 Screening and detection 45t, 230–231
 Staging 234t
 Treatment 233
Chemotherapy 65, 73–82
 Conditioning or Preparative 93–94, *327*
 Consolidation 280, 297, 298, *327–328*
 Induction 280, *331*
 in Bladder cancer 212–213
 in Breast cancer 225–226
 in Central nervous system tumors 256–257
 in Cervical cancer 233
 in Childhood ALL 298t
 in Colorectal cancer 197

in Endometrial cancer 228–229
in Esophageal cancer 187
in Ewing's sarcoma 273
in Fallopian tube cancer 238
in Gastric cancer 189–190
in Hodgkin's disease 288–289
in Kaposi's sarcoma 268
in Leukemias 280, 283, 284
in Liver cancer 202
in Lung cancer 181
in Malignant melanoma 267–268
in Metastatic bone cancer 273
in Multiple myeloma 294
in Neuroblastoma 301
in Ovarian cancer 230
in Pancreatic cancer 201
in Penile cancer 247
in Pituitary cancer 206
in Prostate cancer 246
in Retinoblastoma 302
in Rhabdomyosarcoma 303
in Testicular cancer 249–250
Intensification 297, 298, *331*
Intrathecal *331*
Intravesical *331*
in Vaginal cancer 237
in Wilm's tumor 300
Limb perfusionn 267, *332*
Maintenance 285, 297, *333*
MOPP 77, 77t, *333*
Nadir 81, *334*
Nausea and vomiting re to 101
Pain re to 112t
Principles of 75–76
Safety 79
Toxicity 79
Childhood cancers 65, 296–308
  Acute lymphocytic leukemia 296–
    298, 298t
  Dealing with life-threatening illness
    305, 306
  Incidence 296
  Late effects 306–307
  Neuroblastoma 300–301
  Psychosocial impact 303–305
  Retinoblastoma 301–302
  Rhabdomyosarcoma 302–303
  Wilm's tumor 298–300, 299t
Cholecystojejunostomy 201, *327*
Chondrosarcoma 272, *327*
Citrovorum factor 272, *327*
Clinical trial 78–79, 83, 89
Colon and rectal cancers 44t, 59, 67,
  68t, 191–199
  Detection and Diagnosis 44t, 191–
    193

Follow-up 199
Incidence 191, 192f
Nursing care 197
Pathophysiology 193
Rehabilitation 163t
Risk factors 191
Screening and detection 44t
Staging 193, 194t
Treatment 193–197
Colonoscopy 193
Colony stimulating factor (CSF) 86t,
  88–89, *327*
Colposcopy 233, *327*
Communication
  alt in Head and Neck cancer 173–
    174
Complement Cascade 84, *327*
Computerized Axial Tomography
  (CT) 50, 185, 201, 202, 213, 248,
  255, 271, 287, *327*
Cancer for the Dying 314
Congenital melanocytic nevi 261, *327*
Conization 233, *327*
Continent urinary reservoir (conti-
  nent ileal reservoir) *328*
Corporate Angel Network 314
Corynebacterium parvum (*c. parvum*)
  83, *328*
Costs 93
Counseling
  re to Sexual functioning 148
Craniotomy 255–256, *328*
Cushing's syndrome
  in Lung cancer 177t
Cystectomy 210–212, *328*
  and sexual functioning 145
Cytokines 84, *328*
Cytology studies 52–53
Cytotoxic 77t, *328*
Death
  In childhood cancers 305–306
  Psychosocial aspects 155
Debulking 58–59, *328*
Detection 40–42, 44t–50t, *328*
Diagnostic tests 44–50
  re to pain 112t
Diagnosis 40, 42, *328*
Diethylstilbestrol (DES) 231, *328*
  In Prostate cancer 245
Differentiation 22, *328*
Diffuse histiocytic lymphoma 292,
  328
Disseminated Intravascular Coagula-
  tion (DIC) 137, 278, *328*
Dumping syndrome 123, 189, *328*
Dyspareunia 143t, 144, *328*

Dysphagia 124, 128t, *328*
  in Esophageal cancer 185
  in Head and Neck cancer 168
  in Lung cancer treatment 180
Dysplastic nevi 261, *329*
Dyspnea
  and Lung cancer 108
Education
  Nursing 4, 5
  Patient 61, 81
Electrolyte disturbance 122–123, 124
Emergencies, oncologic 60, 66, 132–140
Employment
  Discrimination 162
  Work and indentity 161–162
Endocrine Cancers
  (*See specific glands*)
Endometrial cancer 67, 228–229
  Clinical Manifestations 228
  Incidence and Etiology 228
  Screening and detection 45t, 228
  Staging 229
  Treatment 228–229
Endoscopic retrograde chloangio-pancreatogram (ERCP) 201, *329*
Endoscopic laser therapy 187, *329*
Epidemiology 15–16, *329*
  Incidence rate 11, 15, *330*
Erythroplasia
  in Head and Neck cancer 167–168
Esophageal cancer 44t–45t, 68t, 184–187
  Clinical presentation 185
  Diagnostic tests 185
  Incidence 184
  Pathology 184–185
  Risk 184
  Screening and detection 44t–45t
  Treatment 185–187
Esophagoscopy 185, *329*
Ewing's sarcoma 272–273
Eyes 69t
  Retinoblastoma 301–302
Extrahepatic bile duct cancer 45t
  Screening and detection 45t
Extravasation 80–81, 81t, *329*
FAB morphology 297, *329*
Fallopian Tube Cancer 237–238
  Clinical Manifestations 237
  Incidence and Etiology 237
  Screening and detection 237–238
  Staging 238t
  Treatment 238
Families
  Communication 155–156

Coping with illness 154, 156–157
  and Pediatric Cancers 303–306
  and Rehabilitation 159
Fatigue 70, 109–110, 109t
Fever
  re to Septic shock 137
Fibrosarcoma 273
Food and Drug Administration 317
Gallbladder cancer 203
  Clinical Manifestations and Diagnosis 203
  Incidence 203
  Risk 203
  Screening and detection 45t
  Treatment 203
Gastric cancer 187–190
  Clinical presentation 188
  Diagnosis 188
  Incidence 187
  Palliative care 190
  Pathology 188
  Risk factors 187
  Treatment 188–189
Gestational trophoblastic disease 238–240, *329*
  Choriocarcinoma 239, *327*
  Clinical manifestations 239
  Diagnosis 231
  Hydatidiform mole 238, *330*
  Invasive mole 239, *331*
  Treatment 239–240
Glioblastoma multiforme 252, *329*
Gliomas 252, *329*
Gonads 69t
Gonadotropin releasing hormone *329*
Graft versus Host Disease 96, 98, *329*
Granulocytopenia 100, 100t
Gray 63, *329*
Guiaic testing 192
Gynecomastia 147, 245, *329*
Hair 68t
Head and neck cancers 65, 67, 68t, 166–174
  Incidence 166
  Laryngectomy 173
  Prevention and detection 166–168
  Primary sites 167t
  Rehabilitation 103t
  Risk factors 166
  Screening 45t–46t
  Treatment 168–170
  Warning signs 167
Hemocult testing 192
Hemoptysis
  in Lung cancer 182
Histology 26, 57, 291, *329*

Hodgkin's disease 65, 77, 92t, 286–290, *329*
  Clinical Presentation 287
  Etiology 286
  Incidence 286
  Nodular schlerosing 287, *330*
  Lymphocyte predominant, 287, *330*
  Lymphocyte depleted 287, *330*
  Mixed cellularity 287, *330*
  Pathophysiology 286–287
  Screening and detection 48t
  Staging 288t
  Treatment 287–290
Hormonal therapy 78
  in Breast cancer 225–226
  in Prostate cancer 245–246
Hormone Receptor Assay 219, *330*
Hospice 155
Human Chorionic Gonadotropic (HCG) 51, 239–240, *330*
Human-leukocyte antigen (HLA) 91–92, 93f, 96, *330*
Humoral immunity 84, 85f, *330*
Hyperalimentation 129–131, 130t, *330, 331, 337*
  Indications for 130t
Hypercalcemia 123, 135–136, *330*
  and Lung cancer 177t
  and Multiple myeloma 294
  Symptoms of 136t
I Can Cope 312
  and Breast cancer 227
  and Rehabilitation 164
Ilial conduit 210, 211f, 212f, *330*
Immune system 83–84
Immunosuppression 77t
Immunotherapy 84, 214, *330*
Incidence 10, 12t, 31, 33t, *330*
  and Age 16
  and Gender 20, 33t
  and Race 20
  (See specific cancers)
Incontinence
  re to Prostate treatment 243
Infection 56, 97, 240, 284, 295
Infertility
  and Testicular cancer 145
Interdisciplinary Processes
  and Rehabilitation 160–161
Interferons 86t, 87–88, *331*
  Alpha 87, 214, 268, *331*
  Beta 87, *331*
  Gamma, 86t, 87, 268, *331*
Interleukin II 86, 88, 214, 268, *331*
International Association of Laryngectomies 312

International Society of Nurses in Cancer Care 316
International Union Against Cancer 316
Investigational therapy 78–79
In vitro fertilization *331*
Kaposi's sarcoma 36, 268
  Pathology 268
  Treatment 268
Kidney cancer 68t, 88, 89, 213–214
  Clinical manifestations and diagnosis 213
  Incidence and risk 213
  Patterns of spread 213
  Screening and detection 46t
  Treatment 214
Lactose deficiency 127, *331*
Late effects 306–307
Latency period 25, *331*
Leukemia 46t–47t, 92t, 276–285, *331–332*
  Acute lymphocytic (ALL) 277, 280, *332 (See also pediatric ALL 296–298)*
  Acute nonlymphocyctic (ANLL) 277, 280, *322*
  Acute myelocytic (AML) 278, *332*
  Clinical manifestations 278, 279f
  Chronic lymphocytic (CLL) 278, 282–283, 282f
  Chronic myelocytic (CML) 278, 283, *332*
  Diagnosis 279
  Etiology 276
  Hairy-cell (HCL) 278, *332*
  Incidence 276
  Pathophysiology 276–278, 277f
  Screening and detection 46t–47t
  Supportive care 283–284
  T-cell Chronic lymphocytic 278, *332*
Leukemia Society of America 314
Leukophoresis *332*
Leukoplakia 167, *332*
Leukostasis 278, *332*
Libido, loss of 147–148
Liver cancer 202–203
  Clinical Manifestations and diagnosis 202
  Incidence 202
  Prognosis 203
  Risk 202
  Screening and detection 47t
  Treatment 202–203
Liver dysfunction 88
Long-term effects 97–98

Lost Chord Club 174
Lung cancer 16, 65, 67, 92t
  and Dyspnea 108
  and Rehabilitation 163t
  Clinical Manifestations 178
  Cough 111
  Diagnosis 178
  Incidence 175
  Non-small cell carcinoma 177, *336*
  Nursing care 181-182
  Prognosis 175
  Risk factors 175
  Screening and detection 47t-48t
  Sites of metastasis 177
  Small cell carcinoma 177, *336*
  Treatment 179-181
  Types 175-176
Lymphadenectomy *332*
  in Prostate cancer 245
Lymphangiography 51, *332*
Lymphocyte 86t, *332*
Lymphokines 85t, *333*
Lymphokine activated killer cells
  (LAK cells) 88, 214, *333*
Lymphoma 36, 48t, 59, *333*
  (see also Hodgkin's disease)
  Non-Hodgkin's lymphoma 48t, 65,
    88, 92t
  Screening and detection 48t
Macrophages 84, 85t, 86t, 89, *333*
Magnetic Resonance Imaging (MRI)
  50, 206, 213, 255, *333*
Make a Wish Foundation of America
  310
Make Today Count 311
Malignant 23, 23t, 28t, *333*
Malignant Melanoma 267-268
  Pathology 267
  Treatment 267-268
Malnutrition
  Causes ofd 121, 125
Mammography 218
Melanoma *333*
  Screening and detection 49t
Meningiomas 252, *333*
Metastasis 26, 27t, *333*
Micrometastases 219, *333*
Mohs surgery 266, *333*
Monoclonal antibodies 85-87, *333*
Monokines *333*
MOPP 77, 77t, 288, *333*
Mortality 13t, 17t, 18t, 19t
Mucosal erythroplasia 167,*333*
Mucositis 81, 88, 105, 106t-107t, 285
Multiple Myeloma 92t, 293-295
  Clinical Manifestations 293

Diagnosis 294
Incidence 293
Pathophysiology 293
Screening and detection 48t
Supportive care 295
Treatment 294
Myelosuppression 81, *333*
Nasoenteric feedings 129t
National Cancer Institute 127
National Coalition for Cancer Survi-
  vors 161, 315
National Hospice Organization 315
National Institute for Occupational
  Safety and Health 317
Natural killer cells 84, 85t, *334*
Nausea and vomiting 81, 88, 101-103,
  128t
Neurotoxicity 77t
Non-Hodgkin's lymphomas
  Classifications 292t
  Clinical manifestations 291
  Diagnosis 291
  Incidence 290-291
  Pathophysiology 291
  Treatment 291
Non-seminomatous tumors (testicular) 247, 248f, *334*
Nursing care
  in Bladder cancer 210
  in Bone cancers 273
  in Breast cancer 226-227
  in Breast cancer detection 218
  in Central nervous system tumors
    257-258
  in Colorectal cancer 197
  in Esophageal cancer 186
  in Gynecologic cancers 240-241
  in Head and Neck cancer 170-174
  in Hodgkin's disease 290
  in Lung cancer 181-182
  in Prevention and detection 4, 30,
    38
  in Rehabilitation 163-164
  in Screening 41
  re to Radiation 70-71
  re to Biological response modifiers
    89-90
  re to Surgery 60-61, 61t
Nursing education 4, 5
Nursing research 5
Nutrition 121-131
  Assessment 125, 125t
  in Esophageal cancer 187
  in Head and Neck cancer 171-172
Odynophagia 124, 128t, *334*
  in Head and Neck cancer 168

Ommaya Reservoir 293, *334*
Oncogenes 24-25, 305, *334*
Oncologic emergencies 132-140
  (See also specific emergencies)
Oncology Nursing Certification Corporation 5
Oncology Nursing Society 4, 5, 317
Orchiectomy 245, *334*
OSHA 79
Osteoarthropathy
  and Lung cancer 177t
Osteoblast cells 271, *334*
Osteoradionecrosis 170, *334*
Ostomies
  and Colorectal cancer 195-196,
    197-198, 198t
  and Body image 147-148
  and Rehabilitation 163t
Ovarian cancer 59, 229-230
  Clinical manifestations 229-230
  Diagnosis 230
  Incidence 229
  Screening and detection 45t
  Treatment 230
Ovaries
  Response to radiation 69t
Pain 60, 111-120
  and Pancreatic cancer 201
  as aa Barrier to rehabilitation 160
  Assessment 113-119, 114t
  Bone pain 294, 295
  Diagnostic tests in 112t
  in Nephrectomy 214
  Medications 118t
Palliation 60, 66
  in Esophageal cancer 187
  in Gastric cancer 188
  in Prostate cancer 246
Pancreatic cancer 200-202
  Clinical manifestations and diagnosis 200
  Incidence 200
  Risk factors 200
  Screening and detection 48t
  Treatment 201-202
Pancreatoduodenectomy *(Whipple)*
  201, *334*
Papanicolaou smear 40, 52, 230-231,
  232f, *334*
Parenteral nutrition 130, 130t, *337*
  Indications for 130t
  (See also hyperalimentation)
Parotid and submandibular cancers
  Screening and detection 46t
Patient
  Communication 156

Coping 156-157
Pediatric cancers
  (See Childhood cancers)
  (See also specific cancers)
Pelvic exenteration 145, 233, *334*
Penile cancer 246-247
  Diagnosis 246
  Treatment 246-247
Pericardial effusion 136-137
Pheochromocytoma 206, *334*
Philadelphia Chromosome 283, *335*
Pituitary cancer 206
  Clinical Manifestations of excess
    secretions 206t
  Diagnosis 206
  Treatment 206-207
Plasma cells *335*
Pluropotent stem cells 276, 277f, *335*
Prevalence rate 11, *325*
Prevention 25, 30, 38, 59
  Primary 30
  Secondary 31, 40
  Tertiary 31
Prophylactic treatment 66
Prostate cancer 65, 67, 242-246
  and penile implants 145
  and Sexual functioning 145
  Clinical Manifestations 242
  Incidence 242
  Palliation 246
  Screening and detection 48t, 242-243
  Staging 244
  Treatment 243, 245
Prostate specific antigen (PSA) 242,
  325
Prosthetics 56, 223, 225
Proto-oncogenes 24, *335*
Pruritus 109
Psychological aspects
  of Pain 111, 113
Psychosocial Support 150-158
  in Childhood cancer 303-305
  Communication 156
  Coping 156-157
  Psychotherapy 151
  re to Cancer diagnosis 152
  re to Cancer treatment 152-153
  Support aspects 150-151
Radiology *329*
Radiation Therapy 63-72
  CNS prophylaxis 297
  Fractions 64
  in Bladder cancer 212
  in Breast cancer 225

in Central nervous system tumors 256
in Cervical cancer 233
in Colorectal cancer 196
in Esophageal cancer 186–187
in Fallopian tube cancer 238
in Gallbladder cancer 203
in Gastric cancer 189
in Hodgkin's disease 288, 289f
in Kidney cancer 214
in Liver cancer 200–203
in Lung cancer 180, 181
in Malignant melanoma 268
in Metastatic bone cancer 273
in Multiple myeloma 294
in Ovarian cancer 230
in Pancreatic cancer 201
in Penile cancer 247
in Pituitary cancer 207
in Prostate cancer 243
in Testicular cancer 249
in Thyroid cancer 204
Intraoperative 196
in Vaginal cancer 237
Pain associated with 112t
Principles of treatment 75–76
Safety 70
Radionuclide 51, *335*
Radiosensitivity 64
Reach to Recovery 164, 220, 226–227, 312
Reconstruction 59–60, 225
Recurrence
Fear of 153–154
in Bladder cancer 210
in Breast cancer 227
in Colorectal cancer 199
in Gestational trophoblastic disease 240
Rehabilitation 159–167
Barriers to 160
Goal setting 159
in bone cancer 274
Team approach to 160–161
Work and Identity 161–162
Relative risk 33–34, *335*
Renal insufficiency 97
Resources 310–317
Respiratory system 69t
Risk 33–35
factors re to 32t
Factors re to Colorectal cancer 191
Ronald McDonald Houses 315
Sarcoma 27, 49t, 335
Ewing's sarcoma *335*

Fibrosarcoma *335*
Kaposi's sarcoma *335*
Osteogenic sarcoma *335*
Screening and detection 49t
Schwannomas 252, *335*
Screening 40–42, 44–50t, *335*
Second malignancies
in Hodgkin's disease 290
SEER 11, 20
Self-esteem 147–148
Self-examination 41
(See specific sites)
Seminomas (testicular) 247, 248f, *336*
Seroma 223, *336*
Septic shock 138–139
Sexual functioning
Alterations in 141, 144
and Chemotherapy 146
and Gynecological cancers 241
and Hodgkin's disease 290
and Hormonal therapy 147
and Prostate cancer 245
and Radiation therapy 146
and Surgery 144–146
and Testicular cancer 248–249
Loss of libido 147–148
Treatment related problems in males 142t
Treatment related problems in females 143t
Sexuality 141–149, 241
Sigmoidoscopy 192, *336*
Skin
and Ultraviolet rays 36–37
Care during radiation 71
Response to radiation 68t
Self-examination 264f–266f
Toxicities due to radiation 70
Skin cancers 36–37, 65, 68t, 259–269
and Radiation therapy 65
Basal cell carcinomas 263–267
Incidence 259, 260t
Prevention and detection 261–262, 262f
Risk 259
Screening and detection 49t
Squamous cell carcinomas 263–267
Treatment 263–267
Smoking
and Esophageal cancer 184
and Lung cancer 175
and Pancreatic cancer 200
Cessation 176t
Society for the Right to Die 315
Society of Otorhinolaryngology and Head and Neck Nurses 174

Spinal cord compression 133–135, *336*
Staging 26, 42–43, 57–58, *336*
Sterility 81
Stomach cancer 49t, 68t
Screening and detection 49t
Subtotal esophagogastrectomy 189, *336*
Superior vena cava syndrome 132–133, *336*
Support 6, 336
professional networks 157–158
Surgery 56–62, 65
and Adrenocortical cancer 205
and Bladder cancer 212
and Breast cancer 222–225
and Central nervous system tumors 255–256
and Cervical Cancer 233
and Colorectal cancer 193–196, 195t
and Endometrial cancer 228
and Esophageal cancer 185–186
and Fibrosarcoma 273
and Gallbladder cancer 203
and Gastric cancer 188–189
and Hodgkin's disease staging 287
and Kidney cancer 214
and Liver cancer 202
and Lung cancer 178–180
and Metastatic bone cancer 273
and Osteosarcoma 271–272
and Ovarian cancer 230
and Pain 112t
and Pancreatic cancer 201
and Penile cancer 246
and Prostate cancer 243
and Testicular cancer 248–249
and Thyroid cancer 204
and Vaginal cancer 237
Cryosurgery 59
Laser 59
Principles 57
Stereotactic 256, *336*
Survival 14t, 164
Survivorship 153–154, *336*
Symptom management 100–110
and psychosocial effect 154
Syndrome of inappropriate anti-di-uretic hormone (SIADH) 137–138, *336*
and Lung cancer 177t
Syngeneic bone marrow transplanta-tion 91, *336*
T-cells 84, 85t, 86t, 277, *336*
Antigens 277

Cytotoxic 84, 85t, *336*
Helper 84, 85t, *336*
Teaching
Patient 61, 81
Terminal illness
Psychosocial aspects 154
Testicular cancer 59, 92t, 247–250
and infertility 145
and sexuality 145
Classification 247
Clinical presentation 247
Risk 247
Screening and detection 49t–50t, 247
Staging 249
Treatment 248–250
TNM stanging classification 26, 43, 43t, *336*
Therapy *337*
Combination or multimodal 65, 77
(See also specific modalities)
Thermography 51, *336*
Thrombocytopenia 100, 102t, *337*
Thyroid cancer 50t, 65, 67, *337*
Anaplastic *337*
Follicular *337*
Medullary *337*
Papillary *337*
Tolerance 117, *337*
Total abdominal hysterectomy 228
With Bilateral salpingectomy and oophorectomy *337*
TOUCH 311
Tracheostomy 171
Transurethral resection of prostate (TURP) 242–243, *337*
Tumor 23, *337*
Tumor lysis syndrome 139, 285, *337*
Tumor markers 51
Alpha-fetoprotein (AFP) *325*
AFPO and gastric cancer 188
AFP and Testicular cancer 248
Carcinoembryonic antigen (CEA) 51, *326*
CEA and Colorectal cancer 193
CEA and gastric cancer 188
Human Chorionic Gonadotropin (HCG) *51*
HGC and testicular cancer 248
Tumor necrosis factor (TNF) 86t, 89, *337*
Tumor registries 11
Tumoricidal dose 64, *337*
Ultrasound 51, 239, *337*
Transrectal in Prostate cancer 243

Undifferentiated or anaplastic 22–23, *337*
United Ostomy Association 197, 315
Ureteral cancer
  Screening and detection 50t
Ureterosigmoidostomy 210, *338*
Vaginal cancer 236–237
  Clinical manifestations 236
  Incidence and etiology 236
  Screening and detection 237
  Treatment 237
Venography 51
Veno-occlusive disease 97, *338*
Venous access devices 80t, 80–81
Vulvar cancer 235–236
  Clinical Manifestations 235
  Diagnosis 235

  Incidence and etiology 235
  Staging 236t
  Treatment 235–236
Vulvectomy 235, *338*
Warning signs 41, 43t
Weight loss
  and Colorectal cancer 192
  and Esophageal cancer 185
Wilm's tumor 298–300
Wound management
  in Bladder cancer 210
  in Head and Neck cancer 172–173
  in Vulvectomy 236
Xeroderma pigmentosa 261, *338*
Xerostoma 124, *338*
Y-me 311